CONDITIONED REFLEXES

AN INVESTIGATION OF

THE PHYSIOLOGICAL ACTIVITY

OF THE

CEREBRAL CORTEX

BY

I. P. PAVLOV, FOR. MEM. R.S.

TRANSLATED AND EDITED

BY

G. V. ANREP, M.D., D.Sc.

DOVER PUBLICATIONS, INC.
NEW YORK

Published in Canada by General Publishing Company, Ltd., 30 Lesmill Road, Don Mills, Toronto, Ontario.

Published in the United Kingdom by Constable and Company, Ltd., 10 Orange Street, London WC 2.

This new Dover edition, first published in 1960, is an unabridged and unaltered republication of the translation first published in 1927 by the Oxford University Press. It is published by special arrangement with the Oxford University Press.

Standard Book Number: 486-60614-7

Library of Congress Catalog Card Number: 60-2546

Manufactured in the United States of America

Dover Publications, Inc.
180 Varick Street
New York 14, N.Y.

TO

THE MEMORY OF

MY SON

VICTOR

IVAN PAVLOV

EDITOR'S PREFACE

PROFESSOR PAVLOV in his preface to this English edition regards it as lucky for his book that the task of preparation fell into my hands ; but I consider that the luck was mine, because it was the best way I had of showing my personal regard for my old teacher. Although I had personal contact with the work, the task was not easy, especially on account of the extreme importance of this new field of investigation, not only for physiology itself, but also for all the biological sciences.

Since the present is the first complete discussion rendered out of the Russian into one of the more familiar European tongues, technical terms had to be devised which should in some measure impart that fluency to the discussion which one finds in the Russian text. A terminology has therefore been adopted which, after having received the advantage of full consideration and advice from my friends and colleagues at University College, London, I believe to answer the purpose sufficiently well.

Professor Pavlov allowed me, for the sake of clarity, to introduce some modifications and additions into the text in order to make the reading lighter for those English and American readers unfamiliar with the original literature in this field. This I have done sparingly, being careful only to expand, but in no sense to alter, the original meaning.

The preparation of the English edition was helped by a grant from the Royal Society, which was sufficient

to cover the draft translation of Lectures I-XII; but
at this stage, owing to the difficulty of finding really
suitable translators, and desiring not to burden the
Royal Society unduly with further costs of translation,
I resolved to undertake the revision of the draft translation and the complete translation of the remaining
lectures myself. This, with the willing help of Mr.
R. A. Nash, a research student in my laboratory, I was
able to accomplish. I desire to thank him, and also to
express my grateful thanks to my friend Mr. E. L. Ball,
who critically read the whole of our manuscript in both
the draft and finished copies.

G. V. A.

CAMBRIDGE.

AUTHOR'S PREFACE

I AM deeply sensible of my good fortune that this book should appear in the English language through the assistance of the Royal Society of London. Without their material help the presentation of the book in its English form could not in the first place have been attempted. I desire to express to them my deepest gratitude.

I count it a great stroke of luck for the book that the preparation of the English edition was carried out entirely under the supervision of, and in part made by, my young friend Dr. Anrep, formerly an active collaborator in the work described in its pages. Dr. Anrep's task has not been an easy one, and it has been fraught with responsibility, as practically at every step he has had to adapt a vast new terminology. I wish to give him also my hearty thanks.

I. P. P.

PETROGRAD, 14*th* *July*, 1926.

PREFACE TO
THE RUSSIAN EDITION

In the spring of 1924, in a series of lectures delivered at the Military Medical Academy in Petrograd to an audience of medical men and biologists, I attempted to give a full and systematized exposition of our researches upon the activities of the cerebral hemispheres in the dog—researches which had then been in progress for nearly twenty-five years. These lectures were taken down by a stenographer with a view to subsequent publication. On looking through the manuscript I found the lectures not entirely satisfactory, and began, therefore, to recast them. This occupied over eighteen months of my leisure, during the whole of which period investigation was being vigorously pushed forward in the laboratories under my direction. As a result of this continued experimentation some of the deductions and interpretations drawn in my lectures had to be considerably modified. However, in the book as it stands at present I intentionally allowed the chapters to remain as they left my hands at the first revision, incorporating in the later lectures the new material as it came to hand. In this manner the reader is placed in a position to obtain a much clearer idea of the natural growth of the subject.

In the lectures I have restricted my exposition to the purely experimental material, avoiding all reference to the literature of the subject. A complete treatment of the literature would have increased the labour of my task excessively. Moreover, my intention was the simple one of treating the subject as an entity from my own personal viewpoint. I am fully aware that not a few of our observations have been in the nature of a confirmation of facts established by other authors. The question of priority has been considered of relatively small account, since I am fully convinced that the subject lends a sufficient scope for the full development of initiative of all workers interested in solving its problems. At the same time we are convinced that this method of research is destined, in the hands of other workers, and with new modifications in the mode of experimentation, to play a yet more considerable part in the study of the physiology of the nervous system.

I have to express my warmest thanks to all my fellow-workers who joined their labour with mine in our common task. If I instigated, directed and correlated all our labour, I was myself continually influenced by the vigilance and the resourcefulness of my co-workers. In all cases of team work where there is a continuous interplay of many minds, it is scarcely possible to draw any definite line, saying what belongs to one and what to another. Each, however, has the satisfaction and joy of having borne his part in the common structure.

I. P. P.

PETROGRAD, 12*th July*, 1926.

CONTENTS

LECTURE I

The development of the objective method in investigating the physiological activities of the cerebral hemispheres.—Concept of Reflex.—Variety of Reflexes.—Signal-reflexes, the most fundamental physiological characteristic of the hemispheres.

THE cerebral hemispheres stand out as the crowning achievement in the nervous development of the animal kingdom. These structures in the higher animals are of considerable dimensions and exceedingly complex, being made up in man of millions upon millions of cells—centres or foci of nervous activity—varying in size, shape and arrangement, and connected with each other by countless branchings from their individual processes. Such complexity of structure naturally suggests a like complexity of function, which in fact is obvious in the higher animal and in man. Consider the dog, which has been for so many countless ages the servant of man. Think how he may be trained to perform various duties, watching, hunting, etc. We know that this complex behaviour of the animal, undoubtedly involving the highest nervous activity, is mainly associated with the cerebral hemispheres. If we remove the hemispheres in the dog [Goltz[1] and others[2]], the animal becomes not only incapable of performing these duties but also incapable even of looking after itself. It becomes in fact a helpless invalid, and cannot long survive unless it be carefully tended.

In man also the highest nervous activity is dependent upon the structural and functional integrity of the cerebral hemispheres. As soon as these structures become damaged and their functions impaired in any way, so man also becomes an invalid. He can no longer proceed with his normal duties, but has to be kept out of the working world of his fellow men.

In astounding contrast with the unbounded activity of the cerebral hemispheres stands the meagre content of present-day physiological knowledge concerning them. Up to the year 1870,

[1] F. Goltz, "Der Hund ohne Grosshirn," Pflüger's *Archiv*, V. li. p. 570, 1892.

[2] M. Rothmann, "Der Hund ohne Grosshirn." *Neurologisches Central-blatt*, V. xxviii. p. 1045, 1909.

in fact, there was no physiology of the hemispheres ; they seemed to be out of reach of the physiologist. In that year the common physiological methods of stimulation and extirpation were first applied to them [Fritsch and Hitzig [1]]. It was found by these workers that stimulation of certain parts of the cortex of the hemispheres (motor cortex) regularly evoked contractions in definite groups of skeletal muscles : extirpation of these parts of the cortex led to disturbances in the normal functioning of the same groups of muscles. Shortly afterwards it was demonstrated [Ferrier,[2] H. Munk [3]] that other areas of the cortex which do not evoke any motor activity in response to stimulation are also functionally differentiated. Extirpation of these areas leads to definite defects in the nervous activity associated with certain receptor organs, such as the retina of the eye, the organ of Corti, and the sensory nerve-endings in the skin. Searching investigations have been made, and still are being made, by numerous workers on this question of localization of function in the cortex. Our knowledge has been increased in precision and filled out in detail, especially as regards the motor area, and has even found useful application in medicine. These investigations, however, did not proceed fundamentally beyond the position established by Fritsch and Hitzig. The important question of the physiological mechanism of the whole higher and complex behaviour of the animal which is—as Goltz showed—dependent upon the cerebral hemispheres, was not touched in any of these investigations and formed no part of the current physiological knowledge.

When therefore we ask the questions : What do those facts which have up to the present been at the disposal of the physiologist explain with regard to the behaviour of the higher animals ? What general scheme of the highest nervous activity can they give ? or what general rules governing this activity can they help us to formulate ?—the modern physiologist finds himself at a loss and can give no satisfactory reply. The problem of the mechanism of this complex structure which is so rich in function has got hidden away in a corner, and this unlimited field, so fertile in possibilities for research, has never been adequately explored.

[1] Fritsch und E. Hitzig, " Ueber die elektrische Erregbarkeit des Grosshirns." *Archiv für (Anatomie und) Physiologie*, p. 300, 1870.

[2] D. Ferrier, *Functions of the Brain*, London, 1876.

[3] H. Munk, *Ueber die Functionen der Grosshirnrinde*, Berlin, 1890 and 1909.

The reason for this is quite simple and clear. These nervous activities have never been regarded from the same point of view as those of other organs, or even other parts of the central nervous system. The activities of the hemispheres have been talked about as some kind of special psychical activity, whose working we feel and apprehend in ourselves, and by analogy suppose to exist in animals. This is an anomaly which has placed the physiologist in an extremely difficult position. On the one hand it would seem that the study of the activities of the cerebral hemispheres, as of the activities of any other part of the organism, should be within the compass of physiology, but on the other hand it happens to have been annexed to the special field of another science—psychology.

What attitude then should the physiologist adopt ? Perhaps he should first of all study the methods of this science of psychology, and only afterwards hope to study the physiological mechanism of the hemispheres ? This involves a serious difficulty. It is logical that in its analysis of the various activities of living matter physiology should base itself on the more advanced and more exact sciences—physics and chemistry. But if we attempt an approach from this science of psychology to the problem confronting us we shall be building our superstructure on a science which has no claim to exactness as compared even with physiology. In fact it is still open to discussion whether psychology is a natural science, or whether it can be regarded as a science at all.

It is not possible here for me to enter deeply into this question, but I will stay to give one fact which strikes me very forcibly, viz. that even the advocates of psychology do not look upon their science as being in any sense exact. The eminent American psychologist, William James, has in recent years referred to psychology not as a science but as a *hope* of science. Another striking illustration is provided by Wundt, the celebrated philosopher and psychologist, founder of the so-called experimental method in psychology and himself formerly a physiologist. Just before the War (1913), on the occasion of a discussion in Germany as to the advisability of making separate Chairs of Philosophy and Psychology, Wundt opposed the separation, one of his arguments being the impossibility of fixing a common examination schedule in psychology, since every professor had his own special ideas as to what psychology really was. Such testimony seems to show clearly that psychology cannot yet claim the status of an exact science.

If this be the case there is no need for the physiologist to have recourse to psychology. It would be more natural that experimental investigation of the physiological activities of the hemispheres should lay a solid foundation for a future true science of psychology ; such a course is more likely to lead to the advancement of this branch of natural science.

The physiologist must thus take his own path, where a trail has already been blazed for him. Three hundred years ago Descartes evolved the idea of the reflex. Starting from the assumption that animals behaved simply as machines, he regarded every activity of the organism as a *necessary* reaction to some external stimulus, the connection between the stimulus and the response being made through a definite nervous path : and this connection, he stated, was the fundamental purpose of the nervous structures in the animal body. This was the basis on which the study of the nervous system was firmly established. In the eighteenth, nineteenth and twentieth centuries the conception of the reflex was used to the full by physiologists. Working at first only on the lower parts of the central nervous system, they came gradually to study more highly developed parts, until quite recently Magnus,[1] continuing the classical investigations of Sherrington[2] upon the spinal reflexes, has succeeded in demonstrating the reflex nature of all the elementary motor activities of the animal organism. Descartes' conception of the reflex was constantly and fruitfully applied in these studies, but its application has stopped short of the cerebral cortex.

It may be hoped that some of the more complex activities of the body, which are made up by a grouping together of the elementary locomotor activities, and which enter into the states referred to in psychological phraseology as " playfulness," " fear," " anger," and so forth, will soon be demonstrated as reflex activities of the sub-cortical parts of the brain. A bold attempt to apply the idea of the reflex to the activities of the hemispheres was made by the Russian physiologist, I. M. Sechenov, on the basis of the knowledge available in his day of the physiology of the central nervous system. In a pamphlet entitled " Reflexes of the Brain," published in Russian in 1863, he attempted to represent the activities of the cerebral hemispheres as reflex—that is to say, as *determined*.

---

[1] R. Magnus, *Körperstellung*, Berlin, 1924.

[2] C. S. Sherrington, *The Integrative Action of the Nervous System*, London, 1906.

Thoughts he regarded as reflexes in which the effector path was inhibited, while great outbursts of passion he regarded as exaggerated reflexes with a wide irradiation of excitation. A similar attempt was made more recently by Ch. Richet,[1] who introduced the conception of the psychic reflex, in which the response following on a given stimulus is supposed to be determined by the association of this stimulus with the traces left in the hemispheres by past stimuli. And generally speaking, recent physiology shows a tendency to regard the highest activities of the hemispheres as an association of the new excitations at any given time with traces left by old ones (associative memory, training, education by experience).

All this, however, was mere conjecture. The time was ripe for a transition to the experimental analysis of the subject—an analysis which must be as objective as the analysis in any other branch of natural science. An impetus was given to this transition by the rapidly developing science of comparative physiology, which itself sprang up as a direct result of the Theory of Evolution. In dealing with the lower members of the animal kingdom physiologists were, of necessity, compelled to reject anthropomorphic preconceptions, and to direct all their effort towards the elucidation of the connections between the external stimulus and the resulting response, whether locomotor or other reaction. This led to the development of Loeb's doctrine of Animal Tropisms ; [2] to the introduction of a new objective terminology to describe animal reactions [Beer, Bethe and Uexküll[3]] ; and finally, it led to the investigation by zoologists, using purely objective methods, of the behaviour of the lower members of the animal kingdom in response to external stimuli—as for example in the classical researches of Jennings.[4]

Under the influence of these new tendencies in biology, which appealed to the practical bent of the American mind, the American School of Psychologists—already interested in the comparative study of psychology—evinced a disposition to subject the highest nervous activities of animals to experimental analysis under various

[1] Ch. Richet, *Réflexes Psychiques. Réflexes Conditionels. Automatisme Mental.* Pavlov's *Jubilee Volume*, Petrograd, 1925.

[2] J. Loeb, *Studies in General Physiology*, Chicago, 1905.

[3] Beer, Bethe und Uexküll, " Vorschläge zu einer objectivirenden Nomenklatur in der Physiologie des Nervensystems," *Biologisches Centralblatt*, V. xix. p. 517, 1899.

[4] H. S. Jennings, *The Behavior of Lower Organisms*, New York, 1906.

specially devised conditions. We may fairly regard the treatise by Thorndyke, *The Animal Intelligence* (1898),[1] as the starting point for systematic investigations of this kind. In these investigations the animal was kept in a box, and food was placed outside the box so that it was visible to the animal. In order to get the food the animal had to open a door, which was fastened by various suitable contrivances in the different experiments. Tables and charts were made showing how quickly and in what manner the animal solved the problems set it. The whole process was understood as being the formation of an association between the visual and tactile stimuli on the one hand and the locomotor apparatus on the other. This method, with its modifications, was subsequently applied by numerous authors to the study of questions relating to the associative ability of various animals.

At about the same time as Thorndyke was engaged on this work, I myself (being then quite ignorant of his researches) was also led to the objective study of the hemispheres, by the following circumstance : In the course of a detailed investigation into the activities of the digestive glands I had to inquire into the so-called psychic secretion of some of the glands, a task which I attempted in conjunction with a collaborator. As a result of this investigation an unqualified conviction of the futility of subjective methods of inquiry was firmly stamped upon my mind. It became clear that the only satisfactory solution of the problem lay in an experimental investigation by strictly objective methods. For this purpose I started to record all the external stimuli falling on the animal at the time its reflex reaction was manifested (in this particular case the secretion of saliva), at the same time recording all changes in the reaction of the animal.

This was the beginning of these investigations, which have gone on now for twenty-five years—years in which numerous fellow-workers on whom I now look back with tender affection have united with mine in this work their hearts and hands. We have of course passed through many stages, and only gradually has the subject been opened up and the difficulties overcome. At first only a few scattered facts were available, but to-day sufficient material has been gathered together to warrant an attempt to present it in a more or less systematized form. At the present time I am in a

---

[1] E. L. Thorndyke, *The Animal Intelligence, An Experimental Study of the Associative Processes in Animals*, New York, 1898.

position to present you with a physiological interpretation of the activities of the cerebral hemispheres which is, at any rate, more in keeping with the structural and functional complexity of this organ than is the collection of fragmentary, though very important, facts which up to the present have represented all the knowledge of this subject. Work on the lines of purely objective investigation into the highest nervous activities has been conducted in the main in the laboratories under my control, and over a hundred collaborators have taken part. Work on somewhat similar lines to ours has been done by the American psychologists. Up to the present, however, there has been one essential point of difference between the American School and ourselves. Being psychologists, their mode of experimentation, in spite of the fact that they are studying these activities on their external aspect, is mostly psychological—at any rate so far as the arrangement of problems and their analysis and the formulation of results are concerned. Therefore—with the exception of a small group of " behaviourists "—their work cannot be regarded as purely physiological in character. We, having started from physiology, continue to adhere strictly to the physiological point of view, investigating and systematizing the whole subject by physiological methods alone. As regards other physiological laboratories a few only have directed their attention to this subject, and that recently ; nor have their investigations extended beyond the limits of a preliminary inquiry.

I shall now turn to the description of our material, first giving as a preliminary an account of the general conception of the reflex, of specific physiological reflexes, and of the so-called " instincts." Our starting point has been Descartes' idea of the nervous reflex. This is a genuine scientific conception, since it implies necessity. It may be summed up as follows : An external or internal stimulus falls on some one or other nervous receptor and gives rise to a nervous impulse ; this nervous impulse is transmitted along nerve fibres to the central nervous system, and here, on account of existing nervous connections, it gives rise to a fresh impulse which passes along outgoing nerve fibres to the active organ, where it excites a special activity of the cellular structures. Thus a stimulus appears to be connected of necessity with a definite response, as cause with effect. It seems obvious that the whole activity of the organism should conform to definite laws. If the animal were not in exact correspondence with its environment it would, sooner or later, cease to exist. To give a biological example : if, instead of being attracted to food, the animal were repelled by it, or if instead of running from fire the animal threw itself into the fire, then it would quickly perish. The animal must respond to changes in the environment in such a manner that its responsive activity is directed towards the preservation of its existence. This conclusion holds also if we consider the living organism in terms of physical and chemical science. Every material system can exist as an entity only so long as its internal forces, attraction, cohesion, etc., balance the external forces acting upon it. This is true for an ordinary stone just as much as for the most complex chemical substances ; and its truth should be recognized also for the animal organism. Being a definite circumscribed material system, it can only continue to exist so long as it is in continuous equilibrium with the forces external to it : so soon as this equilibrium is seriously disturbed the organism will cease to exist as the entity it was. Reflexes are the elemental units in the mechanism of perpetual equilibration. Physiologists have studied and are studying at the present time these numerous machine-like, inevitable reactions of the organism—reflexes existing from the very birth of the animal, and due therefore to the inherent organization of the nervous system.

Reflexes, like the driving-belts of machines of human design, may be of two kinds—positive and negative, excitatory and inhibitory. Although the investigation of these reflexes by physiologists has been going on now for a long time, it is as yet not nearly finished. Fresh reflexes are continually being discovered. We are ignorant of the properties of those receptor organs for which the effective stimulus arises inside the organism, and the internal reflexes themselves remain a field unexplored. The paths by which nervous impulses are conducted in the central nervous system are for the most part little known, or not ascertained at all. The mechanism of inhibitions confined within the central nervous system remains quite obscure : we know something only of those inhibitory reflexes which manifest themselves along the inhibitory efferent nerves. Furthermore, the combination and interaction of different reflexes are as yet insufficiently understood. Nevertheless physiologists are succeeding more and more in unravelling the mechanism of these machine-like activities of the organism, and may reasonably be expected to elucidate and control it in the end.

To those reflexes which have long been the subject of physiological investigation, and which concern chiefly the activities of separate organs and tissues, there should be added another group of inborn reflexes. These also take place in the nervous system, and they are the inevitable reactions to perfectly definite stimuli. They have to do with reactions of the organism as a whole, and comprise that general behaviour of the animal which has been termed " instinctive." Since complete agreement as regards the essential affinity of these reactions to the reflex has not yet been attained, we must discuss this question more fully. We owe to the English philosopher, Herbert Spencer, the suggestion that instinctive reactions are reflexes. Ample evidence was later advanced by zoologists, physiologists, and students of comparative psychology in support of this. I propose here to bring together the various arguments in favour of this view. Between the simplest reflex and the instinct we can find numerous stages of transition, and among these we are puzzled to find any line of demarcation. To exemplify this we may take the newly hatched chick. This little creature reacts by pecking to any stimulus that catches the eye, whether it be a real object or only a stain in the surface it is walking upon. In what way shall we say that this differs from the inclining of the head, the closing of the lids, when something flicks past its eyes ? We should call this last a defensive reflex, but the first has been termed a feeding instinct : although in pecking nothing but an inclination of the head and a movement of the beak occurs.

It has also been maintained that instincts are more complex than reflexes. There are, however, exceedingly complex reflexes which nobody would term instincts. We may take vomiting as an example. This is very complex and involves the co-ordination of a large number of muscles (both striped and plain) spread over a large area and usually employed in quite different functions of the organism. It involves also a secretory activity on the part of certain glands which is usually evoked for a quite different purpose.

Again, it has been assumed that the long train of actions involved in certain instinctive activities affords a distinctive point of contrast with the reflex, which is regarded as always being built on a simple scale. By way of example we may take the building of a nest, or of dwellings in general, by animals. A chain of incidents is linked together : material is gathered and carried to the site chosen ; there it is built up and strengthened. To look upon this as reflex we must assume that one reflex initiates the next following—or, in other words, we must regard it as a chain-reflex. But this linking up of activities is not peculiar to instincts alone. We are familiar with numerous reflexes which most certainly fuse into chains. Thus, for example, if we stimulate an afferent nerve, *e.g.* the sciatic nerve, a reflex rise of blood pressure occurs ; the high pressure in the left ventricle of the heart, and first part of the aorta, serves as the effective stimulus to a second reflex, this time a depressor reflex which has a moderating influence on the first. Again, we may take one of the chain reflexes recently established by Magnus. A cat, even when deprived of its cerebral hemispheres, will in most cases land on its feet when thrown from a height. How is this managed ? When the position of the otolithic organ in space is altered a definite reflex is evoked which brings about a contraction of the muscles in the neck, restoring the animal's head to the normal position. This is the first reflex. With the righting of the head a fresh reflex is evoked, and certain muscles of the trunk and limbs are brought into play, restoring the animal to the standing posture. This is the second reflex.

Some, again, object to the identification of instincts with reflexes on this ground : instincts, they say, frequently depend upon the internal state of an organism. For instance, a bird only builds its nest in the mating season. Or, to take a simpler case, when an animal is satiated with eating, then food has no longer any attraction and the animal leaves off eating. Again, the same is true of the sexual impulse. This depends on the age of the organism, and on the state of the reproductive glands ; and a considerable influence is exerted by hormones (the products of the glands of internal secretion). But this dependence cannot be claimed as a peculiar property of " instincts." The intensity of any reflex, indeed its very presence, is dependent on the irritability of the centres, which in turn depends constantly on the physical and chemical properties of the blood (automatic stimulation of centres) and on the interaction of reflexes.

Last of all, it is sometimes held that whereas reflexes determine only the activities of single organs and tissues, instincts involve the activity of the organism as a whole. We now know, however, from the recent investigations of Magnus and de Kleijn, that standing, walking and the maintenance of postural balance in general, are all nothing but reflexes.

It follows from all this that instincts and reflexes are alike the inevitable responses of the organism to internal and external stimuli, and therefore we have no need to call them by two different terms. Reflex has the better claim of the two, in that it has been used from the very beginning with a strictly scientific connotation.

The aggregate of reflexes constitutes the foundation of the nervous activities both of men and of animals. It is therefore of great importance to study in detail all the fundamental reflexes of the organism. Up to the present, unfortunately, this is far from being accomplished, especially, as I have mentioned before, in the case of those reflexes which have been known vaguely as "instincts." Our knowledge of these latter is very limited and fragmentary. Their classification under such headings as "alimentary," "defensive," "sexual," "parental" and "social" instincts, is thoroughly inadequate. Under each of these heads is assembled often a large number of individual reflexes. Some of these are quite unidentified ; some are confused with others ; and many are still only partially appreciated. I can demonstrate from my own experience to what extent the subject remains inchoate and full of gaps. In the course of the researches which I shall presently explain, we were completely at a loss on one occasion to find any cause for the peculiar behaviour of an animal. It was evidently a very tractable dog, which soon became very friendly with us. We started off with a very simple experiment. The dog was placed in a stand with loose loops round its legs, but so as to be quite comfortable and free to move a pace or two. Nothing more was done except to present the animal repeatedly with food at intervals of some minutes. It stood quietly enough at first, and ate quite readily, but as time went on it became excited and struggled to get out of the stand, scratching at the floor, gnawing the supports, and so on. This ceaseless muscular exertion was accompanied by breathlessness and continuous salivation, which persisted at every experiment during several weeks, the animal getting worse and worse until it was no longer fitted for our researches. For a long time we remained puzzled over the unusual behaviour of this animal. We tried out experimentally numerous possible interpretations, but though we had had long experience with a great number of dogs in our laboratories we could not work out a satisfactory solution of this strange behaviour, until it occurred to us at last that it might be the expression of a special *freedom reflex*, and that the dog simply could not remain quiet when it was constrained in the stand.

This reflex was overcome by setting off another against it—the reflex for food. We began to give the dog the whole of its food in the stand. At first the animal ate but little, and lost considerably in weight, but gradually it got to eat more, until at last the whole ration was consumed. At the same time the animal grew quieter during the course of the experiments : the freedom reflex was being inhibited. It is clear that the freedom reflex is one of the most important reflexes, or, if we use a more general term, reactions, of living beings. This reflex has even yet to find its final recognition. In James's writings it is not even enumerated among the special human " instincts." But it is clear that if the animal were not provided with a reflex of protest against boundaries set to its freedom, the smallest obstacle in its path would interfere with the proper fulfilment of its natural functions. Some animals as we all know have this freedom reflex to such a degree that when placed in captivity they refuse all food, sicken and die.

As another example of a reflex which is very much neglected we may refer to what may be called the *investigatory reflex*. I call it the " What-is-it ? " reflex. It is this reflex which brings about the immediate response in man and animals to the slightest changes in the world around them, so that they immediately orientate their appropriate receptor organ in accordance with the perceptible quality in the agent bringing about the change, making full investigation of it. The biological significance of this reflex is obvious. If the animal were not provided with such a reflex its life would hang at every moment by a thread. In man this reflex has been greatly developed with far-reaching results, being represented in its highest form by inquisitiveness—the parent of that scientific method through which we may hope one day to come to a true orientation in knowledge of the world around us.

Still less has been done towards the elucidation of the class of negative or inhibitory reflexes (instincts) which are often evoked by any strong stimulus or even by weak stimuli, if unusual. Animal hypnotism, so-called, belongs to this category.

As the fundamental nervous reactions both of men and of animals are inborn in the form of definite reflexes, I must again emphasize how important it is to compile a complete list comprising all these reflexes with their adequate classification. For, as will be shown later on, all the remaining nervous functions of the animal organism are based upon these reflexes. Now, although the possession of such reflexes as those just described constitutes the fundamental condition for the natural survival of the animal, they are not in themselves sufficient to ensure a prolonged, stable and normal existence. This can be shown in dogs in which the cerebral hemispheres have been removed. Leaving out of account the internal reflexes, such a dog still retains the fundamental external reflexes. It is attracted by food ; it is repelled by nocuous stimuli ; it exhibits the investigatory reflex, raising its head and pricking up its ears to sound. In addition it exhibits the freedom reflex, offering a powerful resistance to any restraint. Nevertheless it is wholly incapable of looking after itself, and if left to itself will very soon die. Evidently something important is missing in its present nervous make-up. What nervous activities can it have lost ? It is easily seen that, in this dog, the number of stimuli evoking reflex reaction is considerably diminished ; those remaining are of an elemental, generalized nature, and act at a very short range. Consequently the dynamic equilibrium between the inner forces of the animal system and the external forces in its environment has become elemental as compared with the exquisite adaptability of the normal animal, and the simpler balance is obviously inadequate to life.

Let us return now to the simplest reflex from which our investigations started. If food or some rejectable substance finds its way into the mouth, a secretion of saliva is produced. The purpose of this secretion is in the case of food to alter it chemically, in the case of a rejectable substance to dilute and wash it out of the mouth. This is an example of a reflex due to the physical and chemical properties of a substance when it comes into contact with the mucous membrane of the mouth and tongue. But, in addition to this, a similar reflex secretion is evoked when these substances are placed at a distance from the dog and the receptor organs affected are only those of smell and sight. Even the vessel from which the food has been given is sufficient to evoke an alimentary reflex complete in all its details ; and, further, the secretion may be provoked even by the sight of the person who brought the vessel, or by the sound of his footsteps. All these innumerable stimuli falling upon the several finely discriminating distance receptors lose their power for ever as soon as the hemispheres are taken from the animal, and those only which have a direct effect on mouth and tongue still retain their power. The great advantage to the organism of a capacity to react to the former stimuli is evident, for it is in virtue of their action that food finding its way into the mouth immediately encounters plenty of moistening saliva, and rejectable substances, often nocuous to the mucous membrane, find a layer of protective saliva already in the mouth which rapidly dilutes and washes them out. Even greater is their importance when they evoke the motor component of the complex reflex of nutrition, *i.e.* when they act as stimuli to the reflex of seeking food.

Here is another example—the reflex of self-defence. The strong carnivorous animal preys on weaker animals, and these if they waited to defend themselves until the teeth of the foe were in their flesh would speedily be exterminated. The case takes on a different aspect when the defence reflex is called into play by the sights and sounds of the enemy's approach. Then the prey has a chance to save itself by hiding or by flight.

How can we describe, in general, this difference in the dynamic balance of life between the normal and the decorticated animal ? What is the general mechanism and law of this distinction ? It is pretty evident that under natural conditions the normal animal must respond not only to stimuli which themselves bring immediate benefit or harm, but also to other physical or chemical agencies— waves of sound, light, and the like—which in themselves only *signal* the approach of these stimuli; though it is not the sight and sound of the beast of prey which is in itself harmful to the smaller animal, but its teeth and claws.

Now although the *signalling stimuli* do play a part in those comparatively simple reflexes we have given as examples, yet this is not the most important point. The essential feature of the highest activity of the central nervous system, with which we are concerned and which in the higher animals most probably belongs entirely to the hemispheres, consists not in the fact that innumerable signalling stimuli do initiate reflex reactions in the animal, but in the fact that under different conditions these same stimuli may initiate quite different reflex reactions; and conversely the same reaction may be initiated by different stimuli.

In the above-mentioned example of the salivary reflex, the signal at one time is one particular vessel, at another time another ; under certain conditions one man, under different conditions another —strictly depending upon which vessel had been used in feeding and which man had brought the vessel and given food to the dog. This evidently makes the machine-like responsive activities of the organism still more precise, and adds to it qualities of yet higher perfection. So infinitely complex, so continuously in flux, are the conditions in the world around, that that complex animal system which is itself in living flux, and that system only, has a chance to establish dynamic equilibrium with the environment. Thus we see that the fundamental and the most general function of the hemispheres is that of reacting to signals presented by innumerable stimuli of interchangeable signification.

LECTURE II

Technical methods employed in the objective investigation of the functions of the cerebral hemispheres.—Response to signals as reflex action.—Unconditioned and conditioned reflexes.—Necessary conditions for the development of conditioned reflexes.

In the previous lecture I gave an account of the reasons which led us to adopt, for the investigation of the functions of the cerebral hemispheres, the purely objective method used for investigating the physiological activity of the lower parts of the nervous system. In this manner the investigation of the cerebral hemispheres is brought into line with the investigations conducted in other branches of natural science, and their activities are studied as purely physiological facts, without any need to resort to fantastic speculations as to the existence of any possible subjective state in the animal which may be conjectured on analogy with ourselves. From this point of view the whole nervous activity of the animal must be regarded as based firstly on inborn reflexes. These are regular causal connections between certain definite external stimuli acting on the organism and its necessary reflex reactions. Such inborn reflexes are comparatively few in number, and the stimuli setting them in action act close up, being as a rule the general physical and chemical properties of the common agencies which affect the organism. The inborn reflexes by themselves are inadequate to ensure the continued existence of the organism, especially of the more highly organized animals, which, when deprived of their highest nervous activity, are permanently disabled, and if left to themselves, although retaining all their inborn reflexes, soon cease to exist. The complex conditions of everyday existence require a much more detailed and specialized correlation between the animal and its environment than is afforded by the inborn reflexes alone. This more precise correlation can be established only through the medium of the cerebral hemispheres ; and we have found that a great number of all sorts of stimuli always act through the medium of the hemispheres as temporary and interchangeable signals for the comparatively small number of agencies of a general character which determine the inborn reflexes, and that this is the only means by which a most delicate adjustment of the organism to the environment can be established. To this function of the hemispheres we gave the name of " signalization."

Before passing on to describe the results of our investigation it is necessary to give some account of the purely technical side of the methods employed, and to describe the general way in which the signalizing activity of the hemispheres can be studied. It is obvious that the reflex activity of any effector organ can be chosen for the purpose of this investigation, since signalling stimuli can get linked up with any of the inborn reflexes. But, as was mentioned in the first lecture, the starting point for the present investigation was determined in particular by the study of two reflexes—the food or " alimentary " reflex, and the " defence " reflex in its mildest form, as observed when a rejectable substance finds its way into the mouth of the animal. As it turned out, these two reflexes proved a fortunate choice in many ways. Indeed, while any strong defence reflex, e.g. against such a stimulus as a powerful electric current, makes the animal extremely restless and excited ; and while the sexual reflexes require a special environment—to say nothing of their periodic character and their dependence upon age—the alimentary reflex and the mild defence reflex to rejectable substances are normal everyday occurrences.

It is essential to realize that each of these two reflexes—the alimentary reflex and the mild defence reflex to rejectable substances —consists of two distinct components, a motor and a secretory. Firstly the animal exhibits a reflex activity directed towards getting hold of the food and eating it or, in the case of rejectable substances, towards getting rid of them out of the mouth ; and secondly, in both cases an immediate secretion of saliva occurs, in the case of food, to start the physical and chemical processes of digestion and, in the case of rejectable substances, to wash them out of the mouth. We confined our experiments almost entirely to the secretory component of the reflex : the allied motor reactions were taken into account only where there were special reasons. The secretory reflex presents many important advantages for our purpose. It allows of an extremely accurate measurement of the intensity of reflex activity, since either the number of drops in a given time may be counted or else the saliva may be caused to displace a coloured fluid in a horizontally placed graduated glass tube. It would be much more difficult to obtain the same accuracy of measurement for any motor reflex, especially for such complex motor reactions as accompany reflexes to food or to rejectable substances. Even by using most delicate instruments we should never be able to reach such precision in measuring the intensity of the motor component of the reflexes as can easily be attained with the secretory component. Again, a very important point in favour of the secretory reflexes is the much smaller tendency to interpret them in an anthropomorphic fashion—*i.e.* in terms of subjective analogy. Although this seems a trivial consideration from our present standpoint, it was of importance in the earlier stages of our investigation and did undoubtedly influence our choice.

For the purpose of registering the intensity of the salivary reflex all the dogs employed in the experiments are subjected to a preliminary minor operation, which consists in the transplantation of the opening of the salivary duct from its natural place on the mucous membrane of the mouth to the outside skin. For this purpose the terminal portion of the salivary duct is dissected and freed from the surrounding tissue, and the duct, together with a small portion of the mucous membrane surrounding its natural opening, is carried through a suitable incision, to the outside of the cheek in the case of the parotid gland, or under the chin in the case of the submaxillary gland. In this new position the duct is fixed by a few stitches which are removed when the wound has healed. As a result of the operation the saliva now flows to the outside, on to the cheek or chin of the animal, instead of into the mouth, so that the measurement of the secretory activity of the gland is greatly facilitated. It is only necessary for this purpose to adjust a small glass funnel over the opening of the duct on to the skin, and for this we find a special cement prepared according to a formula of Mendeléeff [1] most useful. As an alternative, very suitable and accurate as a recording apparatus is a hemispherical bulb which also can be hermetically sealed on to the skin. From the bulb project two tubes, one pointing up and the other pointing down. The latter tube is used for drawing off the saliva which collects during each observation, while the former tube connects by air transmission with a horizontal graduated glass tube filled with coloured fluid. As the saliva flows into the hemispherical bulb the coloured fluid is displaced along the graduated tube, where

[1] *Mendeléeff's cement :* Colophonium, 50 grammes ; ferric oxide, 40 grammes ; yellow beeswax, 25 grammes.

the amount of secretion can be read off accurately. Further, it is not difficult to fix up an automatic electrically-recording device which will split up the displaced fluid into drops of exactly equal volume and reduce any lag in the movement of the fluid to a minimum.[1]

To come to the general technique of the experiments, it is important to remember that our research deals with the highly specialized

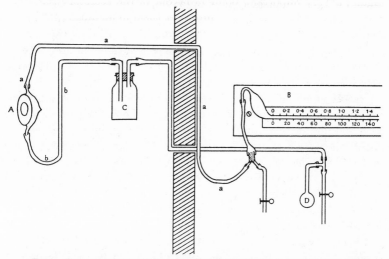

FIG. 1.—The apparatus used for recording the salivary secretion in experiments on conditioned reflexes. *A*, hemispherical bulb which is fixed over the fistula. *aaa*, connecting tube leading through the partition separating the animal's room from the experimenter and connecting the bulb *A* to the registering apparatus, *B*. *bb*, tube connecting the bulb with bottle, *C*.

After each observation a vacuum is created in the bottle *C* by depression of the rubber balloon *D* ; the saliva accumulating in *A* is thus sucked away. During the observation *A* is automatically disconnected from *C* and connected with the registering apparatus. During the aspirations of the saliva from bulb *A* the latter is automatically disconnected from the registering apparatus.

activity of the cerebral cortex, a signalizing apparatus of tremendous complexity and of most exquisite sensitivity, through which the

---

[1] In almost all the experiments quoted in these lectures the amount of salivary secretion is, for the sake of uniformity, given in drops. It was, however, only in the very earliest period of the research—before the separation of the experimenter from the animal was made—that the actual number of drops falling from a small funnel fixed over the fistula was counted, and only a few of these experiments are given. In the great majority of the experiments the salivary secretion was measured by the displacement of water in a graduated tube or by the electric recorder, allowing a much greater accuracy of measurement. The readings so obtained have been converted, in the tables, into drops. Thus, in some experiments it will be noticed that the number of drops is given to an accuracy of one-tenth.

animal is influenced by countless stimuli from the outside world. Every one of these stimuli produces a certain effect upon the animal, and all of them taken together may clash and interfere with, or else reinforce, one another. Unless we are careful to take special precautions the success of the whole investigation may be jeopardized, and we should get hopelessly lost as soon as we began to seek for cause and effect among so many and various influences, so intertwined and entangled as to form a veritable chaos. It was evident that the experimental conditions had to be simplified, and that this simplification must consist in eliminating as far as possible any stimuli outside our control which might fall upon the animal, admitting only such stimuli as could be entirely controlled by the experimenter. It was thought at the beginning of our research that it would be sufficient simply to isolate the experimenter in the research chamber with the dog on its stand, and to refuse admission to anyone else during the course of an experiment. But this precaution was found to be wholly inadequate, since the experimenter, however still he might try to be, was himself a constant source of a large number of stimuli. His slightest movements—blinking of the eyelids or movement of the eyes, posture, respiration and so on—all acted as stimuli which, falling upon the dog, were sufficient to vitiate the experiments by making exact interpretation of the results extremely difficult. In order to exclude this undue influence on the part of the experimenter as far as possible, he had to be stationed outside the room in which the dog was placed, and even this precaution proved unsuccessful in laboratories not specially designed for the study of these particular reflexes. The environment of the animal, even when shut up by itself in a room, is perpetually changing. Footfalls of a passer-by, chance conversations in neighbouring rooms, slamming of a door or vibration from a passing van, street-cries, even shadows cast through the windows into the room, any of these casual uncontrolled stimuli falling upon the receptors of the dog set up a disturbance in the cerebral hemispheres and vitiate the experiments. To get over all these disturbing factors a special laboratory was built at the Institute of Experimental Medicine in Petrograd, the funds being provided by a keen and public-spirited Moscow business man. The primary task was the protection of the dogs from uncontrolled extraneous stimuli, and this was effected by surrounding the building with an isolating trench and employing other special structural devices. Inside the building all the research rooms (four to each floor) were isolated from one another by a cross-shaped corridor ; the top and ground floors, where these rooms were situated, were separated by an intermediate floor. Each research room was carefully partitioned by the use of sound-proof materials into two compartments—one for the animal, the other for the experimenter. For stimulating the animal, and for registering the corresponding reflex response, electrical methods or pneumatic transmission were used. By means of these arrangements it was possible to get something of that stability of environmental conditions so essential to the carrying out of a successful experiment.

Another point should be mentioned—although in this respect the means at our disposal still leave something to be desired. In analysing the exceedingly complex influence of the external environment upon the animal, the experimenter must be able to exercise full control over all the conditions obtaining during the course of any experiment. He should therefore have at his disposal various instruments for affecting the animal by different kinds of stimuli, singly or combined, so as to imitate simple natural conditions. But we were often handicapped by the conditions in which we had to work and by the shortcomings of the instruments at our disposal, for we always found that the cerebral hemispheres were sensitive to far finer gradations of stimulus than we could furnish.

It is possible that the experimental conditions I have described may raise somewhere the objection of being abnormal and artificial. However it is hardly likely, in view of the infinite variety of stimuli met with under natural conditions, that we shall hit on one that is quite unprecedented in the life of the animal. Moreover, in dealing with any phenomenon of vast complexity it is absolutely necessary to isolate the different single factors involved, so as to study them independently, or in arbitrary groups in which we can keep the individual units under control. But as a matter of fact the same objection and the same answer apply equally to the whole of animal physiology. For instance, the methods of vivisection and of the study of isolated organs and tissues, which aim at the same isolation of different individual functions, have been constantly employed, and we may safely say that the greater part of the achievements of physiology are due to the successful application of such methods of control. In our experiments it is the whole animal which is placed under a limited number of rigidly defined conditions, and only by this method is it possible to study the reflexes independently of one another.

The foregoing remarks give an idea of our general aim and of the technical side of our methods. I propose to introduce you to the first and most elementary principles of the subject matter of our research by means of a few demonstrations :

Demonstration.—The dog used in the following experiment has been operated upon as described previously. It can be seen that so long as no special stimulus is applied the salivary glands remain quite inactive. But when the sounds from a beating metronome are allowed to fall upon the ear, a salivary secretion begins after 9 seconds, and in the course of 45 seconds eleven drops have been secreted. The activity of the salivary gland has thus been called into play by impulses of sound—a stimulus quite alien to food. This activity of the salivary gland cannot be regarded as anything else than a component of the alimentary reflex. Besides the secretory, the motor component of the food reflex is also very apparent in experiments of this kind. In this very experiment the dog turns in the direction from which it has been customary to present the food and begins to lick its lips vigorously.

This experiment is an example of a central nervous activity depending on the integrity of the hemispheres. A decerebrate dog would never have responded by salivary secretion to any stimulus of the kind. It is obvious also that the underlying principle of this activity is signalization. The sound of the metronome is the signal for food, and the animal reacts to the signal in the same way as if it were food ; no distinction can be observed between the effects produced on the animal by the sounds of the beating metronome and showing it real food.

Demonstration.—Food is shown to the animal. The salivary secretion begins after 5 seconds, and six drops are collected in the course of 15 seconds. The effect is the same as that observed with the sounds of the metronome. It is again a case of signalization, and is due to the activity of the hemispheres.

That the effect of sight and smell of food is not due to an inborn reflex, but to a reflex which has been acquired in the course of the animal's own individual existence, was shown by experiments carried out by Dr. Zitovich in the laboratory of the late Prof. Vartanov. Dr. Zitovich took several young puppies away from their mother and fed them for a considerable time only on milk. When the puppies were a few months old he established fistulae of their salivary ducts, and was thus able to measure accurately the secretory activity of the glands. He now showed these puppies some solid food—bread or meat—but no secretion of saliva was evoked. It is evident, therefore, that the sight of food does not in itself act as a direct stimulus to salivary secretion. Only after the puppies have been allowed to eat bread and meat on several occasions does the sight or smell of these foodstuffs evoke the secretion.

The following experiment serves to illustrate the activity of the salivary gland as an inborn reflex in contrast to signalization :

Demonstration.—Food is suddenly introduced into the dog's mouth ; secretion begins in 1 to 2 seconds. The secretion is brought about by the physical and chemical properties of the food itself acting upon receptors in the mucous membrane of the mouth and tongue. It is purely reflex.

This comparatively simple experiment explains how a decerebrate dog can die of starvation in the midst of plenty, for it will only start eating if food chances to come into contact with its mouth or tongue. Moreover, the elementary nature of the inborn reflexes, with their limitations and inadequacy, are clearly brought out in these experiments, and we are now able to appreciate the fundamental importance of those stimuli which have the character of *signals*.

Our next step will be to consider the question of the nature of signalization and of its mechanism from a purely physiological point of view. It has been mentioned already that a reflex is an inevitable reaction of the organism to an external stimulus, brought about along a definite path in the nervous system. Now it is quite evident that in signalization all the properties of a reflex are present. In the first place an external stimulus is required. This was given in our first experiment by the sounds of a metronome. These sounds falling on the auditory receptor of the dog caused the propagation of an impulse along the auditory nerve. In the brain the impulse was transmitted to the secretory nerves of the salivary glands, and passed thence to the glands, exciting them to active secretion. It is true that in the experiment with the metronome an interval of several seconds elapsed between the beginning of the stimulus and the beginning of the salivary secretion, whereas the time interval for the inborn reflex secretion was only 1 to 2 seconds. The longer latent period was, however, due to some special conditions of the experiment, as will come out more clearly as we proceed. But generally speaking the reaction to signals under natural conditions is as speedy as are the inborn reflexes. We shall be considering the latent period of signalization in fuller detail in a further lecture.

In our general survey we characterized a reflex as a necessary reaction following upon a strictly definite stimulus under strictly defined conditions. Such a definition holds perfectly true also for signalization; the only difference is that the type of the effective reaction to signals depends upon a greater number of conditions. But this does not make signalization differ fundamentally from the better known reflexes in any respect, since in the latter, variations in character or force, inhibition and absence of reflexes, can also be traced to some definite change in the conditions of the experiment.

Thorough investigation of the subject shows that accident plays no part whatever in the signalizing activity of the hemispheres, and all experiments proceed strictly according to plan. In the special laboratory I have described, the animal can frequently be kept under rigid experimental observation for 1 to 2 hours without a single drop of saliva being secreted independently of stimuli applied by the observer, although in the ordinary type of physiological laboratory experiments are very often distorted by the interference of extraneous and uncontrolled stimuli.

All these conditions leave no grounds for regarding the phenomena which we have termed " signalization " as being anything else than reflex. There is, however, another aspect of the question which at a first glance seems to point to an essential difference between the better known reflexes and signalization. Food, through its chemical and physical properties, evokes the salivary reflex in every dog right from birth, whereas this new type claimed as reflex—" the signal reflex "—is built up gradually in the course of the animal's own individual existence. But can this be considered as a fundamental point of difference, and can it hold as a valid argument against employing the term " reflex " for this new group of phenomena ? It is certainly a sufficient argument for making a definite distinction between the two types of reflex and for considering the signal reflex in a group distinct from the inborn reflex. But this does not invalidate in any way our right logically to term both " reflex," since the point of distinction does not concern the character of the response on the part of the organism, but only the mode of formation of the reflex mechanism. We may take the telephonic installation as an illustration. Communication can be effected in two ways.

My residence may be connected directly with the laboratory by a private line, and I may call up the laboratory whenever it pleases me to do so ; or on the other hand, a connection may have to be made through the central exchange. But the result in both cases is the same. The only point of distinction between the methods is that the private line provides a permanent and readily available cable, while the other line necessitates a preliminary central connection being established. In the one case the communicating wire is always complete, in the other case a small addition must be made to the wire at the central exchange. We have a similar state of affairs in reflex action. The path of the inborn reflex is already completed at birth ; but the path of the signalizing reflex has still to be completed in the higher nervous centres. We are thus brought to consider the mode of formation of new reflex mechanisms. A new reflex is formed inevitably under a given set of physiological conditions, and with the greatest ease, so that there is no need to take the subjective states of the dog into consideration. With a complete understanding of all the factors involved, the new signalizing reflexes are under the absolute control of the experimenter ; they proceed according to as rigid laws as do any other physiological processes, and must be regarded as being in every sense a part of the physiological activity of living beings. I have termed this new group of reflexes **conditioned reflexes** to distinguish them from the inborn or **unconditioned reflexes**. The term " conditioned " is becoming more and more generally employed, and I think its use is fully justified in that, compared with the inborn reflexes, these new reflexes actually do depend on very many conditions, both in their formation and in the maintenance of their physiological activity. Of course the terms " conditioned " and " unconditioned " could be replaced by others of arguably equal merit. Thus, for example, we might retain the term " inborn reflexes," and call the new type " acquired reflexes " ; or call the former " species reflexes " since they are characteristic of the species, and the latter " individual reflexes " since they vary from animal to animal in a species, and even in the same animal at different times and under different conditions. Or again we might call the former " conduction reflexes " and the latter " connection reflexes."

There should be no theoretical objection to the hypothesis of the formation of new physiological paths and new connections within the cerebral hemispheres. Since the especial function of the central nervous system is to establish most complicated and delicate correspondences between the organism and its environment we may not unnaturally expect to find there, on the analogy of the methods used by the technician in everyday experience, a highly developed connector system superimposed on a conductor system. The physiologist certainly should not object to this conception seeing that he has been used to employing the German conception of "Bahnung," which means a laying down of fresh physiological paths in the centres. Conditioned reflexes are phenomena of common and widespread occurrence : their establishment is an integral function in everyday life. We recognize them in ourselves and in other people or animals under such names as "education," "habits," and "training ; " and all of these are really nothing more than the results of an establishment of new nervous connections during the post-natal existence of the organism. They are, in actual fact, links connecting definite extraneous stimuli with their definite responsive reactions. I believe that the recognition and the study of the conditioned reflex will throw open the door to a true physiological investigation probably of all the highest nervous activities of the cerebral hemispheres, and the purpose of the present lectures is to give some account of what we have already accomplished in this direction.

We come now to consider the precise conditions under which new conditioned reflexes or new connections of nervous paths are established. The fundamental requisite is that any external stimulus which is to become the signal in a conditioned reflex must overlap in point of time with the action of an unconditioned stimulus. In the experiment which I chose as my example the unconditioned stimulus was food. Now if the intake of food by the animal takes place simultaneously with the action of a neutral stimulus which has been hitherto in no way related to food, the neutral stimulus readily acquires the property of eliciting the same reaction in the animal as would food itself. This was the case with the dog employed in our experiment with the metronome. On several occasions this animal had been stimulated by the sound of the metronome and immediately presented with food—*i.e.* a stimulus which was neutral of itself had been superimposed upon the action of the inborn alimentary reflex. We observed that, after several repetitions of the combined stimulation, the sounds from the metronome had acquired the property of stimulating salivary secretion and of evoking the motor reactions characteristic of the alimentary reflex. The first demonstration was nothing but an example of such a conditioned stimulus in action. Precisely the same occurs with the mild defence reflex to rejectable substances. Introduction into the dog's mouth of a little of an acid solution brings about a quite definite responsive reaction. The animal sets about getting rid of the acid, shaking its head violently, opening its mouth and making movements with its tongue. At the same time it produces a copious salivary secretion. The same reaction will infallibly be obtained from any stimulus which has previously been applied a sufficient number of times while acid was being introduced into the dog's mouth. Hence a first and most essential requisite for the formation of a new conditioned reflex lies in a coincidence in time of the action of any previously neutral stimulus with some definite unconditioned stimulus. Further, it is not enough that there should be overlapping between the two stimuli ; it is also and equally necessary that the conditioned stimulus should begin to operate before the unconditioned stimulus comes into action.

If this order is reversed, the unconditioned stimulus being applied first and the neutral stimulus second, the conditioned reflex cannot be established at all. Dr. Krestovnikov performed these experiments with many different modifications and controls, but the effect was always the same. The following are some of his results :

In one case 427 applications were made in succession of the odour of vanillin together with the introduction of acid into the dog's mouth, but the acid was always made to precede the vanillin by some 5 to 10 seconds. Vanillin failed to acquire the properties of a conditioned stimulus. However, in the succeeding experiment, in which the order of stimuli was reversed, the odour, this time of amyl acetate, became an effective conditioned stimulus after only 20 combinations. With another dog the loud buzzing of an electric bell set going 5 to 10 seconds after administration of food failed to establish a conditioned alimentary reflex even after 374 combinations, whereas the regular rotation of an object in front of the eyes of the animal, the rotation beginning before the administration of food, acquired the properties of a conditioned stimulus after only 5 combinations. The electric buzzer set going before the administration of food established a conditioned alimentary reflex after only a single combination.

Dr. Krestovnikov's experiments were carried out on five dogs, and the result was always negative when the neutral stimulus was applied, whether 10 seconds, 5 seconds or only a single second after the beginning of the unconditioned stimulus. During all these experiments not only the secretory reflex but also the motor reaction of the animal was carefully observed, and these observations always corroborated one another. We thus see that the first set of conditions required for the formation of a new conditioned reflex encompasses the time relation between the presentation of the unconditioned stimulus and the presentation of that agent which has to acquire the properties of a conditioned stimulus.

As regards the condition of the hemispheres themselves, an alert state of the nervous system is absolutely essential for the formation of a new conditioned reflex. If the dog is mostly drowsy during the experiments, the establishment of a conditioned reflex becomes a long and tedious process, and in extreme cases is impossible to accomplish. The hemispheres must, however, be free from any other nervous activity, and therefore in building up a new conditioned reflex it is important to avoid foreign stimuli which, falling upon the animal, would cause other reactions of their own. If this is not attended to, the establishment of a conditioned reflex is very difficult, if not impossible. Thus, for example, if the dog has been so fastened up that anything causes severe irritation, it does not matter how many times the combination of stimuli is repeated, we shall not be able to obtain a conditioned reflex. A somewhat similar case was described in the first lecture—that of the dog which exhibited the *freedom reflex* in an exaggerated degree. It can also be stated as a rule that the establishment of the first conditioned reflex in an animal is usually more difficult than the establishment of succeeding ones. It is obvious that this must be so, when we consider that even in the most favourable circumstances the experimental conditions themselves will be sure to provoke numerous different reflexes—*i.e.* will give rise to one or other disturbing activity of the hemispheres. But this statement must be qualified by remarking that in cases where the cause of these uncontrolled reflexes is not found out, so that we are not able to get rid of them, the hemispheres themselves will help us. For if the environment of the animal during the experiment does not contain any powerful disturbing elements, then practically always the extraneous reflexes will with time gradually and spontaneously weaken in strength.

The third factor determining the facility with which new conditioned reflexes can be established is the health of the animal. A good state of health will ensure the normal functioning of the cerebral hemispheres, and we shall not have to bother with the effects of any internal pathological stimuli.

The fourth, and last, group of conditions has to do with the properties of the stimulus which is to become conditioned, and also with the properties of the unconditioned stimulus which is selected. Conditioned reflexes are quite readily formed to stimuli to which the animal is more or less indifferent at the outset, though strictly speaking no stimulus within the animal's range of perception exists to which it would be absolutely indifferent. In a normal animal the slightest alteration in the environment—even the very slightest sound or faintest odour, or the smallest change in intensity of illumination—immediately evokes the reflex which I referred to in the first lecture as the investigatory reflex—" What is it ? "— manifested by a very definite motor reaction. However, if these neutral stimuli keep recurring, they spontaneously and rapidly weaken in their effect upon the hemispheres, thus bringing about bit by bit the removal of this obstacle to the establishment of a conditioned reflex. But if the extraneous stimuli are strong or unusual, the formation of a conditioned reflex will be difficult, and in extreme cases impossible.

It must also be remembered that in most cases we are not acquainted with the history of the dog before it came into the laboratory, and that we do not know what sort of conditioned reflexes have been established to stimuli which appear to be of the simplest character. But in spite of this we have, in a large number of cases, found it possible to take a strong stimulus which evoked some strong unconditioned response of its own, and still succeed in converting it into a conditioned stimulus for another reflex. Let us take for example a nocuous stimulus, such as a strong electric current or wounding or cauterization of the skin. These are obviously stimuli to vigorous unconditioned defence reflexes. The organism responds by a violent motor reaction directed towards removal of the nocuous stimulus or to its own removal from it. But we may, nevertheless, make use even of these stimuli for the establishment of a new conditioned reflex. Thus in one particular experiment a strong nocuous stimulus —an electric current of great strength—was converted into an alimentary conditioned stimulus, so that its application to the skin did not evoke the slightest defence reaction. Instead, the animal exhibited a well-marked alimentary conditioned reflex, turning its head to where it usually received the food and smacking its lips, at the same time producing a profuse secretion of saliva. The following is a record taken from a research by Dr. Eroféeva :

Time	Distance of secondary coil in cms.	Part of Skin Stimulated	Secretion of Saliva in drops during 30 secs.	Motor Reaction
4.23 p.m.	4	usual place	6	In all cases the motor reaction displayed was that character-istic of an alimen-tary reflex ; there was no slightest trace of any motor defence reflex.
4.45 ,,	4	,, ,,	5	
5.7 ,,	2	new place	7	
5.17 ,,	0	,, ,,	9	
5.45 ,,	0	,, ,,	6	

After each stimulation the dog was allowed to eat food
for a few seconds.

Similar results were obtained from dogs in which cauterization or pricking of the skin deep enough to draw blood was made to acquire the properties of an alimentary conditioned stimulus. These experiments have been apt to upset very sensitive people ; but we have been able to demonstrate, though without any pretension of penetrating into the subjective world of the dog, that they were labouring under a false impression. Subjected to the very closest scrutiny, not even the tiniest and most subtle objective phenomenon usually exhibited by animals under the influence of strong injurious stimuli can be observed in these dogs. No appreciable changes in the pulse or in the respiration occur in these animals, whereas such changes are always most prominent when the nocuous stimulus has not been converted into an alimentary conditioned stimulus. Such a remarkable phenomenon is the result of diverting the nervous impulse from one physiological path to another. This transference is dependent, however, upon a very definite condition —namely, upon the relative strengths of the two unconditioned reflexes.

Successful transformation of the unconditioned stimulus for one reflex into the conditioned stimulus for another reflex can be brought about only when the former reflex is physiologically weaker and biologically of less importance than the latter. We are led to this conclusion from a consideration of Dr. Eroféeva's experiments.

A nocuous stimulus applied to the dog's skin was transformed into a conditioned stimulus for the alimentary reflex. This, we consider, was due to the fact that the alimentary reflex is in such cases stronger than the defence reflex. In the same way we all know that when dogs join in a scuffle for food they frequently sustain skin wounds, which however play no dominant part as stimuli to any defence reflex, being entirely subordinated to the reflex for food. Nevertheless there is a certain limit—there are stronger reflexes than the alimentary reflex. One is the reflex of self-preservation, of existence or non-existence, life or death. To give only one example, it was found impossible to transform a defence reaction into an alimentary conditioned reflex when the stimulus to the unconditioned defence reaction was a strong electric current applied to skin overlying bone with no muscular layer intervening. This signifies that the afferent nervous impulses set up by injury to the bone, and signalizing far greater danger than those set up by injury to the skin, cannot acquire even a temporary connection with the part of the brain from which the alimentary reflex is controlled. Nevertheless, on the whole, the foregoing considerations emphasize the advantage of using the alimentary reflex for most of our experiments, since in the hierarchy of reflexes this holds a very high place.]

While, as we have seen, very strong and even specialized stimuli can under certain conditions acquire the properties of conditioned stimuli, there is, on the other hand, a minimum strength below which stimuli cannot be given conditioned properties. Thus a thermal stimulus of 45° C. applied to the skin can be made into an alimentary conditioned reflex, whereas at 38° to 39° C. (approximately 2° C. above the skin temperature in the dog) a thermal stimulus is ineffective [experiments of Dr. Solomonov]. Similarly, while with the help of a very strong unconditioned stimulus it is possible to convert a very unsuitable stimulus—for example, one which naturally evokes a different unconditioned reflex—into a conditioned stimulus, it is exceedingly difficult or even impossible with the help of only a weak unconditioned stimulus to transform even a very favourable neutral stimulus into a conditioned stimulus. Even where such a conditioned reflex is successfully established, its occurrence results only in a very small reflex response. Some unconditioned stimuli may be permanently weak, others may display a weakness which is only temporary—varying with the condition of the animal. As an example of the last we may take food. In the hungry animal food naturally brings about a powerful unconditioned reflex, and the conditioned reflex develops quickly. But in a dog which has not long been fed the unconditioned stimulus has only a small effect, and alimentary conditioned reflexes either are not formed at all or are established very slowly.

By complying with all the conditions which I have enumerated —which is not a very difficult task—a new conditioned reflex is infallibly obtained. We apply to the receptors of the animal rigidly defined stimuli ; these stimuli necessarily result in the formation of a new connection in the hemispheres with a consequent development of a typical reflex reaction.

To sum up, we may legitimately claim the study of the formation and properties of conditioned reflexes as a special department of physiology. There is no reason for thinking about all these events in any other way, and it is my belief that in these questions prejudices blunt the intellect and that generally speaking the preconceptions of the human mind stand in the way of any admission that the highest physiological activity of the hemispheres is rigidly determined. The difficulty is mainly due to the tremendous complexity of our subjective states ; and, of course, these cannot yet be traced to their primary causations.

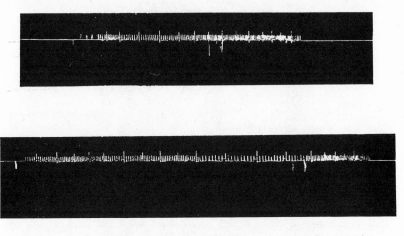

FIG. 2.—The upper tracing is a record of a conditioned salivary reflex to a tone of 637·5 d.v. The tone lasted 30 seconds—began at the first and ended at the second downward mark. The third mark shows the beginning of the unconditioned stimulus. Each mark upwards = 1 drop = 0·01 c.c. Each bigger mark = to each tenth drop. Reflex = 68 drops.

The lower tracing is a similar record, but the tone is continued for 60 seconds. Reflex = 128 drops. (Experiments by Dr. Anrep).

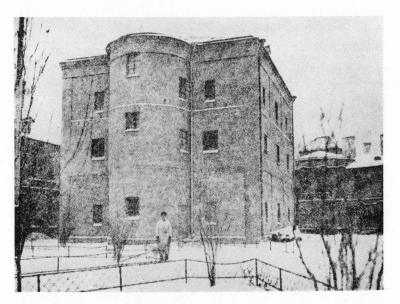

FIG. 3.—The special laboratory built for the study of conditioned reflexes, Institute of Experimental Medicine, Petrograd.

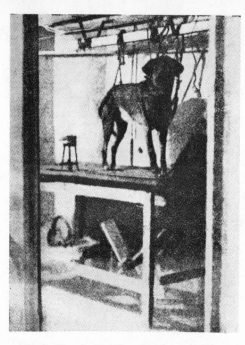

FIG. 4.—The animal's section of the double chamber.

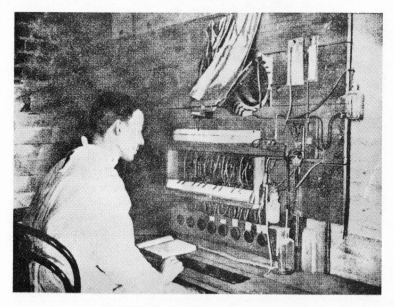

FIG. 5.—Experimenter's section of the double chamber.

LECTURE III

The formation of conditioned reflexes by means of conditioned and direct stimuli.
—Agencies which can be used as conditioned stimuli.—Inhibition of conditioned reflexes : external inhibition.

In the previous cases a conditioned reflex was obtained by linking up the action of a new stimulus with an unconditioned reflex. It is possible, however, to obtain a conditioned reflex less directly, by linking up yet a further stimulus with a conditioned stimulus which is already firmly established. Let us refer again to our experiment with the metronome. The sound of the beats was a conditioned stimulus so firmly and powerfully established as readily to admit of demonstration in face of the large audience present at my lecture. The effect of the metronome even under such unfavourable conditions was complete and precise. With the help of this strong conditioned stimulus it has been found possible to give still another stimulus conditioned properties like the first. For if some new and more or less neutral stimulus is applied in conjunction with the metronome alone—*i.e.* not at the same time giving food—this new stimulus also acquires the character of an alimentary conditioned stimulus [Drs. Zeliony, Foursikov, Frolov].

Conditioned reflexes established in this manner are termed **secondary conditioned reflexes**, and I shall bring to your attention certain precautions which must be observed for the successful establishment of reflexes of this order. The essential condition is that the new stimulus should be withdrawn some seconds before the primary stimulus is applied. With new stimuli of a medium physiological strength this lapse of time must be not less than ten seconds, while for stronger stimuli the interval must be considerably increased. Any shortening of the indicated minimal interval of time leads to a quite different result, typifying a group of extremely delicate and interesting phenomena in the physiology of the hemispheres, which will be treated in the fifth lecture.

I shall describe first an experiment conducted by Dr. Frolov illustrating the development of a secondary conditioned reflex : A dog has two primary alimentary conditioned stimuli firmly established, one to the sound of a metronome and the other to the buzzing of an electric bell. The appearance of a black square in the dog's line of vision is now used as yet a further stimulus, which is to be given the character of a secondary conditioned stimulus. The black square is held in front of the dog for ten seconds, and after an interval of fifteen seconds the metronome is sounded during 30 seconds. In the table given below the square is presented for the tenth time.

Experiment of 15th November, 1924.

Time	Conditioned Stimulus	Secretion of Saliva in Drops
1.49 p.m.	Sound of metronome	13·5
1.57 p.m.	Buzzer	16·5
2.7 p.m.	Black Square	2·5
2 hrs. 7 min. 10 sec. p.m.	[Interval 15 sec.]	3·0
2 hrs. 7 min. 25 sec. p.m.	Sound of metronome	12·0
2.20 p.m.	Buzzer	13·5
2.27 p.m.	Sound of metronome	9·5

The metronome and the buzzer were continued during
30 seconds in each case.

Prior to these experiments the appearance of the black square had no secretory effect at all. As seen from the above table the conditioned reflex of the second order is measured even at this early stage of its development by $5\frac{1}{2}$ drops (2·5 plus 3) during 25 seconds.

It was found impossible in the case of alimentary reflexes to press the secondary conditioned stimulus into our service to help us in the establishment of a new conditioned stimulus of the third order. Conditioned reflexes of the third order can however be obtained with the help of the second order of conditioned reflexes in defence reactions such as that against stimulation of the skin by a strong electric current. But even in this case we cannot proceed further than a conditioned reflex of the third order.

I shall describe the results of an experiment of Dr. Foursikov illustrating a conditioned reflex of the third order : The unconditioned stimulus to a defence reaction in a dog was given by the application of an electric stimulus to the skin over the front paw. A mechanical stimulation of the skin over the hind paw to which the dog was formerly quite indifferent had been converted by the usual procedure into a conditioned stimulus of the first order, while for the establishment of the second order of reflex a sound of bubbling water had been employed. By combining with the sound of bubbling water a tone, previously indifferent, of 760 double vibrations per second, a conditioned stimulus of the third order was now established. In these conditioned reflexes, passing from the first to the third order, the latent period progressively increases. In the same order we pass from the strongest to the weakest conditioned defence reflex. All these conditioned reflexes were maintained by Dr. Foursikov by means of appropriate reinforcement for over a year, but here again many attempts to combine a still further stimulus with the conditioned stimulus of the third order were quite unsuccessful.

So far we have discussed two distinct modes of formation of a conditioned reflex, one in which it is based directly upon an unconditioned reflex and the other in which it is based upon another conditioned reflex which has already been firmly established. There is, however, yet another method of establishing conditioned reflexes. We were led a considerable time ago to perform experiments of the following type : A dog was given a small dose of apomorphine subcutaneously and after one or two minutes a note of a definite pitch was sounded during a considerable time. While the note was still sounding the drug began to take effect upon the dog : the animal grew restless, began to moisten its lips with its tongue, secreted saliva and showed some disposition to vomit. After the experimenter had reinforced the tone with apomorphine several times it was found that the sound of the note alone sufficed to produce all the active symptoms of the drug, only in a less degree [experiments of Dr. Podkopaev]. Unfortunately, Dr. Podkopaev was prevented from pursuing his experiments and extending them by modifications in technique. However, quite recently, Dr. Krylov, of the Tashkent Bacteriological Laboratory, has made some interesting observations bearing on this matter, in the course of certain serological investigations, when he had occasion repeatedly to inject morphine into dogs hypodermically. It is well known that the first effect of a hypodermic injection of morphine is to produce nausea with profuse secretion of saliva, followed by vomiting, and then profound sleep. Dr. Krylov, however, observed when the injections were repeated regularly that after 5 or 6 days the preliminaries of injection were in themselves sufficient to produce all these symptoms—nausea, secretion of saliva, vomiting and sleep. Under these circumstances the symptoms are now the effect, not of the morphine acting through the blood stream directly on the vomiting centre, but of all the external stimuli which previously had preceded the injection of morphine. The connection between the morphine itself and the various signals may in this instance be very remote, and in the most striking cases all the symptoms could be produced by the dogs simply seeing the experimenter. Where such a stimulus was insufficient it was necessary to open the box containing the syringe, to crop the fur over a small area of skin and wipe with alcohol, and perhaps even to inject some harmless fluid before the symptoms could be obtained. The greater the number of previous injections of morphine the less preparation had to be performed in order to evoke a reaction simulating that produced by the drug. Dr. Krylov was able to demonstrate these facts quite easily in my laboratory. In a series of experiments specially adapted to the purpose he showed that the phenomena described are absolutely identical with conditioned reflexes. The experiments readily lend themselves for lecture demonstration.

Demonstration.—The dog has repeatedly been injected with morphine on previous occasions, and is now held quietly on the table by an attendant who has never had anything to do with injecting the morphine. When the experimenter approaches, the dog gets restless and moistens its lips, and as soon as the experimenter touches the animal, severe nausea and profuse secretion of saliva begin.

This experiment provides a clue to the well-known fact that dogs will eat meat the first time it is offered them, after removal of their parathyroids, or after an Eck fistula and tying of the portal vein, but on all subsequent occasions refuse it. Evidently in these cases the appearance and smell of meat produce of themselves a reaction identical with that produced through direct pathological action in the absence of the parathyroids or the portal circulation, by those toxic substances deriving from digestion of the meat.

All this brings us to the important question of the intimate mechanism by which new nervous connections are established in the hemispheres. It is easy to suggest an explanation on the basis of the actual facts as they are known at present. Any unconditioned, or any firmly established conditioned, stimulus undoubtedly evokes a state of nervous activity in some definite part of the brain. Using the generally accepted terminology, let us refer to such areas of the brain as centres, not however thereby implying any idea of anatomical localization. During the period of excitation of such centres all other external stimuli which happen to affect the animal are conducted to these centres, and the paths by which they are conducted through the hemispheres become thereby specially marked out. This is the only possible interpretation of the facts, and upon this interpretation was planned the series of experiments with apomorphine which have just been described as corroborating so thoroughly the experiments of Dr. Krylov with morphine. Arguing that excitations set up in the cells of the cortex were constantly transmitted to the salivary centre when this was reflexly excited to activity by external agencies, we had to expect a precisely similar phenomenon to take place when the centre was stimulated directly (*i.e.* automatically) by changes in the internal environment due to alterations in the composition of the blood. Excitations set up in the cortex would now also be transmitted to the salivary and to the vomiting centres. This assumption was fully justified in the sequel.

The facts dealt with so far reveal another important feature of this mechanism, namely, that such external stimuli as have been from the very birth of the animal transmitted to a definite centre, can, notwithstanding, be diverted and made to follow another route, becoming linked up by the nervous connection to another centre, provided always that this second centre is physiologically more powerful than the first.

This linking up of impulses in different areas of the brain, by the formation of new nervous connections, is the first nervous mechanism we have encountered in our study of the physiology of the hemispheres. The question as to the site where this new nervous connection occurs has not yet been clearly answered. Is it within the cortex exclusively, or does it take place between the cortex and the subcortical areas ? Both possibilities are conceivable. In the latter case it must be assumed that when two points, one in the cortex, the other in a subcortical area, are simultaneously excited by different stimuli, a path is established for the transmission of the excitation direct from the former point to the latter. If on the other hand the connection takes place entirely within the cortex, it is necessary to assume either that all the receptor organs (including internal receptors) of the organism are represented in the cortex, in which case impulses originating in different organs during their activity would be transmitted to the corresponding cortical point, which would then enter into connection with a point excited by the external stimulus, or else that stimuli which lead to activity of an organ gain direct representation in the cortex independently of the simultaneous excitation of a subcortical area. Of the two last mentioned alternatives I have reason to believe that the latter represents what probably takes place in the intact brain when the hemispheres are in a state of alertness. In any case it appears that the cells predominantly excited at a given time become foci attracting to themselves the nervous impulses aroused by new stimuli—impulses which on repetition tend to follow the same path and so to establish conditioned reflexes.

We must now take some account of the agencies which can be transformed into conditioned stimuli. This is not so easy a problem as appears at first sight. Of course to give a general answer is very simple ; any agent in nature which acts on any adequate receptor apparatus of an organism can be made into a conditioned stimulus for that organism. This general statement, however, needs both amplification and restriction. We can, in the first place, divide up natural agencies into their ultimate component parts as regards their properties as physiological stimuli. Even a very small single component of such agency may acquire in itself the properties of a conditioned stimulus. Such, for example, may be a very small variation in loudness of a tone, or a small and barely distinguishable variation in luminosity, and so on. In this way alone the number of potentially effective stimuli in nature is extended almost indefinitely, although it is also obvious that a limit is set to the fineness of gradation of such stimuli by the degree of sensitivity and perfection of the peripheral receptor organs of the organism. On the other hand, the animal may be affected by the sum total of numerous elementary stimuli acting together as a whole. For example, in distinguishing facial appearance we take into account simultaneously form, dimensions, shades, colours. We behave very much in the same way when making out our direction in a more or less familiar neighbourhood. Such examples of compound stimuli can be multiplied indefinitely, and when we consider the unlimited possibilities of grouping the very great number of single elementary stimuli, we shall arrive at a very formidable figure. Yet in this case also a limit is undoubtedly imposed by the intrinsic structure of the cerebral hemispheres themselves. But I wish at present only to give some idea of the possible number of conditioned stimuli, leaving a more detailed discussion of this important matter to a subsequent lecture.

So far we have considered only one broad group of conditioned stimuli, namely those derived from the appearance of any natural agency. But the disappearance also of such an agency may become the stimulus to a conditioned reflex. Let us take the following example as an illustration. A metronome is sounding continuously in the experimental laboratory when the dog is brought in. The sound of the metronome is now cut out, and immediately an unconditioned stimulus, say food or a rejectable substance, is introduced. After several repetitions of this procedure it is found that the disappearance of the sound has become the stimulus to a new conditioned reflex [Dr. Zeliony and Dr. Makovsky].

Not only can the cessation of a stimulus be made the signal to a conditioned reflex, but also a diminution in its strength, if this diminution is sufficiently rapid. The effect of rate of change of some property of a stimulating agent is well brought out in the following experiment by Dr. Zeliony. The sudden stoppage of a powerful pneumatic tuning fork D–2 had been made into the signal for a conditioned alimentary reflex, which was measured by 32 drops of salivary secretion during the test interval ; but a gradual damping down of this tone over a period of 12 minutes, though ending in complete extinction, did not yield a single drop of saliva. So we see that not only can the appearance of some external agency act as a conditional stimulus, but its disappearance also, or the rapid weakening of its strength. Thus the number of potential stimuli to a conditioned reflex is once more greatly increased.

The next group of conditioned stimuli can be regarded as a variation, or further development, of the type of stimuli with deferred action which has just been discussed. The stimulus this time is not the actual disappearance of an external agent, but the trace left by the action of this agent on the central nervous system after the agent itself has been removed. The procedure of development of such reflexes is as follows. Any convenient external stimulus is applied to the animal and continued for $\frac{1}{2}$ to 1 minute. After another definite interval of 1–3 minutes, food or a rejectable substance is introduced into the mouth. It is found that after several repetitions of this routine the stimulus will not itself evoke any reaction ; neither will its disappearance ; but the appropriate reaction will occur after a definite interval, the after-effect of the excitation caused by the stimulus being the operative factor. We have to distinguish this type of reflex from the type described previously, in which the unconditioned stimulus coincided for part of its duration with the conditioned stimulus. The type described in this paragraph is termed a trace conditioned reflex.

I shall describe here an experiment by Dr. Grossman with trace conditioned reflexes : A tactile stimulation of the skin was employed as a stimulus for the trace reflex to injection of acid. The tactile stimulus was applied during one minute and acid was introduced into the mouth after a further period of one minute.

Experiment of 18th February, 1909.

Time	Conditioned Stimulus	Salivary Secretion in Drops	
		During 1 min. of Stimulation	During 1 min. of Pause
12.40 p.m.	Mechanical stimu-	0	0·5
12.50 ,,	lation of the skin	0	10
1.15 ,,	during one minute	0	11
1.27 ,,	in every case.	0	14

The conditioned stimulus was always reinforced by
introduction of acid at the end of the pause.

Trace reflexes may be of different character, depending on the length of pause between the termination of the conditioned stimulus and the appearance of the unconditioned stimulus. When the pause is short, being a matter of only a few seconds, then the trace left by the conditioned stimulus is still fresh, and the reflex is what we may term a short-trace reflex. On the other hand, if a considerable interval, one minute or more, is allowed to elapse between the termination of the conditioned and the beginning of the unconditioned stimulus we have a long-trace reflex. It is important to distinguish all these cases on account of the essential peculiarities exhibited by long-trace reflexes.

We come now to the last of those agents which can be transformed into a conditioned stimulus, and this one is peculiar in that it originates apparently quite regularly and spontaneously. Its operation depends on the fact that every stimulus must leave a trace on the nervous system for a greater or less time—a fact which has long been recognized in physiology under the name of after effect. The further agency I wish to introduce to you is no less real, but the clear apprehension of its nature is apt to present some difficulty.

First of all I shall describe an experiment of a general nature. One dog was given food at regular intervals of time ; another had acid introduced into the mouth at the same intervals. After this had gone on for a little time it was found that food or acid was no longer necessary to produce the alimentary or mild defence reflex, but that these reflexes appeared spontaneously at the regular intervals of time. This may be illustrated by the following detailed experiment of Dr. Feokritova : A dog is placed in the stand and given food regularly every thirtieth minute. In the control experiments any-one feeding after the first few is omitted, and it is found that despite the omission a secretion of saliva with a corresponding alimentary motor reaction is produced at about the thirtieth minute. Sometimes this reaction occurs exactly at the thirtieth minute, but it may be one or two minutes late. In the interval there is not the least sign of any alimentary reaction, especially if the routine has been repeated a good number of times. When we come to seek an interpretation of these results, it seems pretty evident that the duration of time has acquired the properties of a conditioned stimulus.

⌐ The experiment just described may be performed with the following modification. The animal can be given food regularly every thirtieth minute, but with the addition, say, of the sound of a metronome a few seconds before the food. The animal is thus stimulated at regular intervals of thirty minutes by a combination of two stimuli, one of which is the time factor and the other the beats of the metronome. In this manner a conditioned reflex is established to a compound stimulus consisting of the sound plus the condition of the hemispheres at the thirtieth minute, when both are reinforced by food. Further, if the sound is now applied not at the thirtieth minute after the preceding feeding, but, say, at the fifth or eighth minute, it entirely fails to produce any alimentary conditioned reflex. If it is applied slightly later it produces some effect ; applied at the twentieth minute the effect is greater ; at the twenty-fifth minute greater still. At the thirtieth minute the reaction is of course complete. If the sound is never combined with food except when applied at the full interval, in time it ceases to have any effect even at the twenty-ninth minute and will only produce a reaction at the thirtieth minute—but then a full reaction. An illustration is given from experiments by Dr. Feokritova : A dog is given food every half-hour, each feeding being preceded by the sound of a metronome, which is continued for thirty seconds; the effect of the metronome is tested at the twenty-ninth minute.

Experiment, 20th December, 1911.

Time	Conditioned Stimulus applied 30 secs. previously	Amount of Saliva secreted in drops during 30 seconds
3.30 p.m.	Sound of metronome	10
4.00 p.m.	,, ,,	7
4.29 p.m.	,, ,,	**0**
4.30 p.m.	,, ,,	7

Of course in the establishment of a conditioned reflex of this type any length of time interval can be employed. No experiments, however, were made with longer intervals than half an hour.⟩

What is the physiological meaning of these time intervals in their rôle as conditioned stimuli ? Only a tentative approach can be made to a definite answer to such a question at present : Time is measured from a general point of view by registering different cyclic phenomena in nature, such for instance as the rising and setting of the sun or the vibration of the pendulum of a clock. But many cyclic phenomena take place inside the animal's body. In the course of 24 hours the brain receives a very considerable number of stimuli, becomes fatigued, and again restored through sleep. The alimentary canal is periodically filled or emptied ; and, in fact, changes in practically all the component tissues and parts of the organism are capable of influencing the cerebral hemispheres. This continuous cycle of direct and indirect influences upon the nervous activity constitutes the physiological basis for the estimation of duration of time. We may consider the following simple case of physiological registration of short intervals of time by the hemispheres. It is well known that a fresh stimulus—we will take for example an olfactory stimulus—produces a very definite nervous excitation. This, however, gradually and progressively weakens. The physiological state of the nervous elements, under the influence of the continued stimulation, without doubt undergoes a series of simultaneous and successive changes. The same is true for the reverse condition : When a stimulus is withdrawn the change is perceived for some time very acutely, but quite soon its influence diminishes until we are no longer aware of it. Here again the physiological condition of the nerve cells is, doubtless, undergoing the reverse series of changes. From this point of view we can give an interpretation of the establishment of conditioned reflexes to an interruption of a stimulus, and to a trace of a stimulus, as well as, apparently, to a duration of time. In the experiment described the administration of food was accompanied and followed by a definite activity in a large number of organs, which all underwent a series of definite cyclic changes. All these changes were reflected in the cerebral hemispheres where they fell on appropriate receptive fields, and a definite phase of these changes acquired the properties of the conditioned stimulus.

To conclude this part of our discussion I shall suggest the following modification and amplification of our definition of agencies which can become conditioned, viz. that innumerable individual fluctuations in the external and internal environment of the organism may, each and all of them, singly or collectively, being reflected in definite changes in the cells of the cerebral cortex, acquire the properties of a conditioned stimulus.

We shall now follow out another important group of phenomena. Hitherto we have been dealing with reflexes of a positive character —i.e. reflexes which ultimately gave rise to positive reactions, both motor and secretory, all of them associated with various processes of excitation in the nervous system. There is, however, another manifestation of nervous activity which is in no way inferior in physiological and vital importance to that positive manifestation which has just been considered. I refer to nervous inhibition. When we come to investigate the highly complex functions of the cerebral hemispheres, we naturally expect to come across inhibitory phenomena, for these are very constantly and very intimately mixed up with the positive phenomena of nervous excitation. But before dealing with these I consider it advisable to give a brief description of inhibition of centres as observed in the field of unconditioned reflexes.

The present state of physiological knowledge enables us to recognize under normal conditions two types of central inhibition. These may be termed direct and indirect, or internal and external respectively. On the one hand we are familiar with the direct inhibitory action of certain afferent nerves, or of certain physical and chemical properties of the blood, upon definite nervous centres controlling respiration, circulation, locomotion and so on. On the other hand the central nervous system supplies numerous cases of indirect inhibition. In the latter cases inhibition of the activity of a given centre is brought about as the result of an activity of some other centre, which activity has arisen in its turn as a result of excitation from some afferent nerve or from some change in the composition of the blood. Instances of other kinds of inhibition are provided by those complex unconditioned reflexes generally known as "instincts." Thus many insects, especially when in the larval stage, become immobilized and drop down at the slightest touch. This is obviously a case of direct inhibition of the entire nervous apparatus of locomotion. Another example may be taken from the newly hatched chick, which manifests straightway a pecking reflex to the visual stimulus of small objects or patches of light and shade. If, however, a strongly irritant and injurious substance gets taken up, the pecking reflex becomes inhibited immediately and is replaced by a defence reaction leading to a rejection of the irritating substance. This is a result of an interaction of two active centres, and is an example of external inhibition.

Conditioned reflexes are also subject to these two types of central inhibition. Since the indirect or external inhibition of conditioned reflexes does not differ in the least from the corresponding inhibition of unconditioned reflexes I shall take this first. The following is a very simple case, and one of common occurrence in our earlier experiments. The dog and the experimenter would be isolated in the experimental room, all the conditions remaining for a while constant. Suddenly some disturbing factor would arise—a sound would penetrate into the room ; some quick change in illumination would occur, the sun going behind a cloud ; or a draught would get in underneath the door, and maybe bring some odour with it. If any one of these extra stimuli happened to be introduced just at the time of application of the conditioned stimulus, it would inevitably bring about a more or less pronounced weakening or even a complete disappearance of the reflex response, depending on the strength of the extra stimulus. The interpretation of this simple case does not present much difficulty. The appearance of any new stimulus immediately evokes the investigatory reflex and the animal fixes all its appropriate receptor organs upon the source of disturbance, pricking up its ears, fastening its gaze upon the disturbing agency, and sniffing the air. The investigatory reflex is excited and the conditioned reflex is in consequence inhibited.

These extra stimuli have also another important influence. Every stimulus, however rapidly it may disappear, is effective not only while it lasts, but also for some time after its cessation while its after-effect lasts. On account of this, if the conditioned stimulus is applied shortly after the extra stimulus, the reflex reaction will be partly inhibited. Different extra stimuli, whether accidental or deliberate, produce after-effects of different length. Some may still have a powerful after-effect after 2 or 3 minutes, others after 10 or 12 minutes, and still others after several days. These longer after-effects occur especially with alimentary, and gustatory stimuli in general, and in many experiments they have to be taken seriously into account. The effect of exciting an extra reflex will, of course, vary according as the conditioned reflex has only freshly been formed or has already been firmly established. It is obvious that an old-established reflex is not likely to be so easily inhibited as a recent one. In our old laboratory the neglect to provide against external stimuli often led to a curious complication when I visited some of my co-workers. Having by himself established a new conditioned reflex, working in the room with the dog, the experimenter would invite me for a demonstration, and then everything would go wrong and he would be unable to show anything at all. It was I who presented the extra stimulus : the investigatory reflex was immediately brought into play : the dog gazed at me, and smelled at me, and of course this was sufficient to inhibit every recently established reflex. Another example is very similar. If one experimenter had worked with a dog and established some firm and stable conditioned reflexes, conducting numerous experiments with them, when he handed the animal over to another experimenter to work with, all the reflexes disappeared for a considerable time. The same happened when the dog was changed over from one research room to another.

In the case of extra stimuli, which awaken specialized reflex responses, the resulting inhibition is extremely profound. Examples of such extra stimuli are, the sight or sound of game for sporting dogs, of cats for some dogs, rustling under the floor for others, and so on. Not only such specialized stimuli, but also any very strong or unusual stimulus exhibits a prolonged and pronounced inhibitory after-effect. With respect to strong or unusual stimuli dogs can be divided into two groups. Some respond in a manner which may be termed positive, i.e. aggressively—barking furiously and baring their teeth. Others exhibit a defence reaction of a passive nature—they try to get free and run away or they stand like lumps of stone absolutely motionless ; and sometimes they will shiver violently and crouch down in the stand ; or they may urinate, a most unusual occurrence for dogs while in the stand. In these dogs inhibition predominates. This case can also be classified as a type of **indirect** or **external inhibition** of conditioned reflexes, for the inhibition originates primarily in other parts of the brain than that where the reflex response is initiated.

All the cases of external inhibition which have just been discussed are of a temporary nature, and on this account the stimuli producing these effects are termed **temporary inhibitory stimuli.** If they act upon the animal repeatedly and are not reinforced with any unconditioned or conditioned stimulus, sooner or later they become lost upon the organism and lose all their inhibitory properties.

An experiment providing an admirable illustration of this condition occurred during the first two lectures, without the audience being aware of it. The dog used for the experiment with the metronome (p. 22) had been kept in the lecture theatre during the whole of one lecture previous to the demonstration, while one of my co-workers repeatedly tried the experiment. As a matter of fact the experiment was at first a failure, the reflex being inhibited, and the animal only freed itself gradually from the inhibitory influence of the unfamiliar surroundings.

Some years ago, when I was delivering a series of lectures on conditioned reflexes, I had to proceed in a similar manner for demonstration of experiments. The dogs were placed in the lecture theatre from the very beginning of the course of lectures, and my co-workers constantly repeated the experiments preliminary to the actual lecture demonstration, and only with this precaution could the experiments be successfully conducted. In this series of lectures, unfortunately, the present unavoidable and unforeseen circumstances have deprived me of these facilities; I shall have to restrict myself to occasional demonstrations, keeping chiefly to a description of experiments and researches conducted in our laboratories.

In addition to the **temporary external inhibition,** a second type of external inhibition can be distinguished. This may be termed **permanent external inhibition,** since it does not weaken through repetition, but constantly maintains its strength. An example may be found in the reaction to acid. If the dog is given food, even some considerable time before the conditioned stimulus to the acid is applied, this reflex cannot be obtained. What happens is that the alimentary centres inhibit the reaction to acid for a considerable time after they themselves are set into activity, and this happens always, no matter how often the experiment may be repeated. It is therefore a permanent external inhibition which does not undergo any sort of spontaneous extinction. Such cases are not at all rare. If a conditioned reflex is established to introduction of acid, any careless administration—too much acid, or too concentrated, or applied too often—produces a severe irritation of the buccal mucous membrane and produces a permanent inhibition of conditioned reflexes which lasts until the pathological condition is removed. Again, the dog may have some laceration of the skin which may be constantly irritated by the supporting loops of the stand. The defence reflex will then become dominant while the conditioned reflexes, and especially the mild defence reflex to acid, will be inhibited. Many more examples of this nature could be quoted. I will give one or two more. In one case an experiment may be running quite smoothly, and suddenly all conditioned reflexes begin to fail, and finally disappear altogether. The dog is taken out, allowed to urinate, and then all the reflexes return to normal. Evidently stimulation of the centre for micturition had inhibited the conditioned reflexes. Another example may be chosen in the season when the females are in heat. If the males have been housed near the females before the experiment, it is found that all their conditioned reflexes are inhibited in greater or less degree. It is obvious in this case that the inhibition derives from the sexual centres in the hemispheres. In face of such numerous potential sources of inhibition we see that our term of " conditioned " reflexes is very appropriate. Yet these conditions can readily be controlled, and the disquieting factors can be eliminated. All of them produce external inhibition, and I should like to give a final summing up of their character : No sooner does any extra nervous excitation occur in the central nervous system than it immediately makes its presence felt in diminishing or abolishing conditioned reflexes, but temporarily only, as long as the causative stimulus or its after-effect is present.

LECTURE IV

Internal inhibition of conditioned reflexes : (a) Extinction.

TOWARDS the end of the last lecture I discussed external inhibition of conditioned reflexes, as exhibited in numerous cases of temporary clashing between conditioned reflexes and other extra excitatory processes in the brain, and we saw how this clashing led to weakening, more or less profound, and sometimes even to the disappearance of the conditioned reflexes.

In the second type of inhibition, which may be termed **internal inhibition,** the positive conditioned stimulus itself becomes, under definite conditions, negative or inhibitory ; it now evokes in the cells of the cortex a process of inhibition instead of the usual excitation. Conditions favouring the development of conditioned reflexes of the negative or inhibitory type are of frequent occurrence, and these reflexes are met with not less frequently than reflexes of the positive or excitatory type.

The most striking difference between external and internal inhibition is that, whereas under the conditions described in the preceding lecture external inhibition is produced on the very first application of an extra stimulus, internal inhibition on the other hand always develops progressively, quite often very slowly, and in many cases with difficulty.

I shall start by describing that form of internal inhibition which was first encountered in our researches, and shall trace the growth of our present conception of its nature.

Demonstration.—The following is an example of an experiment illustrating the first group of internal inhibitions.

We are taking for this experiment the same dog that was used in the second lecture for the conditioned reflex to the sound of the metronome. In testing the reflex the metronome is sounded for 30 seconds during which the secretion of saliva is measured in drops, and at the same time the interval between the beginning of the stimulus and the beginning of the salivary secretion is recorded. This interval is customarily called the latent period, although as will be seen later some other term might more usefully have been employed. Stimulation by the metronome is not followed in this particular experiment by feeding, *i.e.* contrary to our usual routine the conditioned reflex is not reinforced. The stimulus of the metronome is repeated during periods of 30 seconds at intervals of two minutes. The following results are obtained :

Latent Period in Seconds	Secretion of Saliva in Drops during 30 seconds
3	10
7	7
5	8
4	5
5	7
9	4
13	3

The continuation of this experiment must be left over until later on in the lecture when it will be possible to add a further important detail. One detail, however, already stands out quite clearly, namely that repeated application of a conditioned stimulus which is not followed up by reinforcement leads to a weakening of the conditioned reflex. If the experiment had been pushed further there would have come a stage when the reflex would entirely disappear. This phenomenon of a rapid and more or less smoothly progressive weakening of the reflex to a conditioned stimulus which is repeated a number of times without reinforcement may appropriately be termed **experimental extinction of conditioned reflexes**. Such a term has the advantage that it does not imply any hypothesis as to the exact mechanism by which the phenomenon is brought about.

Abundant evidence has been collected in our laboratories relating to experimental extinction of conditioned reflexes, but before I can discuss this it is necessary to make a few remarks about the terminology which will be employed. Formerly we made a distinction between " natural " and " artificial " conditioned reflexes, " natural " reflexes being those which appeared to be formed spontaneously as a result of the natural association of, for example, the sight and smell of food with the eating of food itself, or of the procedure of introducing acid or some rejectable substance with the acid or the rejectable substance itself, while " artificial " reflexes were those which could be formed as a result of artificially associating with the food or rejectable substance stimuli which in the ordinary course of events have nothing in common with food or the rejectable substance. At the present time, however, we know that there is not the slightest difference in properties between all these reflexes. I mention this fact here because the numerous experiments of the earlier period of our work were carried out with the " natural " conditioned reflexes, and it is from these that I shall draw many examples in the present lecture. All the numerous artificial stimuli which we now use every day in our experiments were important to us at the time of those experiments because they provided easily controlled, exact, and regularly reproducible stimuli, and because they could be applied to check the correctness of our conception of the mechanism by which natural conditioned reflexes are formed. At present the artificial stimuli predominate in importance because of the vast field of research they have unfolded to us and because they came ultimately to provide the most important material for our investigation.

The progress of experimental extinction is often subject to fluctuation. The fluctuations of an otherwise smooth curve may be brought about both by external and internal factors. To obtain a smooth curve of extinction of a conditioned reflex it is necessary to maintain the unreinforced conditioned stimulus rigidly constant in character and strength ; the environing experimental conditions also must remain absolutely constant. Very wide fluctuations in the reflex undergoing experimental extinction are apt to occur in the case of a natural conditioned stimulus, for example the presentation of food, which may be held at one time further away from the animal than at another, or which may be held stationary or slightly moving. With an artificial conditioned stimulus, on the other hand, it is quite easy to obtain an exact repetition of the stimulus and so to avoid this cause of disturbance in the curve of extinction. With regard to variations in the experimental conditions it is only natural that any marked changes in the environment, such, for example, as any introduction of strong extra stimuli which would produce external inhibition, should also affect the smoothness of the curve of experimental extinction. Such strong stimuli abruptly diminish all conditioned reflexes, including of course reflexes undergoing extinction, but the reflexes reappear when the disturbing stimuli are removed. Even greater interest attaches to the effect of extra stimuli of small intensity. Such stimuli produce a temporary weakening, not of the reflex, but of the progress of the experimental extinction. An example can be seen in the fifth repetition of the conditioned stimulus in our lecture demonstration (p. 49). The rise in the reaction from 5 drops to 7 drops definitely coincided with some small disturbance produced by the audience. This effect of extra stimuli of small intensity is of great importance for the physiology of the hemispheres, and we shall return to it later in this lecture.

Even with stimuli of constant strength, and with constant environing conditions, fluctuations in the curve of experimental extinction are sometimes observed. These fluctuations are of rhythmic character and are evidently due to some internal factors. These factors affect directly the nervous processes involved in experimental extinction, and we shall come across examples on frequent occasions in the further course of our discussion.

The rate of experimental extinction, measured by the period of time during which a given stimulus must be applied at definite regular intervals without reinforcement before the reflex response becomes zero, depends on numerous conditions. First among these come any individual peculiarities of the nervous organization of the animal. Under the same set of external conditions some animals will have the conditioned reflexes rapidly extinguished, while in others the whole process will be much delayed. In excitable dogs the reflexes are mostly slow of extinction, but in quiet animals extinction is rapid. Clearly also the extent to which a reflex has gained a firm footing is an important point : a reflex which has only recently been established is likely to be less firmly grounded than an older one and is likely to suffer extinction the more quickly. The rapidity of extinction depends also in a great measure upon the intensity of the unconditioned reflex underlying the conditioned one which is undergoing experimental extinction.

In this connection the following experiments by Dr. Babkin are of interest :

An unconditioned reflex to a given quantity of a 1% extract of quassia introduced into the dog's mouth produces on an average of ten experiments 1·71 c.c. of salivary secretion. A conditioned reflex established on the basis of this unconditioned one produces 0·3 c.c. during one minute of stimulation. A definite quantity of 0·1% aqueous solution of hydrochloric acid evokes in the same dog an unconditioned reflex measuring on an average of five experiments

5·2 c.c. The corresponding conditioned reflex gives 0·9 c.c. during one minute of stimulation. The conditioned stimuli are " natural " ones, namely, the presentation of quassia or of acid, as the case may be, at some distance from the animal. Every other condition of the experiment is maintained rigidly constant. The following table illustrates the experimental extinction of each of the two conditioned reflexes in this animal.

Extinction of the Conditioned Reflex to Hydrochloric Acid. Secretion of Saliva in c.cs. during one minute	Extinction of the Conditioned Reflex to Extract of Quassia. Secretion of Saliva in c.cs. during one minute
1·00 c.c.	0·35 c.c.
0·60 c.c.	0·10 c.c.
0·40 c.c.	0·00 c.c.
0·30 c.c.	
0·15 c.c.	
0·20 c.c.	
0·10 c.c.	
0·00 c.c.	

Yet another important factor in determining the rate of experimental extinction is the length of pause between successive repetitions of the stimulus without reinforcement. The shorter the pause the more quickly will extinction of the reflex be obtained, and in most cases a smaller number of repetitions will be required. The conditions may be illustrated from an experiment by Dr. Babkin :

The conditioned stimulus was provided by meat powder presented to the dog at a distance for one minute ; the stimulus was repeated several times in succession, and was of course not reinforced. The five series of extinctions given below were carried out on the same animal in a single day. Between separate extinctions the dog was given a rest, and the reflex was reinforced by feeding with meat powder.

Stimulation applied at intervals of two minutes.

Time	Amount of Saliva secreted during one minute in c.cs.
11.46 a.m.	0·6
11.49 ,,	0·3
11.52 ,,	0·1
11.55 ,,	0·2
11.58 ,,	0·15
12.01 p.m.	0·0

Stimulation applied at intervals of four minutes.

Time								Amount of Saliva secreted during one minute in c.cs.
12.10 p.m.	-	-	-	-	-	-	-	0·7
12.15 ,,	-	-	-	-	-	-	-	0·4
12.20 ,,	-	-	-	-	-	-	-	0·3
12.25 ,,	-	-	-	-	-	-	-	0·1
12.30 ,,	-	-	-	-	-	-	-	0·0

Stimulation applied at intervals of eight minutes.

1.47 p.m.	-	-	-	-	-	-	-	0·4
1.56 ,,	-	-	-	-	-	-	-	0·3
2.05 ,,	-	-	-	-	-	-	-	0·2
2.14 ,,	-	-	-	-	-	-	-	0·15
2.23 ,,	-	-	-	-	-	-	-	0·1
2.32 ,,	-	-	-	-	-	-	-	0·2
2.41 ,,	-	-	-	-	-	-	-	0·0

Stimulation applied at intervals of sixteen minutes.

3.23 p.m.	-	-	-	-	-	-	-	0·6
3.40 ,,	-	-	-	-	-	-	-	0·6
3.57 ,,	-	-	-	-	-	-	-	0·5
4.14 ,,	-	-	-	-	-	-	-	0·3
4.31 ,,	-	-	-	-	-	-	-	0·1
4.48 ,,	-	-	-	-	-	-	-	0·2
5.05 ,,	-	-	-	-	-	-	-	0·1
5.22 ,,	-	-	-	-	-	-	-	0·1

Stimulation applied at intervals of two minutes.

5.27 p.m.	-	-	-	-	-	-	-	0·6
5.30 ,,	-	-	-	-	-	-	-	0·3
5.33 ,,	-	-	-	-	-	-	-	0·3
5.36 ,,	-	-	-	-	-	-	-	0·2
5.39 ,,	-	-	-	-	-	-	-	0·1
5.42 ,,	-	-	-	-	-	-	-	0·05
5.45 ,,	-	-	-	-	-	-	-	0·0

To sum up :

With an interval of 2 minutes extinction was obtained in 15 minutes.
,,   ,,   4   ,,   ,,   ,,   20   ,,
,,   ,,   8   ,,   ,,   ,,   54   ,,
,,   ,,   16   ,,   ,,   incomplete in 2 hours.
,,   ,,   2   ,,   ,,   occurred in 18 minutes.

The final condition which influences the rate of experimental extinction is the number of times the given reflex has been subjected to extinction in the same animal. After each fresh extinction of a conditioned reflex the number of unreinforced conditioned stimuli required to produce the next experimental extinction is less, until in the end a zero reaction results in some dogs from only a single application of the unreinforced conditioned stimulus.

A circumstance of especial interest is that experimental extinction of any single conditioned reflex results, not only in a weakening of that particular conditioned reflex which is directly subjected to the extinction (*primary extinction*), but also in a weakening of other conditioned reflexes which were not directly subjected to extinction (*secondary extinction*). This latter phenomenon involves not only those conditioned reflexes which were based upon a common unconditioned reflex with the primarily extinguished one (*homogeneous conditioned reflexes*), but also those which were based upon a different unconditioned reflex (*heterogeneous conditioned reflexes*). Sometimes secondary extinction reaches a profound degree, involving even the unconditioned reflexes. The latter case is illustrated by the following experiment of Dr. Perelzweig :

A given quantity of hydrochloric acid produced on an average in a dog a salivary secretion of 6 c.c. After several extinctions of the corresponding conditioned defence reflex, in which the conditioned stimulus was tactile, application of the acid itself produced only 3·8 c.c. Even more striking results were obtained in connection with the secondary extinction of homogeneous conditioned reflexes, and our experiments were mainly concerned with these.

In every case of secondary extinction the degree to which the primary experimental extinction is carried is of first importance. A primary experimental extinction of a conditioned reflex which is carried to its final stages smooths out the many small points of difference between secondary extinctions of different conditioned reflexes, but a primary extinction which is carried to only a moderate degree leaves these small differences well pronounced. It may be stated, other things being equal, that the extent to which homogeneous conditioned reflexes undergo secondary extinction is determined by their relative physiological strengths. The strength of a conditioned reflex, in its turn, depends on whether it has long been established, on the number of times it has been refreshed by reinforcement, and on whether or not the reinforcement has been discontinued, and for how long. The extent of secondary extinction depends also on whether, and on how often, the reflex has previously been subjected to experimental extinction, and on whether or not it is reinforced immediately before the primary extinction is begun.

The greater the strength of the conditioned reflex as compared with the reflex which is subjected to primary extinction, the less does it undergo secondary extinction ; on the other hand, if the stronger reflex is subjected to primary experimental extinction the weaker conditioned reflex undergoes complete secondary extinction. The following experiments bearing on this subject were performed by Dr. Babkin :

A dog has three conditioned reflexes to acid, one depending on the sound of a buzzer, a second on the sound of a metronome and a third on a tactile stimulation of the skin. Every conditioned stimulus was continued always for 30 seconds. The first experiment shows the relative strengths of the reflexes.

Time	Conditioned Stimulus	Salivary Secretion in drops during 30 seconds	
3.24 p.m.	Metronome	5	All the
3.41 ,,	Buzzer	8	conditioned
4.05 ,,	Tactile	4	reflexes were
4.41 ,,	Metronome	12	reinforced by
4.51 ,,	Buzzer	13	acid.

In the following experiment a primary extinction of the reflex to the metronome was produced by repeating the stimulus at intervals of three minutes.

Time	Conditioned Stimulus	Salivary Secretion in drops during 30 seconds	
12.07 p.m.	Metronome	13	
12.10 ,,	,,	7	
12.13 ,,	,,	5	
12.16 ,,	,,	6	
12.19 ,,	,,	3	None of the
12.22 ,,	,,	2·5	stimuli were
12.25 ,,	,,	0	reinforced.
12.28 ,,	,,	0	
12.31 ,,	Tactile	0	
12.34 ,,	Metronome	0	
12.37 ,,	Buzzer	2·5	

On primary extinction of the conditioned reflex of medium strength the weaker tactile reflex also was completely extinguished, while the stronger reflex (to buzzer) was still partly active. These results were corroborated by further experiments in which the order of testing the secondarily extinguished reflexes was reversed.

The same dependence of the degree of extinction upon the strength of the conditioned reflexes is seen when the conditioned reflex undergoing extinction is one to a compound stimulus composed of several distinct elements which can be applied either simultaneously or else independently. Primary extinction of the reflex to the compound stimulus is always accompanied by secondary extinction of the reflexes to its individual components. Supposing there are two components of equal physiological strength, then the primary extinction of the one leads to simultaneous secondary extinction of the other, while the reflex to the compound stimulus is usually considerably diminished. Where, however, the two components of the compound stimulus are unequal in strength, primary extinction of the stronger reflex leads to a complete extinction of the reflex to the weaker component, while extinction of the weaker (unless carried beyond zero) leads only to a partial weakening of the reflex to the stronger component. The primary extinction of the stronger reflex leads also to a complete extinction of the reflex to the compound stimulus. The question of interrelation between the different individual components in a compound stimulus will be discussed further in a future lecture.

In the meantime we must endeavour to find a correct interpretation of the phenomenon of experimental extinction, and we shall find it important in this connection to give attention to a case in which the weaker of the two components in a conditioned reflex is completely overshadowed by the stronger, the weaker when tested separately producing no positive reflex effect. When in such a case the weaker stimulus is applied singly several times in succession, without reinforcement, there results, nevertheless, an extinction not only of the reflex to the stronger stimulus, but also of the reflex to the compound stimulus. An experiment by Dr. Perelzweig can be taken to illustrate this point :

A compound conditioned reflex has been established on a basis of the defence reflex to acid. The individual components of the compound stimulus are a tactile stimulus and a thermal stimulus of 0° C. In the experiment given below the animal is stimulated by

the compound stimulus and by its components separately. In every
case the stimulus is applied during one minute.

Time	Conditioned Stimulus	Secretion of Saliva in c.cs.	
12.0 noon	Compound	1·0	
12.25 p.m.	Compound	1·0	Reflex reinforced.
12.55 p.m.	Compound	1·4	
2.7 p.m.	Thermal	0·0	
2.30 p.m.	Thermal	0·0	Reflex not reinforced.
2.55 p.m.	Thermal	0·0	
3.25 p.m.	Tactile	0·0	
3.40 p.m.	Compound	0·05	Reflex reinforced.
4.5 p.m.	Compound	1·0	
4.25 p.m.	Tactile	1·0	

This experiment shows that the application of the thermal component,
which by itself was ineffective, led when repeated three times without
reinforcement to a complete secondary extinction of the stronger
tactile component and to a practically complete extinction of the
reflex to the compound stimulus.

Hitherto, when referring to the degree of extinction, we have
only spoken of the extinction as being partial or as being complete,
but we shall now have to extend our conception. Not only must we
speak of partial or of complete extinction of a conditioned reflex,
but we must also realize that extinction can proceed beyond the
point of reducing a reflex to zero. We cannot therefore judge the
degree of extinction only by the magnitude of the reflex or its
absence, since there can still be a silent extinction beyond the zero.
This statement rests upon the fact that a continued repetition of
an extinguished stimulus beyond the zero of the positive reflex
deepens the extinction still further. Such an extension of our conception serves fully to elucidate the experiment just described, and
it explains why the seemingly inactive thermal component when
subjected to experimental extinction led to such a profound secondary
extinction of the stronger tactile component. The importance of
considering the degree of extinction in all experiments thus becomes
evident. The methods of determining the degree of extinction when
it goes beyond zero will be explained in connection with the question
which will next be discussed.

We shall consider what happens to the conditioned reflexes after
they have been subjected to experimental extinction and inquire

whether they ever regain their original strength. Left to themselves extinguished conditioned reflexes spontaneously recover their full strength after a longer or shorter interval of time, but this of course does not apply to conditioned reflexes which are only just in process of formation. Such reflexes, being weak and irregular, may require for their recovery after extinction a fresh reinforcement by the underlying unconditioned reflex. However, all those conditioned reflexes which have been fully established invariably and spontaneously return sooner or later to their full strength. This provides one way of determining the depth of extinction ; it is measured, other conditions being equal, by the time taken for spontaneous restoration of the extinguished reflex to its original strength. Such time interval may vary for the different reflexes from a few minutes to a number of hours. I shall give a few experiments in illustration. The first is an experiment by Dr. Babkin :

Presentation of meat powder a short distance away at intervals of three minutes ; the reflex is not reinforced.

Time								Secretion of Saliva in c.cs.
11.33 a.m.	-	-	-	-	-	-	-	1·0
11.36 ,,	-	-	-	-	-	-	-	0·6
11.39 ,,	-	-	-	-	-	-	-	0·3
11.42 ,,	-	-	-	-	-	-	-	0·1
11.45 ,,	-	-	-	-	-	-	-	0·0
11.48 ,,	-	-	-	-	-	-	-	0·0

Interval of 2 hours.

1.50 p.m.	-	-	-	-	-	-	-	0·15

The second experiment is by Dr. Eliason :

Meat powder is presented a short distance away at intervals of ten minutes ; the reflex is not reinforced.

Time								Secretion of Saliva in drops
1.42 p.m.	-	-	-	-	-	-	-	8
1.52 ,,	-	-	-	-	-	-	-	3
2.2 ,,	-	-	-	·	-	-	-	0

Interval of 20 minutes.

2.22 p.m.	-	-	-	-	-	-	-	7

It will be interesting now to return to the demonstration given in the earlier part of this lecture and to examine whether there is any spontaneous recovery of the reflex to the metronome which was partially extinguished just twenty-three minutes ago.

Continuation of Demonstration.—The dog is again subjected to the stimulus of the metronome for 30 seconds : the latent period of the conditioned reflex now comes out at 5 seconds and the salivary secretion is 6 drops. At the last reading the latent period was 13 seconds and the salivary secretion 3 drops. Considerable recovery has therefore taken place spontaneously during the lecture.

The great differences in rapidity of restoration of extinguished reflexes depend on a number of factors. The most important factor is the depth of the preceding extinction. The individual character of an animal and its type of general nervous organization also play an important part. Much depends also on the intensity of the conditioned reflex which was subjected to experimental extinction ; and finally, upon how often the experimental extinction has been repeated. In every case, however, it is possible to accelerate the restoration of an extinguished conditioned reflex. For this purpose it is only necessary to apply the unconditioned stimulus on which the conditioned reflex was built up, either singly, or together with the extinguished conditioned stimulus. This method produces a more or less rapid restoration, according as the conditioned reflex has been extinguished to a greater or less degree. If the extinction has not been carried very far, a single application of the unconditioned stimulus is often sufficient to restore the reflex to full strength ; but if the extinction has been made profound, repeated reinforcements are necessary. This means of accelerating the recovery of the extinguished reflex affords another method of measuring the depth of extinction. The further question whether the acceleration in the restoration of an extinguished conditioned reflex is greater when the unconditioned reflex is applied singly, or when it is applied in the form of reinforcement cannot be discussed at present, as it is still under investigation (see Lecture XXII).

All this description of facts about extinction may have proved rather wearisome to the reader, owing to the absence of any underlying uniformity. Nevertheless they served an important purpose in that through a careful consideration of them we were enabled gradually to come upon a solution of the fundamental question as to the intimate nature of experimental extinction. By ruling out one interpretation after another we arrived at the conclusion that extinction must be regarded as a special form of inhibition. That it cannot be regarded as an irreparable destruction of the conditioned reflex, due to disruption of the respective nervous connections, is evidenced by the fact that the extinguished reflexes spontaneously regenerate in course of time. Another possible explanation also suggests itself : may it not be that the experimental extinction is brought about simply by fatigue in some part of the neuro-secretory apparatus involved in the reflex ? This is ruled out by the following evidence. The secretory elements in the gland do not become fatigued when the conditioned reflexes are being reinforced, although they continue indefinitely during an experiment to produce a full salivary secretion. Moreover, the restoration of an extinguished reflex is greatly accelerated by a fresh application of the unconditioned stimulus, a still further secretory activity of the gland being readily obtained although the reflex has been deeply extinguished. Neither can there be fatigue in the nervous centres of the secretory reflex. It is sufficient to recall the experiment with the conditioned reflex to the compound stimulus which had two cutaneous components—tactile and thermal. The thermal stimulus, which was the weaker, could not by itself produce even the slightest positive effect : yet none the less its repeated application brought about a secondary extinction of the stronger tactile stimulus and even of the compound stimulus itself. The extinction of the ineffective thermal stimulus was at no time accompanied by any kind of positive activity of the nervous elements, and it is difficult to conceive that a part of the central nervous system underwent fatigue without previous activity. Again, it would seem that if we were to admit the possibility of any fatigue in the nervous centres, we could expect only the reflex to the thermal stimulus to become fatigued, but we find also an extinction of the reflex to the tactile stimulus which was not brought into activity at any time during the repeated stimulation of the thermal receptors. Thus by a process of elimination we are forced to the conclusion that experimental extinction is based on inhibition, and if we look at the facts which have been described, in the light of this conclusion nearly all of them become perfectly intelligible.

The spontaneous rhythmic fluctuations in the reflexes sometimes observed during the process of experimental extinction can now easily be explained as a manifestation of the struggle which is taking place between the nervous processes of excitation and inhibition before one or other of them gains the mastery. Similarly it becomes quite easy to understand the part played by the individuality of the animal. We have all observed for ourselves how the inhibitory processes in the nervous system of human beings are seldom of the same intensity in any two people, and numerous examples in the further course of these lectures will make it clear that a precisely similar variation obtains in the nervous system of animals.

It is clear that the more vigorous a conditioned reflex, or in other words the greater the intensity of the excitatory process, the more intense must be the inhibitory process in order to overcome it, and therefore the greater the number of unreinforced repetitions necessary to bring about complete extinction. Again, it was seen that a repetition of the non-reinforced conditioned stimulus was necessary to produce a sufficient summation of the inhibitory after-effect for complete experimental extinction, and it is reasonable to suppose that the shorter the intervals between successive repetitions of the stimulus the more quickly will the required intensity of the inhibitory process be obtained. This also was found to be the case. As a result of repetitions of experimental extinction on the same animal the zero level of a fresh extinction of the reflex is reached more rapidly. This shows that inhibition like excitation is facilitated by repetition. The fact itself is well known from observation of ourselves and others, but abundant experimental evidence for animals will be afforded during the further course of our study of conditioned reflexes.

The influence exerted by experimental extinction on reflexes other than the one undergoing extinction, including unconditioned reflexes as well as homogeneous and heterogeneous conditioned reflexes, must be regarded as the result of a spreading of the inhibitory process from its point of initiation through the entire nervous structure of the hemispheres. This process will be fully discussed in one of the later lectures.

We have now to consider in detail still another important feature which has already been noted in passing, but was left unexplained, namely the frequent deviations observed in the curve of experimental extinction. These deviations represent sudden rapid strengthenings in the intensity of the reflex which is undergoing extinction, and they depend on the introduction of any accidental stimuli into the experimental environment. Some extraneous sound or shadow finding its way into the room produces at once a rapid strengthening of the reflex, and of course a similar effect is produced by different extra stimuli which we ourselves apply on purpose in order to study this phenomenon experimentally.

I shall describe first of all an observation which for a long time we were at a loss to interpret. A natural conditioned reflex to meat powder, which, as we know from control experiments, after extinction recovers its initial value spontaneously in something between a half and one hour, is again extinguished to zero. This time, however, instead of waiting for the spontaneous recovery of the reflex a weak solution of acid is immediately introduced into the dog's mouth, and after the termination of the secretion produced by the acid (about five minutes) meat powder is again presented at a short distance. This time although nothing like half an hour has elapsed the conditioned alimentary reflex is found to be almost completely restored. At first sight the accelerated recovery of the extinguished reflex seems paradoxical, since we know already that positive conditioned reflexes are always quite definitely specific—a definite stimulus rigidly evoking a definite reaction—but in this case a stimulus to an extinguished conditioned alimentary reflex has had its full strength restored through the single application of a stimulus to a heterogeneous unconditioned reflex, namely the defence reflex to acid. And there can be no doubt that although the secretory component of the two reflexes is effected through the same glands yet they are distinctly heterogeneous in nature, since the defence reflex to acid differs sharply from the alimentary reflex to food both as regards the composition of the saliva secreted and as regards the character of the motor response. Without attempting for the present to give any explanation we can designate this observation from a purely matter of fact point of view as consisting of a sudden removal by an extraneous reflex of the inhibitory process set up by experimental extinction.

The whole group of cases of which the above is an illustration have one common feature. In all of them the removal of the inhibition is only temporary, persisting no longer than the extra stimulus responsible for the removal of inhibition and its after-effect.

It is interesting to mention in this connection a disagreement which arose among the members of the staff in our laboratory before the fact of the restorative effect of acid upon an extinguished alimentary conditioned reflex had been indubitably established. Some of the workers admitted this restorative effect without question, while others disputed it. However, the experimental side of the question turned out to be right in both cases. The cause of the discrepancy was clearly brought out in Dr. Zavadsky's researches. It appeared that previous observers had overlooked the fact that their conditions of experimentation were not fully identical. Those workers who accepted the restorative effect had tested the extinguished conditioned alimentary reflex immediately or only a few moments after the salivary secretion in response to the acid had ceased, while the others had tested the extinguished reflex after allowing a considerable interval of time to elapse. Realizing the difference in the experimental procedure of the two sets of workers Dr. Zavadsky was able in his experiments to obtain all the different stages that had been reported by other workers. Two of his experiments, performed on the same day, are given below.

Time	Stimulus applied during one minute	Salivary Secretion in drops during one minute.	
		From submaxillary gland	From Parotid gland
2.28 p.m.	Meat powder pre-	16	12
2.40 ,,	sented at a dis-	9	6
2.52 ,,	tance out of	7	4
3.5 ,,	reach of the	5	2
3.18 ,,	animal.	0	0
3.20 ,,	Acid introduced into the dog's mouth. The flow of saliva consequent on this ceased at 3 hrs. 23 min. 50 sec. p.m.		
3.31 ,,	Meat powder presented at a distance.	1	0

The time interval between the end of the secretion produced by acid and the subsequent testing of the extinguished reflex was in the above experiment 7 minutes 10 seconds.

Time	Stimulus applied during one minute	Salivary Secretion in drops during one minute.	
		From submaxillary gland	From Parotid gland
3.34 p.m.	{ Meat powder consumed.		
3.46 ,,	{ Meat powder presented at a distance.	10	8
3.47 ,,	{ Meat powder consumed.		
4.5 ,,		9	7
4.15 ,,	Meat powder presented at a distance.	7	6
4.25 ,,		4	3
4.35 ,,		1	0
4.45 ,,		0	0
4.51 ,,	Acid introduced into the dog's mouth. The resulting salivary secretion ceased at 4 hrs. 54 min. 20 sec. p.m.		
4.55 p.m.	{ Meat powder presented at a distance.	7	5

The time interval between the end of the secretion produced by acid and the subsequent testing of the extinguished reflex was in this experiment 40 seconds.

Seven minutes after the salivary secretion to acid had ceased the restoration of the conditioned alimentary reflex was minimal, only one gland showing any activity. When, however, the reflex was tested only 40 seconds after the salivary secretion to acid had ceased, a considerable restoration of the alimentary conditioned reflex was found, involving both glands.

By this and similar experiments the temporary nature of the restoration of an extinguished reflex in response to other extra stimuli was easily demonstrated. The restorative effect was in no way confined to the administration of acid but was produced also by any other extra stimulus. A further example from Dr. Zavadsky's experiments illustrates this general case. The experiment was conducted on another dog.

| Time | Stimulus applied during one minute | Amount of Saliva in drops during one minute. | |
		From submaxillary gland	From Parotid gland
1.53 p.m.	⎱ Meat powder pre- ⎰	11	7
1.58 ,,	⎰ sented at a dis- ⎱	4	2
2.3 ,,	⎰ tance. ⎱	0	0
2.8 ,,	Same + tactile stimulation of skin.	3	1
2.13 ,,	Same + knocks under the table.	2	1
2.18 ,,	Meat powder at a distance.	0	0
2.20 ,,	Prof.Pavlov enters the room containing the dog, talks, and stays for two minutes.		
2.23 ,,	Meat powder at a distance.	5	2
2.28 ,,	Same.	0	0

NOTE.—Previously to this experiment it had been repeatedly shown that neither the tactile nor the auditory stimulus, nor the entry of Prof. Pavlov into the experimental room, produced any secretory effect at all.

This experiment leaves no doubt that the extinguished alimentary conditioned reflex is restored both by the actual presence of the extra stimulus (tactile and auditory), and by its after-effect (after-effect of stimulus of my entering the room).

In all the experiments which have just been described the restoration of the extinguished reflexes lasts only for a few minutes, depending on the duration of the extra stimulus and its after-effect. In the case, however, of certain special extra stimuli already mentioned in connection with external inhibition, stimuli which are of a protracted nature, the restorative effect is felt throughout the whole course of experimental extinction, which is therefore never smoothly progressive and can never be brought down to and kept at the zero level of the reflex.

We have now to discuss another important observation bearing on the same point. During the whole period of our work we observed on many occasions the simultaneous existence of several different reflexes, leading of course to an interaction between them which resulted either in predominance of one or another reflex or in their mutual neutralization. Thus, if we make a tactile stimulation of the skin the stimulus to a conditioned reflex, it frequently happens that we are bothered with an interference from the unconditioned reflex response to the cutaneous stimulus itself, in the form of the scratch reflex or some sort of quivering reflex. This may, in rare cases, be so troublesome that the conditioned reflex never reaches a stable value. Exactly the same thing happens sometimes with musical tones of exceedingly high pitch, it being in some dogs impossible to overcome the difficulty of the resulting sharp motor response. All such powerful unconditioned stimuli exercise an external inhibitory influence which perpetually interferes with all positive conditioned reflexes. But it is obvious that these persistent extra reflexes should exert a still more powerful disturbing influence upon the normal course of the inhibitory processes underlying extinction, since inhibition is in every respect more labile than excitation. I shall be giving a number of examples substantiating this statement in a further lecture, when the whole matter will be subjected to a rigorous experimental analysis. All the considerations put forward in this lecture permit us to regard the temporary restoration of the reflex which is in process of extinction, or which is already extinguished, as based upon the removal of an inhibitory process. We therefore describe this phenomenon as a dis-inhibition, a term we shall always use in the future when we wish to denote a temporary removal of inhibition.

The next question is, whether any distinction can be drawn between the case of the restoration of an extinguished conditioned reflex resulting from fresh applications of the appropriate unconditioned stimulus, and the case which has just been termed dis-inhibition. Our experiments show that undoubtedly such a distinction does exist. In the first case, when restoration is effected by the special unconditioned stimulus underlying the reflex which has undergone extinction, such restoration is permanent. In the second case, however, when the restoration is effected under the influence of any alien stimulus, such restoration is only temporary. As to the actual reason for this difference it is not possible to say very much upon the experimental evidence available up to the present. There is, however, no doubt that in the first case, just as has already been shown in the second, we are dealing with a removal of inhibition. Any hypothesis of an irreparable destruction of the conditioned reflex in the process of experimental extinction cannot possibly stand for a moment, since in every case of extinction the reflex invariably becomes spontaneously restored in a longer or shorter time.

The question of the difference in the mode of restoration in these two cases probably goes much deeper, involving the intimate nature of the nervous process underlying dis-inhibition. Regarding the nervous mechanism of dis-inhibition we cannot hope at present to approach anything like a fundamental conception, since as yet we know little about the real nature either of the inhibitory process, or of the excitatory process, or of their mutual relations.

I should like, however, specially to direct your attention to one very important feature which repeatedly enforces notice. We have seen that the very same extra stimuli, which, when they evoke strong extraneous reflexes, produce external inhibition of the positive conditioned reflexes, produce, when their effect is weak from the start or weakened by repetition, dis-inhibition of the conditioned reflexes which were made to undergo extinction. Many examples of this will appear in the next lecture. We are now afforded some justification for regarding dis-inhibition, as we did a short while ago, as being the " inhibition of an inhibition." By this we do not pretend, however, to explain the underlying mechanism of dis-inhibition.

The main conclusion of our discussion of the experimental evidence described in this lecture can be summed up briefly as follows. A stimulus to a positive conditioned reflex can under certain definite conditions readily be transformed into a stimulus for a negative or inhibitory conditioned reflex ; this transformation is fairly rapid, smooth and progressive. It becomes obvious therefore that in our further study of the function of the cerebral hemispheres we shall necessarily be dealing not only with positive but also with negative or inhibitory conditioned reflexes.

LECTURE V

THE fourth lecture was devoted entirely to the study of the first type of internal inhibition, which was termed **experimental extinction**. In extinction the positive conditioned stimulus is temporarily transformed into a negative or inhibitory one by the simple method of repeating it several times in succession without reinforcement. In the present lecture we shall consider the second type of internal inhibition, which has also been investigated in some detail.

The method of experimentation is as follows. A positive conditioned stimulus is firmly established in a dog by means of the usual repetitions with reinforcement. A new stimulus is now occasionally added, and whenever the combination is applied, which may be at intervals sometimes extending to hours or days, it is never accompanied by the unconditioned stimulus. In this way the combination is gradually rendered ineffective, so that the conditioned stimulus when applied in combination with the additional stimulus loses its positive effect, although when applied singly and with constant reinforcement it retains its full powers.

We have been accustomed in our investigations to designate this phenomenon by the name of **conditioned inhibition**, although this cannot be regarded as especially appropriate since the development of experimental extinction also is subject to equally rigid conditions. The use of this term, in fact, can only be justified by historical considerations. Since we were concerned in this case with the participation of an additional stimulus, the whole phenomenon was confused at first with external inhibition. It was only later when its character of internal, as distinct from external, inhibition became firmly established that the prefix " conditioned " was added. As will be shown further on, this form of inhibition might more appropriately have been termed " differential inhibition."

The process of development of conditioned inhibition **presents** especial interest. While illustrating the varied complexity of the phenomena involved, it demonstrates at the same time the value of the experimental method as providing a satisfactory means for the analysis of this very complexity into simple general principles. For this reason we shall discuss conditioned inhibition in considerable detail.

The first point of importance in the establishment of a conditioned inhibition is its dependence on time relations between the applications of the two stimuli in the inhibitory combination. Conditioned inhibition is developed with comparative ease in all those cases where the duration of the positive stimulus overlaps that of the additional stimulus. In our experiments it is usual to start the additional stimulus a few seconds (generally from 3 to 5) before the positive stimulus, but provided there is an overlap it is immaterial whether the commencement of the additional stimulus precedes, coincides with, or even follows by a few seconds, that of the positive stimulus. If, on the other hand, the additional stimulus is removed as soon as the positive stimulus is applied, so that the two stimuli never coincide, the development of the conditioned inhibition may be a matter of considerable difficulty, and accompanied by restlessness and various defence reactions of the animal. If, finally, a pause of several seconds is introduced between the termination of the additional stimulus and the beginning of the positive stimulus no inhibition develops at all. On the contrary, in the majority of cases, when this pause reaches a duration of about ten seconds, the additional stimulus itself acquires the properties of a positive stimulus. This has been discussed already as the general method of formation of positive conditioned reflexes of the second order. It is only with exceptionally powerful additional stimuli, such for example as a powerful motor-car hooter, that the pause can be increased to so much as twenty seconds and a conditioned inhibition still be developed. An example from the work of Dr. Frolov will serve to illustrate the latter case :

A motor-car hooter was allowed to act for 10 seconds, when, after a pause of a further 10 seconds, the alimentary conditioned stimulus of a metronome was applied. The first application of the hooter did not in the least diminish the magnitude of the succeeding reflex reaction. When, however, the same combination had been repeated several times in succession, and always without reinforcement, the reflex began gradually to diminish.

This diminution persisted even when the pause was lengthened to 20 seconds.

Experiment of 28th December, 1924.
Second application of the motor-car hooter.

Time	Stimulus			Duration of Stimulation in seconds	Salivary Secretion in drops	Remarks
1.41 p.m.			Metronome	30	9	Reinforced.
1.48 ,,	Inhibitory Combination	{	Hooter	10	0	} Not reinforced.
			Pause	20	0	
			Metronome	30	6	

Experiment of 21st January, 1925.
Thirteenth application of hooter.

Time	Stimulus			Duration of Stimulation in seconds	Salivary Secretion in drops	Remarks
1.58 p.m.			Metronome	30	8·5	Reinforced.
2.9 ,,	Inhibitory Combination	{	Hooter	10	0	} Not reinforced.
			Pause	20	0	
			Metronome	30	1	

We thus find that the time interval between the two stimuli required to produce either conditioned inhibition, or alternatively a positive conditioned reflex of the second order, varies according to the intensity of the additional stimulus. This contingency of the ultimate significance of the additional stimulus upon the time relations is interesting as evidence of an encounter between the antagonistic processes of excitation and inhibition.

The following interpretation of the complete difference in the final character assumed by the additional stimulus under so slight a difference in the experimental conditions seems best to agree with the experimental results : When the additional stimulus or its fresh trace left in the hemispheres coincides with the action of the positive stimulus, there must result some sort of special physiological fusion of the effect of the stimuli into one compound excitation partly differing from and partly resembling the positive one. It will be shown in the seventh lecture, that in response to closely related stimuli, such as neighbouring tones or tactile stimulation of adjacent places of the skin, the same events take place as in the development of conditioned inhibition. If one stimulus with the help of the usual procedure is given positive conditioned properties, the neighbouring stimuli belonging to the group also give at first a positive conditioned reaction, whereas later, on their systematic repetition without reinforcement, they lose their excitatory properties and acquire inhibitory properties instead. This result corresponds exactly with the successful development of conditioned inhibition in the experiment mentioned at the beginning of this lecture. When, however, the additional stimulus is separated from the application of the positive conditioned stimulus by a longer interval, the union in the hemispheres into a single compound excitation does not materialize ; instead, the stimuli act upon the hemispheres as two distinctly separate events, and the additional stimulus acquires new properties as a positive conditioned stimulus of the second order. The older conditioned stimulus acts in this case in exactly the same capacity as an unconditioned stimulus in the usual method of establishing conditioned reflexes of the first order. A strong stimulus has a prolonged after-effect ; it is, therefore, still capable of being fused by the hemispheres with the conditioned stimulus into a special new compound even after a long interval of time. It is easy to understand from this point of view that in the establishment of conditioned inhibition the interval which can be made between the end of the additional stimulus and the beginning of the positive conditioned stimulus must depend directly upon the strength of the additional stimulus. Whether our interpretation be the correct one or not, the phenomena are encouraging to the experimenter in that in every case he can discern a remarkable regularity in these very complex activities of the cortex.

In addition to the usual results obtained as described above, mention must be made of certain very rare phenomena obtained with some apparently normal animals and with animals in which surgical interference with the hemispheres had produced a condition of obviously increased excitability of the nervous system. In these cases even perfectly synchronous applications of the additional and of the positive conditioned stimuli led not to conditioned inhibition but to the development of a definite positive conditioned reflex of the second order. This generally persisted for a very long time, but later it often happened that the secondary conditioned reflex and also conditioned inhibition were both present simultaneously.

Such a case is represented in the following experiment of Dr. Kasherininova :

Tactile stimulation of the skin was used in this dog as the conditioned stimulus for the defence reflex to acid, and a metronome served for the additional stimulus in an inhibitory combination which, of course, was never reinforced. The twenty-fifth application of the inhibitory combination evoked a secretion of only 3 drops of saliva during one minute, whereas the conditioned stimulus applied singly evoked a secretion of 29 drops during one minute. After thirty-four repetitions of the inhibitory combination the stimulus of the metronome applied singly elicited a salivary secretion of 8 drops, although prior to its participation in the inhibitory combination it had no excitatory effect whatsoever. It is clear, therefore, that the metronome coupled with the tactile stimulus exerted a strong inhibitory influence, but it acquired at the same time some of the excitatory properties of the tactile stimulus, so that when used alone it behaved as a conditioned stimulus of the second order. Though cases such as that just described have been observed but rarely, it is quite possible that a transitory acquisition of weak excitatory properties of the second order is of no infrequent occurrence in the development of conditioned inhibition.

The course of development of conditioned inhibition is not always the same. In some cases the first addition of a new stimulus to the positive conditioned stimulus immediately results in a diminution, or even in a complete disappearance, of the conditioned reflex. With successive repetitions of the combination the reflex comes back nearly to its original level and then again falls slowly to zero. In other cases the first few combinations result in an augmentation of the reflex as compared with the normal isolated action of the conditioned stimulus, and only subsequently does the reflex gradually diminish to zero. In yet a third group it is found that an initial diminution in the strength of the reflex is followed by a phase of augmentation above normal and then again the reflex slowly falls to a permanent zero. All these different phases which are observed during the establishment of the conditioned inhibition depend entirely upon the intensity of the extraneous reflex which is evoked in the animal by the additional stimulus. The initial diminution of the reflex which occurs in one group during the first few applications of the combination is due undoubtedly to external inhibition. When the additional stimulus applied singly evokes in the dog a strong investigatory reflex it is found that its addition to the positive conditioned stimulus exerts an inhibitory influence from the very start. When on the other hand the stimulus evokes only a mild investigatory reflex, the preliminary phase of diminution of the reflex is absent and the first applications of the combination produce an increase in the reflex. This increase is undoubtedly due to dis-inhibition, since—as we may state now in anticipation of a future discussion—the positive effect of the majority of conditioned stimuli in our experimental reflexes is almost invariably preceded by a phase of internal inhibition. The inhibitory process is removed by the investigatory reflex, provided that the latter is not sufficiently strong also to influence the excitatory component of the conditioned reflex. The third group of cases, in which the initial diminution in strength of the reflex is followed by an increase above normal, depends on the gradual weakening through repetition of the extraneous reflex produced by the additional stimulus. The external inhibition brought about by the investigatory reaction is at first strong enough to inhibit the conditioned reflex, but, on weakening, produces only dis-inhibition and so increases the strength of the reflex response. Several examples of this will be given at the end of the present lecture.

It is obvious that any agent in nature may be used as a stimulus for the development of a conditioned inhibition, supposing of course that the organism is provided with the requisite organs for the perception of such an agent. The records of actual experiments will afford numerous illustrations of the different types of stimuli employed.

As was mentioned before, not only the actual stimulus but also its trace in the hemispheres can be used for the development of conditioned inhibition. The trace must, however, in all cases be as recent as possible. The establishment of conditioned inhibition when the interval between the stimuli is more prolonged can be brought about only by the use of exceptionally strong additional stimuli. Once, however, the inhibitory combination has been firmly established the pause between the end of the additional stimulus and the beginning of the positive conditioned stimulus may be extended even to so much as one minute without the inhibitory effect of the combination being impaired.

Some experiments have been made in which the time interval was itself employed as a stimulus for internal inhibition.

The following experiment by Dr. Krjyshkovski illustrates such case :

A definite tone served as a positive conditioned stimulus to acid, while a tactile stimulation of the skin served for the additional stimulus in the inhibitory combination. The inhibitory combination in this dog had been habitually applied for some other special purpose at the 19th-20th minute after the last introduction of acid. This led to the result that at the 19th-20th minute only a minimal salivary secretion was produced by the action of the positive conditioned stimulus when it was applied singly.

Interval between the successive applications of the Reinforced Conditioned Stimulus in minutes	Salivary Secretion in drops during one minute
13	9
12	14
19	0
33	11
19	3
33	8

In these experiments the interval of 19 to 20 minutes had itself acquired sufficient inhibitory properties to abolish or greatly reduce the effect of the conditioned stimulus.

The rate of development of conditioned inhibition as well as its completeness (absolute or relative inhibition) also depends upon a number of conditions. Of first importance in this connection is the individuality of the animal, the excitable or inhibitable character of its nervous organization. In some dogs the establishment of a conditioned inhibition takes a long time and never becomes absolute ; in other dogs an inhibition becomes completely and firmly established after very few repetitions of the inhibitory combination.

A further important factor is the intensity of the additional stimulus employed in the inhibitory combination. For example, in an experiment by Dr. Mishtovt, a metronome was used for a positive conditioned stimulus to acid, while a thermal stimulation of the skin was employed as the additional stimulus. It was found that with the thermal stimulus at a temperature of 4 to 5° C. the first indication of a conditioned inhibition could be observed only after the 30th application of the inhibitory combination, and the inhibition was not yet complete even after 145 applications. With the use, however, of a thermal stimulus at a temperature of 1° C., in an experiment performed on the same animal after an interval of four months, only twelve repetitions of the inhibitory combination were required to establish complete inhibition.

The rate of formation of conditioned inhibition depends, again, on the character and the relative intensity of the additional stimulus in comparison with the conditioned stimulus. In some dogs it was found impossible to establish complete inhibition by the addition of a thermal stimulus at 45° C., when the sound of a metronome served as the positive conditioned stimulus. When, however, a visual stimulus was employed as the positive conditioned stimulus in a similar combination, a conditioned inhibition could be readily produced [experiment by Dr. Foursikov].

Finally, it should be mentioned that, although other factors may remain constant, the first establishment of a conditioned inhibition in a dog takes more time than any succeeding one.

I have not up to the present given any conclusive evidence that the phenomenon of conditioned inhibition is really in the nature of an inhibition at all, and is not merely a passive disappearance of the positive conditioned reflex owing to the compound stimulus remaining habitually unreinforced. The proof that the phenomenon actually does represent a real inhibition will be gradually brought out as we proceed with our study of the experimental evidence.

It will be of interest, first of all, to study the nature and ultimate function of the additional stimulus on which conditioned inhibition depends. This can, of course, be determined only by trying out the action of the additional stimulus in different modifications of the experiment. Tested singly after the conditioned inhibition has been fully established it produces no positive effect at all. The action of the additional stimulus can be tested, however, by applying it in combination with some other positive conditioned stimulus with which it has never previously been associated. In such a case the inhibitory properties of the additional stimulus become clearly revealed, the result being an immediate diminution in the positive reflex response. This is true not only in the case of homogeneous reflexes, but also in the case of heterogeneous reflexes, and the inhibitory effect may extend even to the unconditioned reflexes themselves. These facts are clearly exhibited in the following experiment by Dr. Leporsky :

Three alimentary conditioned reflexes have been established in the dog used for this experiment, the three stimuli being the flash of a lamp, a rotating object, and the tone C sharp of a pneumatic tuning fork. Two independent conditioned inhibitions of the reflex to rotation have also been firmly established, one by the use of tactile stimulation of the skin and the other by the use of a metronome.

In the first experiment the flash of the lamp is for the first time accompanied by a tactile stimulation of the skin :

Time	Stimulus applied during 1 minute	Amount of Saliva in drops during 1 minute
1.38 p.m.	Rotating Object.	16
1.50 ,,	Flash of lamp.	17
2.14 ,,	Flash of lamp + tactile stimulus.	2
2.25 ,,	Routine reinforcement of rotating object by feeding	—
2.43 ,,	Rotating object + tactile stimulus (the usual inhibitory combination)	0

In the second experiment the tone C sharp is for the first time accompanied by the metronome.

Time	Stimulus applied during 1 minute	Amount of Saliva in drops during 1 minute
1.30 p.m.	Tone + metronome	3
1.40 ,,	Tone	20
1.54 ,,	Rotating object	18
2.3 ,,	Routine reinforcement of rotating object by feeding	—
2.23 ,,	Rotating object + metronome (the usual inhibitory combination)	0

It will be seen that the additional stimulus when applied for the first time in the new combination produced a diminution almost to zero in the conditioned reflex response. It follows, therefore, that when an additional stimulus is used with an alien homogeneous conditioned reflex its inhibitory property becomes thereby immediately revealed. This same property is seen also when the additional stimulus is combined for the first time with a heterogeneous conditioned reflex, a case which is illustrated in the following experiment :

A dog has a conditioned alimentary reflex which has been established by the use of the metronome, while the addition of a whistle provides a powerful inhibitory combination. Besides this a conditioned reflex to acid has been established in response to tactile stimulation of the skin. The metronome and the tactile stimuli belong therefore to heterogeneous conditioned reflexes, and the positive effect of one of them (*i.e.* the metronome) is completely inhibited by the sound of the whistle. The whistle is now for the first time combined with the heterogeneous tactile conditioned stimulus [experiment by Dr. Babkin].

Time	Stimulus applied during 1 minute	Salivary Secretion in drops during 1 minute
3.8 p.m.	Tactile	3
3.16 ,,	Tactile	8
3.25 ,,	Tactile + whistle	Less than 1 drop.
3.30 ,,	Tactile	11

In all the foregoing experiments it had, of course, to be shown before any particular additional stimulus was used in combination with an alien positive conditioned stimulus that it would not exercise any effect of external inhibition. With this precaution it seems to me that the experiments justify our conclusion that where a conditioned inhibition has been firmly established the additional stimulus itself acquires inhibitory properties which can be manifested outside the parent combination. The additional stimulus is therefore termed in our investigations **the conditioned inhibitor.**

It is made clear by further experiments that a real inhibitory effect is also produced by the inhibitory combination itself, the inhibitory process persisting as an after-effect which may be detected some considerable time after the stimulus of the inhibitory combination itself has been removed. The inhibitory after-effect exerts its influence not only upon the particular reflex to the conditioned stimulus employed in the combination, but also upon all other conditioned reflexes whether homogeneous or heterogeneous. In this connection we may consider the following experiments :

In the first experiment a rotating object serves as an alimentary conditioned stimulus, and a tone of 30,000 vibrations produced by a Galton's whistle as its conditioned inhibitor [experiment by Dr. Nikolaev].

Time	Stimulus applied during 1 minute	Salivary Secretion in drops during 1 minute
3.5 p.m.	Rotating object	7
3.26 ,,	Rotating object	6
3.38 ,,	Rotating object + tone	0
3.58 ,,	Rotating object	1
4.10 ,,	Rotating object	2

After withdrawal of the stimulation by the inhibitory combination the effect of the positive conditioned stimulus is weakened for several minutes, and only regains its normal strength by degrees.

In the next experiment a rotating object serves as a conditioned stimulus for the defence reflex to acid, and a musical tone serves as a conditioned alimentary stimulus. A tactile stimulus is used as a conditioned inhibitor for the alimentary reflex. [Experiment by Dr. Ponisovsky.]

Time	Stimulus applied during 30 seconds	Salivary Secretion in drops during 30 seconds
12.23 p.m.	Rotating object	5
12.32 ,,	Rotating object	12
12.46 ,,	Tone + tactile stimulus	0
12.48 ,,	Rotating object	1

This experiment demonstrates that the heterogeneous conditioned reflex also becomes diminished as a result of the inhibitory after-effect of the combination.

When the inhibitor is applied by itself alone, and not together with the excitatory stimulus in combination with which it was originally developed, it can also be demonstrated to produce an inhibitory after-effect.

The degree to which positive conditioned reflexes are influenced by the conditioned inhibitor varies inversely as their relative physiological strength. An experiment may be taken from a paper by Dr. Leporsky in illustration of this point :

Three independent conditioned alimentary reflexes have been firmly established to a rotating object, to the flash of several electric lamps, and to a musical tone. A tactile stimulation of the skin has been established as a conditioned inhibitor for each of the three reflexes, so that in combination with any one of them separately it reduces the reflex to zero. All three positive stimuli applied together produce a much greater salivary secretion than any one of them applied singly, showing summation of conditioned reflexes. The experiment shows the effect of the application of the conditioned inhibitor in conjunction with the simultaneous action of all three positive stimuli.

Time	Stimulus during 1 minute	Amount of Saliva in drops during 1 minute
1.40 p.m.	Tone	21
2.0 ,,	Rotating object + tone + flash	32
2.10 ,,	Rotating object	23
2.27 ,,	Simultaneous application of all three positive conditioned stimuli + tactile stimulus	9
2.51 ,,	Rotating object + tactile stimulus	0

The conditioned inhibitor, therefore, although it reduced to zero every one of the positive conditioned reflexes taken singly, could only partially inhibit the reflex secretion evoked by all three acting simultaneously (2.27 p.m.).

Two further details concerning the inhibitory after-effect remain to be considered. The first is the phenomenon of summation of after-effect. If the inhibitory combination is applied not once only, but several times in succession, so much the more will the strength and duration of the inhibitory after-effect be increased. Two experiments of Dr. Chebotareva, carried out on successive days, serve to illustrate the case in point :

A metronome serves as a conditioned alimentary stimulus, and a rotating object as its conditioned inhibitor.

Time	Stimulus during 30 seconds	Amount of Saliva in drops during 30 seconds
First experiment :		
3.32 p.m.	Metronome	5
3.40 ,,	Metronome	6
3.50 ,,	Metronome + rotating object	0
3.52 ,,	Metronome	3
4.4 ,,	Metronome	5
Experiment on the same dog on the succeeding day :		
12.59 p.m.	Metronome	7
1.6 ,,	Metronome	8
1.15 ,,	Metronome + rotating object	1
1.19 ,,	Metronome + rotating object	0
1.25 ,,	Metronome	2
1.32 ,,	Metronome	6

In the first experiment it is seen that the conditioned reflex, which, to start with, was of considerable strength, when tested by a fresh application of the positive conditioned stimulus $1\frac{1}{2}$ minutes after the cessation of a single application of the inhibitory combination (3.52 p.m.), is diminished by half (*i.e.* from 6 drops to 3). In the second experiment, taking place on the following day, the reflex, when tested $5\frac{1}{2}$ minutes after the second of two successive applications of the inhibitory combination (1.25 p.m.), is diminished by three-quarters (*i.e.* from 8 drops to 2).

The second important detail concerning the inhibitory after-effect is that its duration becomes shorter as the experiments proceed from day to day. It may extend in the earlier experiments for something over an hour, but in the course of succeeding experiments gradually becomes reduced to only a few minutes or seconds. The following two experiments of Dr. Nikolaev which were performed, with an interval of over 6 months' continuous experimentation, provide an illustration of the case in question :

A rotating object provides the stimulus to a conditioned alimentary reflex, while a given tone serves as its conditioned inhibitor. In the first experiment the inhibitory after-effect was obvious for over 20 minutes ; six months later, after continual practice, it was absent so soon as $3\frac{1}{2}$ minutes after the single application of the inhibitory combination.

Time	Stimulus during 30 seconds	Salivary Secretion in drops during 30 seconds

Experiment of 2nd June, 1909.

Time	Stimulus during 30 seconds	Salivary Secretion
3.5 p.m.	Rotating object	7
3.26 ,,	Rotating object	6
3.38 ,,	Rotating object + tone	0
3.58 ,,	Rotating object	1
4.10 ,,	Rotating object	2

Experiment of 10th January, 1910. Same dog.

Time	Stimulus during 30 seconds	Salivary Secretion
2.16 p.m.	Rotating object	8
2.37 ,,	Rotating object + tone	0
2.41 ,,	Rotating object	12

The problem of experimental destruction of the inhibitory properties of the conditioned inhibitor applied singly or in its inhibitory combination is very complex and has not yet been fully worked out. I shall mention, therefore, only some of the better established facts. It is obvious that a complete abolition of the inhibitory properties of the combination should most readily be brought about by reversing the technique employed in its formation —*i.e.* by systematically reinforcing the inhibitory combination by the appropriate unconditioned reflex. An experiment by Dr. Krjishkovski will illustrate this process :

A given tone of a pneumatic tuning fork provides a conditioned stimulus to acid, while a tactile stimulation of the skin serves as the conditioned inhibitor.

Time	Stimulus during 1 minute	Salivary Secretion in drops during 1 minute	Routine
10.43 a.m.	Tone	10	Reinforced by acid.
10.57 ,,	Inhibitory combination	0	Every application of the inhibitory combination was followed up by injection of acid into the mouth.
11.9 ,,	,, ,,	0	
11.23 ,,	,, ,,	1	
11.35 ,,	,, ,,	3	
11.49 ,,	,, ,,	5	
12.3 p.m.	,, ,,	10	
12.25 ,,	,, ,,	14	

It is interesting to note that if alternately with every application of the reinforced inhibitory combination we repeat the reinforced positive conditioned stimulus, a very considerable retardation in the progress of destruction of the inhibition is produced. This matter will be subjected to rigorous experimental analysis further on (Lecture XI).

Quite distinct from the above process of gradual weakening of the inhibitory combination is the case in which the disturbance appears suddenly and as suddenly disappears. Extra stimuli belonging to the group of mild *external* inhibitors, as we may term them, influencing the animal during the action of the inhibitory combination instantaneously restore to something of its normal value the positive conditioned reflex which underwent conditioned inhibition. It is evident that external inhibition has brought about the removal of conditioned inhibition, and that we deal again with the phenomenon of dis-inhibition. These relations may be illustrated by the following experiments of Dr. Nikolaev :

Time	Stimulus during 1 minute	Salivary Secretion in drops during 1 minute
	Experiment of 16th December, 1909.	
2.12 p.m.	Rotating object	10
2.30 ,,	Rotating object + tone + metronome	5
2.37 ,,	Rotating object + tone	0
2.53 ,,	Rotating object	7
3.5 ,,	Rotating object + tone	0
3.22 ,,	Rotating object	8
	Experiment of 21st December, 1909.	
2.25 p.m.	Rotating object	12
2.47 ,,	Rotating object + tone + tactile stimulation	3
2.57 ,,	Rotating object + tone	0
3.12 ,,	Rotating object	8
3.21 ,,	Rotating object + tone	0
3.36 ,,	Rotating object	8
	Experiment of 22nd December, 1909.	
2.37 p.m.	Rotating object	9
2.55 ,,	Rotating object + tone + thermal stimulus at 50°C.	7
3 4 ,,	Rotating object + tone	0
3.16 ,,	Rotating object	11
3.31 ,,	Rotating object + tone	0

The stimulus to a conditioned alimentary reflex is provided by a rotating object, while a given tone serves as its conditioned inhibitor. Tactile and thermal stimulations of the skin and the sounds of a metronome serve as different extra stimuli.

The above three experiments show that during the time when the extra stimuli (metronome, tactile, or thermal) were acting upon the animal the conditioned inhibition was partially removed, revealing the underlying excitation.

In connection with these observations considerable interest is attached to the following experiment on the same dog, in which it was the intention to introduce an odour as still another dis-inhibiting agent. For this purpose the dog was transferred into another room fitted with a special box for graduating the intensity of odours. The apparatus itself, in addition to its visual effect and the sound of its electric motor, acted upon the animal by blowing a continuous current of air. All these agencies introduced a whole complex of new extra stimuli into the experiment, even without the addition of the odour. The new complex of extra stimuli dis-inhibited the inhibitory combination, but this effect gradually declined as time went on, disappearing completely in an hour and a half after the experiment was started. The following experiment was performed on the day following the last experiment.

Experiment of 23rd December, 1909.

Time	Stimulus during 1 minute	Amount of Saliva in drops during 1 minute
1.2 p.m.	Rotating object	14
1.18 ,,	Rotating object + tone	9
1.25 ,,	Rotating object + tone	6
1.31 ,,	Rotating object	11
1.40 ,,	Rotating object + tone	4
1.48 ,,	Rotating object + tone	2
1.58 ,,	Rotating object	7
2.6 ,,	Rotating object + tone	1
2.20 ,,	Rotating object	7
2.28 ,,	Rotating object + tone	less than 1 drop.
2.35 ,,	Rotating object	6
2.53 ,,	Rotating object + tone + odour of Camphor	6
3.7 ,,	Rotating object + tone + odour of Camphor	less than 1 drop.

The first application of the camphor dis-inhibited the combination, while on the second application this extra stimulus had already lost its dis-inhibiting effect. This rapid disappearance of the effect of the extra stimuli introduced by the new apparatus, and again by the use of the camphor, is the most usual case with extra stimuli which bring about dis-inhibition. The dog employed in this particular experiment was an old laboratory animal and had previously been subjected to numerous extraneous agencies, so that different changes produced now only a transient effect, the animal speedily becoming indifferent to them. This is why the introduction of new conditions into this experiment produced a dis-inhibition right from the very start and never any inhibition of the positive conditioned reflexes.

Results were quite different in the case of another dog used by Dr. Nikolaev. This dog was fresh to the laboratory and may have possessed also a type of nervous organization which was more easily subjected to inhibition. In this dog a rotating object was used for a conditioned alimentary stimulus, and a tone for its conditioned inhibitor. A metronome provided the extra stimulus.

Experiment of 15th February, 1910.

Time	Stimulation during 30 seconds	Salivary Secretion in drops during 30 seconds
11.25 a.m.	Rotating object	4
11.41 ,,	Rotating object + tone + metronome	0
11.52 ,,	Rotating object	4
12.4 ,,	Rotating object	5
12.14 ,,	Rotating object + metronome	0
12.26 ,,	Rotating object	5

The experiment on the following day gave similar results. On the 18th February, at the beginning of the next experiment, the metronome was applied alone during one minute, the subsequent course of the experiment being shown on the opposite page.

In the experiment of 15th February the sound of the metronome, which served as an extra stimulus, did not produce during its first application the result which would be expected from dis-inhibition (11.41 a.m.). But the very same stimulus of the metronome when applied along with the positive conditioned stimulus used singly produced a complete inhibition (12.14 p.m.). It follows, therefore, that the zero value of the reflex in the first case—inhibitory combination + metronome—was not really due to the internal inhibition remaining undisturbed but was due to external inhibition resulting from a very powerful extraneous reflex in response to the first application of the metronome. As a result of several repetitions of the stimulus of the metronome with the inhibitory combination on the 16th February and an application at the beginning of the experiment of 18th February, the stimulus of the metronome was no longer able to produce so powerful an alien reflex and therefore its inhibitory

Experiment of 18th February, 1910.

Time	Stimulus during 30 seconds	Salivary Secretion in drops during 30 seconds
11.15 a.m.	Rotating object	9
11.32 ,,	Rotating object + tone + metronome	5
11.39 ,,	Rotating object	4
11.54 ,,	Rotating object	3
12.9 p.m.	Rotating object + tone + metronome	2
12.14 ,,	Rotating object	5
12.27 ,,	Rotating object + metronome	3
12.34 ,,	Rotating object	4
12.40 ,,	Rotating object + tone	0

effect upon the positive conditioned component had practically disappeared (12.27 p.m.). However, its dis-inhibitory effect was still retained and could be well seen in the experiment of 18th February (11.32 a.m. and 12.9 p.m.).

The terminology used in the interpretation of the foregoing phenomena may seem to be artificial and arbitrary, but it is not possible at a time when the intimate mechanism is still beyond our powers of analysis to avoid such terms in what is necessarily a schematic representation of the complex nervous processes involved. Our terms serve to describe only the actual state and succession of events.

A dis-inhibition of the inhibitory combination can further be obtained by means of those stimuli which determine a permanent external inhibition (p. 46). The following experiment by Dr. Nikolaev bears out this statement :

A rotating object serves for the conditioned alimentary stimulus, while a tone serves for its conditioned inhibitor.

Time	Stimulus during 1 minute	Salivary Secretion in drops during 1 minute
1.47 p.m.	Rotating object	10
2.0 ,,	Rotating object + tone	0
2.23 ,,	Rotating object	10
2.39 ,,	10 cc. of 5% solution of sodium carbonate introduced in two doses into the dog's mouth	—
2.44 ,,	Rotating object + tone	2.5
2.55 ,,	Rotating object + tone	0
3.2 ,,	Rotating object	6

In this case the inhibitory after-effect of sodium carbonate, given 4 minutes before, caused a definite dis-inhibition of the reflex (2.44 p.m.).

If an inhibitory combination is applied early within the time of the after-effect left by a very strong extra stimulus, for example a concentrated solution of quinine, no dis-inhibition is obtained. This corresponds exactly with the case of the metronome in the experiment on page 84. However, the dis-inhibiting effect of quinine can be exhibited as clearly as in the case of the metronome, simply by throwing in the inhibitory combination at a later stage, when the strength of the after-effect of the action of the quinine has had time to diminish. On account of the complete accord of the two sets of experiments the description of the experiments with quinine need not be given.

All the experimental evidence which has been dealt with in this lecture establishes conclusively that the nervous processes on which conditioned inhibition depends are identical in character with those of extinctive inhibition. The fundamental condition for their development is the same, namely that there shall be no reinforcement by the unconditioned reflex. In both cases the process develops gradually, being strengthened by repetition. Moreover, the inhibitory after-effect does not limit itself to the particular positive conditioned reflex which undergoes experimental extinction or conditioned inhibition, but in both cases extends to other conditioned reflexes as well, including even those which are of heterogeneous origin.

The final point of resemblance is that in both cases the inhibitory process can be rapidly though temporarily removed, the inhibited reflexes undergoing dis-inhibition on account of external inhibition resulting from alien reflexes to extra stimuli of small intensity. The only point of difference is that in extinctive inhibition it is the positive conditioned stimulus taken by itself which changes its positive significance to an inhibitory one, while in the case of conditioned inhibition the positive conditioned stimulus becomes involved in a new complex and changes its character in conjunction with an additional stimulus.

LECTURE VI

Internal inhibition (continued) : (c) Delay.

WE shall now consider the third type of internal inhibition, which has been termed **inhibition of delay.** It is obvious from the previous discussion that a considerable choice is allowed in the establishment of conditioned reflexes as regards the time interval between the beginning of the conditioned stimulus and the moment at which it is reinforced by the unconditioned reflex. This interval can be made very short, 1-5 seconds, or even a fraction of a second, provided that the beginning of the conditioned stimulus precedes the moment of application of the unconditioned stimulus. Alternatively, the length of time of the isolated action of the conditioned stimulus can be made comparatively long, extending over several minutes. The reflexes which develop with these two different methods, *i.e.* with short and with prolonged duration of action of the conditioned stimulus, present great differences with respect to their general properties and their latent periods. These two types of reflex are designated respectively **simultaneous**—or to be more precise, almost simultaneous—reflexes, and **delayed reflexes.** The duration of the isolated action of the conditioned stimulus is of fundamental importance, since, in the first place, it determines, as we shall see later, the eventual character of every conditioned reflex, and secondly, because it forms the basis of development of that type of inhibition which is the subject of our present lecture.

In all conditioned reflexes in which the interval between the beginning of the conditioned stimulus and the moment of its reinforcement is short, say 1-5 seconds, the salivary reaction almost immediately follows the beginning of the conditioned stimulus. On the other hand, in reflexes which have been established with a longer interval between the two stimuli the onset of the salivary response is delayed, and this delay is proportional to the length of the interval between the two stimuli and may even extend to several minutes.

Delayed reflexes can be established in various ways. One way is to start by the preliminary establishment of an almost simultaneous reflex—*i.e.* one in which the conditioned response appears quickly, say 1-3 seconds after the beginning of the conditioned stimulus— and to develop the delay gradually. By retarding the moment of the application of the unconditioned stimulus about five seconds each day a corresponding and progressive delay is easily obtained, and we can stop finally at a convenient interval when the required length of delay has been reached.

Another method of establishing a delayed reflex is to pass directly from an almost simultaneous reflex to one with a long delay, leaving out all intermediate stages. As a result of this modification in technique the mode of formation of the delayed conditioned reflex is considerably altered. The reflex, however well established as a simultaneous reflex, disappears at first altogether—or, to use an expression commonly employed by some of my collaborators, there follows a prolonged period of zeros. Eventually, however, some conditioned secretion of saliva does appear, but not until just before the moment when the unconditioned stimulus is usually applied. On continuing the experiments with the chosen interval of time the secretion progressively increases, and at the same time its commencement shifts further along towards the beginning of the conditioned stimulus and finally settles at a definite intermediate position between the commencement of the conditioned stimulus and its reinforcement.

In both the foregoing methods the experiments start with the establishment of simultaneous reflexes which are then changed either at once or by gradual stages into delayed reflexes. It has been found impracticable, in the great majority of animals, to develop a delayed reflex without first establishing the corresponding simultaneous reflex, since, as will be described in a later lecture, the dogs under these conditions quickly become subjected to drowsiness and sleep so that the experimental formation of conditioned reflexes becomes difficult if not impossible. For this reason the method has received little attention in our investigations.

The following example of a delayed reflex is taken from a paper by Dr. Zavadsky who carried out a considerable number of experiments upon internal inhibition of delay. The sound of a whistle is employed as a conditioned stimulus to acid ; the isolated action of the whistle is continued during an interval of 3 minutes and is then reinforced by acid, the sound being continued for some time longer so as to overlap the action of the unconditioned stimulus.

Time	Conditioned Stimulus	Salivary Secretion in drops during successive periods of 30 seconds of the isolated action of the conditioned stimulus
3.12 p.m.	Whistle	0, 0, 2, 2, 4, 4
3.25 ,,	,,	0, 0, 4, 3, 6, 6
3.40 ,,	,,	0, 0, 2, 2, 3, 6

The rate of formation of a delayed reflex is subject to great variation. In the first place, the individual character of the animal's nervous system plays an important part. In some dogs the establishment of the reflex is rapid, while in others the beginning of the salivary secretion persistently refuses to separate itself from the beginning of the conditioned stimulus, and the development of delay is very slow. In some animals an indication of a developing delay can be observed in the course of a single day and after only a few delayed reinforcements ; in others there is no indication of the conditioned delay even after a month of persistent work. In the type of dog in which the formation of delay is rapid, it is found that the delay frequently passes into sleep at an early stage of the isolated action of the conditioned stimulus. On this account it is necessary when carrying out a systematic investigation with dogs of this character to restrict the experiments to short-delayed reflexes, which means that we must be content with recording only the small secretion of saliva during the comparatively short time of isolated action of the conditioned stimulus as compared with the larger secretion accompanying a prolonged action of the stimulus.

Another influence affecting the development of delay in the conditioned reflex response is the type of conditioned stimulus used. Tactile and thermal stimulation of the skin and visual stimuli lead to a quicker formation of delay than auditory stimuli, but other things being equal, tactile, thermal and visual stimuli give a smaller total conditioned effect. These facts are illustrated in the following experiments by Dr. Iacovleva :

Preliminary to the development of long-delayed reflexes three short-delayed conditioned alimentary reflexes were established by repeating the isolated action of the stimuli during 30 seconds, followed by reinforcement. The stimuli corresponding to the three reflexes were the sound of a metronome, a tactile stimulus, and the flash of a lamp.

Experiment of 9th April, 1924.

Time	Conditioned Stimulus applied during 30 seconds	Latent period in seconds	Salivary Secretion in divisions of the graduated tube during the isolated action of the conditioned stimulus
10.15 a.m.	Lamp	3	30 ⎫ All
10.25 ,,	Tactile	2	30 ⎬ reflexes are
10.35 ,,	Metronome	2	53 ⎭ reinforced.

During the year which intervened between this experiment and the experiment of 24th April, 1925, which is given next, the three reflexes had been used repeatedly in other investigations and had been gradually converted into reflexes of longer delay. The isolated action of the conditioned stimulus had been first prolonged to one minute and then to two minutes, and each reflex had been reinforced an equal number of times.

Time	Conditioned Stimulus applied for two minutes	Latent period in seconds	Salivary Secretion in graduations of tube per 30 secs. during the isolated action of the conditioned stimulus
9.40 a.m.	Metronome	1	40, 32, 30, 26
9.48 ,,	Tactile	36	0, 10, 20, 18
10.10 ,,	Flash	75	0, 0, 13, 20

In the cases of the tactile and visual stimuli the delay is more precise, the reflex response having more perfectly separated itself from the beginning of the conditioned stimulus and being more perfectly related to the time of administration of the unconditioned stimulus.

Another factor which exerts a great influence upon the development of a long-delayed reflex is the amount of practice which has been given to the reflex during the preliminary stage of short delay ;

a long practised short delay sometimes operates as a persistent obstacle to the development of a longer delay.

Finally, I have evidence that the delay for a stimulus of one and the same character develops at a different rate according as the stimulus is continuous or intermittent. In the former case the development of delay is more rapid.

It can be seen that the reflex response in the case of reflexes with a prolonged delay consists of two phases, an initial phase of inactivity and a subsequent phase of activity, and we must now inquire into the nature of these phases. Does this first and comparatively long period of inactivity mean that the excitatory process is undergoing a progressive summation so that it can evoke an obvious activity when it has reached the necessary intensity? Or is the excitatory process sufficiently strong from the beginning, but unable to produce any secretory effect because it is temporarily overcome by some antagonistic process?

The first possibility must be ruled out straightway on the evidence already given with regard to the formation of delayed reflexes, for seeing that in the case of a short delay the conditioned stimulus can evoke a conditioned reflex with great ease, there seems to be no reason why the same stimulus when more prolonged should require a greater period of summation.

Any suggestion that this first phase of inactivity is caused through fatigue can also easily be eliminated. If, owing to the isolated action of the conditioned stimulus, fatigue did develop, we should expect a gradual diminution of the positive effect of the conditioned stimulus: this, however, is not observed. On the contrary, although the beginning of the secretion gets delayed, nevertheless the secretion increases progressively in amount when the delayed reflex is developed by the first method. With the second method, in which the isolated action of the conditioned stimulus is prolonged from the start, although the positive effect disappears at first altogether, it reappears after a while and then the secretion increases steadily until it settles at a constant maximum value.

There remains now only the supposition that the initial phase of inactivity is due to the excitatory process being temporarily inhibited. That this is the correct interpretation is evidenced by the fact that the existence of an excitatory process in a concealed form during the period of delay can easily be demonstrated : if during the inactive phase of a delayed reflex we act upon the animal by some extra stimulus which has not hitherto been associated in any way with an activity of the salivary glands, we shall immediately elicit a secretion of saliva which is frequently copious and which is always accompanied by the motor reaction peculiar to the conditioned stimulus which was used ; in other words, the conditioned reflex becomes revealed throughout the entire duration of the conditioned stimulus in a single positive phase instead of in two phases—negative and positive. The following are some experiments by Dr. Zavadsky bearing upon this question :

Tactile stimulation of the skin is used as a conditioned stimulus for acid. The conditioned stimulus is allowed to act for a period of 3 minutes and is then reinforced, being still continued so as to overlap the action of the acid. The sound of the metronome which is used in the following experiment has had hitherto no relation to any secretory reflexes and has of itself been unable to evoke any secretion of saliva.

Time	Stimulus	Salivary Secretion in drops per 30 secs. during the isolated action of the conditioned stimulus
9.50 a.m.	Tactile	0, 0, 3, 7, 11, 19
10.3 ,,	Tactile	0, 0, 0, 5, 11, 13
10.15 ,,	Tactile + metronome	4, 7, 7, 3, 5, 9
10.30 ,,	Tactile	0, 0, 0, 3, 12, 14
10.50 ,,	Tactile	0, 0, 5, 10, 17, 19

The next example is taken from a further experiment in which a noiselessly rotating object was used as an extra stimulus hitherto neutral with regard to its effect upon the salivary secretion.

Time	Stimulus	Salivary Secretion in drops per 30 secs. during the isolated action of the conditioned stimulus
11.46 a.m.	Tactile	3,* 0, 0, 2, 4, 5
12.02 p.m.	Tactile	0, 0, 0, 2, 6, 9
12.17 ,,	Tactile	0, 0, 0, 2, 7, 9
12.30 ,,	Rotating object + tactile	6, 4, 6, 3, 7, 15
12.52 ,,	Tactile	0, 0, 0, 3, 7, 15

* At the 10th second from the beginning of the tactile stimulus the dog moved its leg, striking against a metal basin.

These experiments of Dr. Zavadsky are important as revealing a new and unexpected phenomenon. The established conditioned stimulus had no positive effect by itself during $1-1\frac{1}{2}$ minutes, but the neutral stimulus which was added to it for the first time immediately disclosed the regular positive conditioned reflex. It is obvious that we have come across a fresh case of dis-inhibition.

During the last three lectures considerable stress has been laid on the phenomenon of dis-inhibition and many examples have been given. I would plead as my excuse the great importance of an adequate conception of the rôle played by this phenomenon in the physiology of the hemispheres, although of course the study of the lower parts of the nervous system presents many instances of analogous phenomena. So far, however, as the interpretation of the intimate mechanism of dis-inhibition goes we are completely in the dark, and it can only be hoped that accumulation of experimental evidence may at some future date throw light on its nature.

I wish now to call your attention again to the first of the two experiments just described. It can clearly be seen that the stimulus of the metronome when added to the tactile stimulus not only elicited a flow of saliva during the initial phase of inactivity, but also caused a considerable diminution in the salivary secretion during the active phase. While the tactile stimulus applied singly elicited a secretion during the second $1\frac{1}{2}$ minutes ranging from 29-46 drops, the addition of the metronome reduced this to 17 drops. There must, therefore, be a double effect on the part of the extra stimulus— dis-inhibitory in the initial phase, usually of inactivity; inhibitory in the succeeding phase, usually of activity.

If different extra stimuli producing external inhibition are allowed to act upon delayed conditioned reflexes, various definite and regular modifications are observed in the course followed by the delay. The extra stimuli which were used in this connection for one experimental animal have been arranged in the following groups according to the influence they exerted upon delay :

I. Thermal stimuli at 5°C. and at 44°C.; a weak odour of camphor.

II. Thermal stimuli at 0·5°C. and at 50°C.

III. Noiselessly rotating objects ; the sound of a metronome ; tactile stimulation of the skin (the conditioned stimulus to the delayed reflex being in this animal a similar tactile stimulation of a different place on the skin) ; a whistle of moderate strength ; the odour of amyl acetate.

IV. Intense odour of camphor ; loud whistle ; sound of an electric buzzer.

Extra stimuli belonging to the first group did not, in this dog, affect either phase of the delayed reflexes. Extra stimuli belonging to the second group exerted an effect only upon the initial phase of the reflex, causing a salivary secretion. Extra stimuli belonging to the third group disturbed both phases of delay : during the first phase a salivary secretion was produced, and during the second phase the secretion which should normally have been present was much diminished. Extra stimuli belonging to the fourth group exercised little or no influence upon the initial phase of the delayed reflex, but completely suppressed the second phase. It may be added that when all due precautions were taken the experiments proceeded as a rule with striking precision.

The following experiments serve to illustrate the grouping of extra stimuli given above :

A tactile stimulation of the skin is used as a conditioned stimulus to acid in a delayed reflex. The conditioned stimulus acts continuously during three minutes before the administration of acid. The extra stimuli employed are : (1) a thermal cutaneous stimulus of 44°C., (2) a thermal cutaneous stimulus of 0·5°C., (3) an odour of amyl acetate, (4) the sound of an electric buzzer.

Time	Stimulus	Salivary Secretion in drops per 30 secs. during the isolated action of the conditioned stimulus
	Experiment of 13th October, 1907.	
10.17 a.m.	Tactile	0, 0, 0, 0, 1, 5
10.32 ,,	Tactile	0, 0, 0, 0, 2, 9
10.45 ,,	Tactile + thermal at 44°C.	0, 0, 0, 1, 2, 10
11.0 ,,	Tactile	0, 0, 0, 0, 1, 10
11.12 ,,	Tactile	0, 0, 0, 1, 5, 9
	Experiment of 15th September, 1907.	
2.28 p.m.	Tactile	0, 0, 0, 0, 2, 8
2.40 ,,	Tactile	0, 0, 0, 5, 20, 17
2.55 ,,	Tactile + thermal stimulus at 0·5°C.	2, 2, 3, 4, 20, 24
3.10 ,,	Tactile	1, 0, 0, 0, 10, 17

Time	Stimulus	Salivary Secretion in drops per 30 secs. during the isolated action of the conditioned stimulus
	Experiment of 18th September, 1907.	
10.12 a.m.	Tactile	0, 0, 2, 7, 9, 11
10.25 ,,	Tactile	0, 0, 1, 7, 11, 17
10.43 ,,	Tactile	0, 0, 0, 5, 8, 11
11.2 ,,	Tactile + odour of amyl acetate	3, 3, 0, 5, 5, 7
11.16 ,,	Tactile	0, 0, 2, 4, 8, 11
	Experiment of 13th September, 1907.	
3.30 p.m.	Tactile	1, 0, 0, 8, 10, 12
3.48 ,,	Tactile + buzzer	0, 0, 0, 0, 0, 0
4.15 ,,	Tactile	0, 0, 0, 0, 2, 8
4.35 ,,	Tactile	0, 0, 0, 3, 5, 10

Absolutely identical results are obtained when the extra stimuli are allowed to act, not throughout the whole of the time of the isolated action of the conditioned stimulus, but only during either the first, inactive phase or the second, active phase. This is illustrated in the following experiments carried out on the same dog and under the same conditions as before.

Time	Stimulus	Secretion of Saliva in drops per 30 secs. during the isolated action of the conditioned stimulus
	Experiment of 23rd July, 1907.	
9.33 a.m.	Tactile	0, 0, 0, 3, 12, 12
9.47 ,,	Tactile	0, 0, 0, 1, 9, 10
10.2 ,,	Tactile + whistle of medium strength during first 1½ minutes	3, 2, 6, 6, 8, 6
10.15 ,,	Tactile	0, 0, 1, 4, 7, 11
	Experiment of 18th August, 1907.	
9.35 a.m.	Tactile	0, 0, 0, 3, 10, 13
9.50 ,,	Tactile	0, 0, 1, 3, 8, 14
10.5 ,,	Tactile + whistle of medium strength during the second 1½ minutes	0, 0, 1, 3, 0, 2
10.20 ,,	Tactile	0, 0, 1, 2, 7, 9

The extra stimulus of the whistle, which belongs to the third group of external inhibitors, when acting during the first phase of the delayed reflex brought about a secretion of saliva, but when acting during the second phase it diminished the secretion. A certain diminution of the secretion is sometimes observed during the second phase of the reflex in experiments where the extra stimulus is applied during the first phase. This must be due to the after-effect of the extra stimulus.

It now remains to interpret the empirical grouping of the extra stimuli, and to determine the reason of their different action upon the delayed reflexes. All the experimental evidence at our disposal indicates that the intensity of the effect which they produce depends on their relative physiological strength and the magnitude of the general reactions by which the animal responds to their independent action. The distribution of extra stimuli among the four groups represents a classification according to such physiological strength. In some cases this can be seen by a casual glance at the list itself, where different intensities of the same stimulus appear in different groups.

The difference in the effects of these extra stimuli is also revealed by the motor reaction of the animal (investigatory reflex). With stimuli belonging to the first group there is frequently no motor reaction at all. As we pass on to stimuli belonging to the remaining groups the reactions become more and more vigorous and prolonged. Moreover, the inhibitory effect of all these extra stimuli, which belong, of course, to the group of external inhibitors, is clearly seen in relation to the second (usually active) phase of the delayed reflexes. The inhibitory effect becomes the more pronounced as we ascend from the first to the fourth group until with stimuli belonging to the latter group complete inhibition is obtained. It is thus obvious that the classification represents stimuli of progressively increasing physiological effect upon the organism, those in the first group exerting the least effect.

In cases where an extra stimulus is allowed to act upon a delayed conditioned reflex repeatedly, it is found that its inhibitory effect upon the second (usually active) phase progressively diminishes. This is a further proof that inhibition and dis-inhibition of delayed reflexes by extra stimuli is closely associated with external inhibition. Two experiments may be given which were performed on the dog employed for the last experiment :

Time	Stimulus	Salivary Secretion in drops per 30 secs. during the isolated action of the conditioned stimulus

Experiment of 13*th November*, 1907.

10.20 a.m.	Tactile	0, 0, 0, 2, 8, 9
10.35 ,,	Tactile + whistle	0, 0, 1, 1, 1, 4
10.47 ,,	,, ,,	1, 1, 1, 0, 1, 2
11.0 ,,	,, ,,	2, 2, 3, 2, 2, 3
11.15 ,,	,, ,,	1, 2, 3, 10, 10, 11
11.27 ,,	,, ,,	2, 2, 2, 5, 2, 12

Experiment of 20*th November*, 1907.

10.35 a.m.	Tactile	0, 0, 0, 8, 10, 11
10.47 ,,	Tactile + metronome	3, 2, 1, 5, 6, 5
11.0 ,,	,, ,,	1, 1, 2, 3, 8, 9
11.15 ,,	,, ,,	0, 0, 1, 2, 8, 14
11.30 ,,	,, ,,	0, 0, 2, 3, 12, 12

It can be seen from these two experiments how the inhibitory effect of the extra stimulus upon the active phase falls gradually with each repetition, the recovery of the delayed reflex being especially regular in the second experiment.

All these experiments, which were carried out on one and the same animal, have been repeated with similar results on many other dogs. The only variation was in the distribution of stimuli among the four groups, which differed slightly for the individual animals. This appears only reasonable when it is recalled that the intensity of the reactions of different animals in response to extraneous stimuli varies to a considerable and sometimes to an extreme degree, depending on the individual character of the nervous system and on the previous history of the animal.

Thus we come to the conclusion that variations in the effect of different extra stimuli upon the delayed reflex are determined by differences in the physiological strength of the stimuli. When the strength of the extra stimulus is insignificant the delayed reflex in either of its two phases remains unaffected. When the strength of the extra stimulus is somewhat increased it is only the initial (usually inactive) phase which becomes affected, being now converted into a phase of activity. With a greater strength of the extra stimulus the second (usually active) phase of the delayed reflex also becomes involved, the secretion being considerably diminished in magnitude, so that it becomes equal to or even smaller than the secretion during the dis-inhibited first phase. Finally, with a maximal intensity of the extra stimulus all conditioned activity disappears, and the delayed reflex is represented throughout both phases by a series of zeros.

As a result of the different effects upon the two phases of the reflex brought about through external inhibition, two facts relating to the central nervous activities stand out clearly. The first is that the extraneous stimulus acting on the positive phase of the reflex inhibits, and acting on the negative phase dis-inhibits, in either case, therefore, reversing the nervous process prevailing at the time. The second is that the inhibitory process is more labile and more easily affected than the excitatory process, being influenced by stimuli of much weaker physiological strength.

The following was a chance, but instructive, observation with regard to the second point. I meant to illustrate a series of public lectures on conditioned reflexes by demonstration of experiments. The lectures were given at a place remote from our laboratories so that the dogs had to be conveyed and set down in surroundings which were quite unfamiliar. All the five or six experiments with positive conditioned reflexes, in the first lecture, were carried out successfully. On the other hand, in the second lecture, the experiments with inhibitory reflexes, again five or six in number and attempted on the same animals as before, did not succeed, all the reflexes having undergone dis-inhibition. Thus the very same extra stimulus of the changed environmental conditions had not the slightest disturbing effect upon the positive conditioned reflexes, but exercised a profound influence upon the inhibitory conditioned reflexes, even though the effect of the extra stimulus was now weakened on account of repetition. These facts will be discussed more fully in a further lecture, in connection with other observations bearing on the interrelations between excitation and inhibition.

Since the first phase of a delayed reflex, like experimental extinction and conditioned inhibition, involves an inhibitory process, we should expect to find between all three a close similarity. It has already been noticed in the cases of extinction and conditioned inhibition of a definitely positive conditioned reflex, that the inhibition spreads spontaneously to other conditioned reflexes, and that the degree of this spreading is determined by the relative physiological intensity of the reflexes. It has further been observed that if the reflexes involved secondarily are physiologically weaker than the reflex in which the inhibition was developed primarily, the accompanying secondary inhibition of these other reflexes is complete ; but that if the reflexes involved secondarily are the stronger only a partial inhibition is obtained. In other words, the intensity of the primary inhibition is found to be exactly proportional to the intensity of the excitatory process on which it is based. This holds good also for inhibition of delay. An alteration in either direction of the strength of the conditioned stimulus causes a sharp disturbance in the established relation between the inhibitory and excitatory phases of the delay. The two following experiments on this point were conducted on the same animal as was employed in the preceding experiments :

Time	Stimulus	Salivary Secretion in drops per 30 secs. during the isolated action of the conditioned stimulus
	Experiment of 25th October, 1907.	
10.4 a.m.	Rhythmic tactile stimulation at the rate of 18-22 per minute	0, 0, 0, 5, 8, 8
10.17 ,,	Rhythmic tactile stimulation at the rate of 18-22 per minute	1, 0, 3, 6, 10, 11
10.30 ,,	Same stimulus at the rate of 10 per minute	0, 0, 0, **0, 3, 10**
10.45 ,,	Same stimulus at the rate of 18-22 per minute	0, 0, 0, 2, 9, 17
11.0 ,,	Same stimulus at the rate of 18-22 per minute	0, 0, 0, 0, 5, 16
	Experiment of 29th October, 1907.	
10.6 a.m.	Rhythmic tactile stimulation 18-22 per minute	0, 0, 0, 0, 0, 3
10.19 ,,	Rhythmic tactile stimulation 18-22 per minute	0, 0, 0, 0, 2, 11
10.38 ,,	Same stimulus at the rate of 38-40 per minute	0, 0, 0, **6, 13, 14**
10.51 ,,	Same stimulus at the rate of 18-22 per minute	0, 0, 0, 0, 0, 7
11.7 ,,	Same stimulus at the rate of 18-22 per minute	0, 0, 0, 0, 5, 16

The experiments show a more definite effect in the case of a diminution in the strength of the conditioned stimulus than in the case of an increase in strength, though both effects are evident.

Just as with extinction and conditioned inhibition, the intensity of the inhibition in delay also depends upon the strength of the unconditioned stimulus. This can easily be shown with conditioned alimentary stimuli, when the delayed reflex is tested in the dog after it had been fed at the usual time and again after a certain period of fast. The following experiment illustrates this point. A whistle of moderate strength is used as a conditioned alimentary stimulus in a conditioned reflex delayed by three minutes.

Experiment of 13th December, 1907.
Previously to the experiment the dog was fed at the usual time.

Time	Stimulus	Salivary Secretion in drops per 30 secs. during the isolated action of the conditioned stimulus
2.40 p.m.	Whistle	0, 0, 0, 0, 2, 6
2.54 ,,	,,	0, 0, 0, 2, 3, 6
3.30 ,,	,,	0, 0, 0, 0, 2, 5

Experiment of 15th December, 1907.
Conducted upon the same dog after two days deprivation of food.

Time	Stimulus	Salivary Secretion in drops per 30 secs. during the isolated action of the conditioned stimulus
3.5 p.m.	Whistle	0, 2, 2, 4, 4, 6
3.20 ,,	,,	2, 5, 3, 3, 4, 6
3.40 ,,	,,	1, 6, 4, 3, 5, 5

Experiments of this kind show that when the physiological significance of the conditioned stimulus is increased through deprivation of food, the inactive or inhibitory phase of the delay almost entirely disappears.

Summation of intensity of the inhibitory after-effect can be observed with inhibition of delay exactly as with extinction and conditioned inhibition. This is clearly evidenced by an experiment such as the following :

A tactile stimulation of the skin serves as a conditioned stimulus in a delayed reflex, the isolated action of this stimulus being

continued during three minutes before the application of the unconditioned.

Time	Stimulus	Salivary Secretion in drops per 30 secs. during the isolated action of conditioned stimulus	Remarks
10.21 a.m.	Tactile stimulation during 4 minutes	0, 0, 0,　0,　3, 10	Reinforced with acid at the end of the 3rd minute of isolated action of the conditioned stimulus.
10.35　,,	Tactile stimulation during 4 minutes	0, 0, 0, 10, 18, 21	
10.50　,,	Tactile stimulation during 4 minutes	0, 0, 0,　8, 17, 23	
11.5　,,	Tactile stimulation during only $1\frac{1}{2}$ minutes	0, 0, 2,　2,　0,　0	
11.10　,,	Tactile stimulation during only $1\frac{1}{2}$ minutes	0, 0, 1,　0,　0,　0	Not reinforced.
11.15　,,	Tactile stimulation during only $1\frac{1}{2}$ minutes	0, 0, 0,　0,　0,　0	
11.21　,,	Tactile stimulation during 4 minutes	0, 0, 0,　1,　3,　5	Reinforced with acid at the end of the 3rd minute of isolated action of the conditioned stimulus.
11.33　,,	Tactile stimulation during 4 minutes	0, 0, 1,　5,　9, 17	
11.45　,,	Tactile stimulation during only $1\frac{1}{2}$ minutes	0, 0, 0,　0,　0,　0	
11.50　,,	Tactile stimulation during only $1\frac{1}{2}$ minutes	0, 0, 0,　0,　0,　0	Not reinforced.
11.55　,,	Tactile stimulation during only $1\frac{1}{2}$ minutes	0, 0, 0,　0,　0,　0	
12 noon	Tactile stimulation during 4 minutes	0, 0, 0,　0,　0, 0,	

The tactile stimulus which normally produced inhibition during the first $1\frac{1}{2}$ minutes of its isolated action, when abbreviated so as not to act during the second $1\frac{1}{2}$ minutes associated with the excitatory phase of the reflex, led to such a strengthening of the inhibition that on its subsequent application for the full three minutes the positive phase of the reflex was either greatly reduced (11.21 a.m.) or else abolished altogether (12 noon).

It remains now to seek an interpretation of the fact that in the case of a delayed reflex, the same stimulus has at first an inhibitory, and later an excitatory, effect. What factor determines these two distinct properties of one and the same stimulus acting under apparently identical conditions ? We shall find no difficulty in correlating this phenomenon with the experimental evidence already considered in these lectures. In the third and fifth lectures a number of agencies were discussed which can be given either excitatory or inhibitory conditioned properties. In particular the factor of duration of time was shown to act as a real physiological stimulus, and experiments were described in which definite time intervals appeared as effective stimuli. I should like especially to recall to your memory the experiment in which the compound stimulus consisted of an external stimulus related to a definite moment of time (p. 41). In this experiment the external stimulus was without any effect until applied in the neighbourhood of the particular moment after the previous administration of acid, but as this particular moment was approached the secretory effect made its appearance and gradually and precisely increased to a maximum. This is exactly the case with delayed reflexes also. In the experiments which have just been described in the present lecture the unconditioned stimulus was added to the external stimulus only at the expiration of 3 minutes ; in other words, the external stimulus itself *plus* its duration for three minutes together constitute the actual compound stimulus which was immediately reinforced, and it was this particular combination and not the nominal conditioned stimulus which acquired conditioned properties. The same nominal stimulus at any time previously to the end of the third minute acted as a component of a different stimulatory compound which remained unreinforced by the unconditioned reflex and therefore became inhibitory, exactly as would any other stimulus if it were not reinforced. The same phenomenon has already been demonstrated in the case of conditioned inhibition, and illustrations even more striking will be given in the next lecture, which is to deal with the fourth type of internal inhibition.

In the case of delayed reflexes the significance of the duration of a stimulus can be observed in a very concrete and simple manner. When the external stimulus selected for the formation of a conditioned reflex is applied during a given interval of time, at each successive moment the stimulus forms part of a definite and distinct stimulatory compound. It is well known how soon we get accustomed to stimuli of smell, sound or illumination. This, of course, means that the nerve cells which are being excited pass through a series of successive physiological changes. In accordance with this it is obvious that if a definite unconditioned reflex is repeatedly evoked coincidently with any one particular physiological state of the cerebral cells, it is this definite state and no other that acquires a definite conditioned significance. In the next lecture it will be shown to how great an extent the discrimination of different intensities of one and the same stimulus can proceed, and how the stimulus evokes at one particular intensity a positive and at another intensity an inhibitory conditioned reflex. We are thus fortunately provided with a great deal of perfectly good experimental evidence which throws light on the phenomenon of internal inhibition involved in delay.

The possibility of the development of a delay has always to be reckoned with in studying conditioned reflexes. We know that in order to determine the intensity of excitation in a simultaneous or a short-delayed conditioned reflex in its numerous and subtle variations under different conditions, it is necessary to apply the appropriate conditioned stimulus singly for a longer or a shorter period of time, combining its action with that of the unconditioned stimulus at the end of this interval. Only in this manner can we get a measurable reflex response. This procedure, even though rarely performed, tends to the development of a more or less prolonged delay, so that along with the excitatory process there originates also an inhibitory one. The investigation thus naturally becomes complicated, for it is now necessary to deal with two simultaneous and antagonistic processes. For example, it is not easy by our usual methods to obtain the true latent period of conditioned reflexes, since what has often been referred to in our description of experiments as the " latent period " represented in actual fact a delay— *i.e.* the interposition of an inhibitory period, which could appropriately be termed the "preliminary inhibitory period," but which is certainly not the true latent period of the reflex.

In order to determine the true latent period of conditioned reflexes it is necessary to use reflexes which are as nearly as possible simultaneous, the unconditioned stimulus succeeding rapidly on the conditioned after an interval of a fraction of a second. It is only by using such reflexes, and then chiefly their motor components, that convincing experimental evidence can be obtained showing that the length of the true latent period of a conditioned reflex is really of the same order as is the true latent period of reflexes in the lower centres of the brain and spinal cord. Such determinations have only recently been introduced into our investigations, as we did not consider the determination of the true latent period of conditioned reflexes to be of fundamental importance for establishing their nature as reflex. The regularity and infallibility with which these reflexes could be evoked constituted in our opinion the main evidence for their reflex nature, and in this connection differences in the period of latency did not seem of much importance since the latent period of lower reflexes also is known to be subject to fairly wide variations depending on the complexity of the central paths and connections involved in the reflex. It may justly be admitted, however, and without prejudice to our conception of the reflex nature of conditioned reflexes, that the nervous connections are of greater complexity in those reflexes which involve the cerebral cortex.

The elucidation of many other problems concerning conditioned reflexes, such, for instance, as that of the actual course of the excitatory process from the moment of its origination, is also rendered difficult by interference from delay. In this respect individual differences in the character of the nervous system may be very helpful. For example, it was shown above that in some animals the delay is developed with difficulty, and that the excitatory process is only slightly, or often not at all, disturbed. The experimenter, in order to diminish the influence of delay, can also take the precaution to abbreviate the isolated action of the conditioned stimulus to the minimum compatible with obtaining a secretion of sufficient magnitude to allow of comparison in different variations of the experiment. On the other hand, there are some problems in the elucidation of which the initial process of inhibition may be turned to advantage, as will be shown in the next lecture. It can clearly be seen how, when inquiring into the properties of conditioned reflexes, the experimenter has to adapt his methods to the character of the animal at his disposal.

The experimental evidence with which we have been dealing in the last three lectures demonstrates the enormous biological importance of internal inhibition of conditioned reflexes. It is by means of internal inhibition that the signalizing activity of the hemispheres is constantly corrected and perfected. To sum up :

If over a given time a signalling, *i.e.* a conditioned, stimulus is repeatedly presented without the accompaniment of the unconditioned stimulus, then the conditioned stimulus becomes meaningless to the organism as calling for an unnecessary expenditure of energy, and the stimulus loses, though generally for only a short time, its physiological significance (experimental extinction).

In exactly the same manner, if a conditioned stimulus is repeatedly applied together with another extraneous stimulus and in the combination is never followed by the unconditioned stimulus, the conditioned stimulus loses its positive excitatory conditioned effect, but only in that particular combination and not when applied singly (conditioned inhibition).

Finally, if a regular interval of sufficient duration is established between the commencement of a conditioned stimulus and its reinforcement by the unconditioned stimulus, the former becomes ineffective during the first part of its isolated action ; during the second part of its action a positive excitatory effect appears, and this increases progressively in intensity as the moment approaches when the unconditioned stimulus has customarily been applied (inhibition of delay).

In the above manner a continuous and most exact adaptation of the organism to its environment is effected, revealing a most delicate adjustment in the antagonistic nervous processes of the higher animals.

As has been clearly demonstrated in the last three lectures the phenomena of extinction, conditioned inhibition and delay all represent the formation of inhibitory conditioned reflexes. Inhibitory conditioned reflexes can, however, also be obtained by a totally different procedure. If an inhibitory stimulus is applied simultaneously and repeatedly for short periods of time together with some neutral stimulus the latter also develops an inhibitory function of its own.

This subject has been specially examined by Dr. Volborth, who started by rendering the extraneous stimuli absolutely neutral, presenting them repeatedly to the animal until they ceased to produce any inhibition of the positive conditioned reflexes or any dis-inhibition of the inhibitory reflexes. He then repeatedly allowed these neutral stimuli to act during short intervals of time either with conditioned reflexes which had just been experimentally extinguished or with the inhibitory combination in a conditioned inhibition. After repeating this procedure several times he tested the action of these hitherto neutral stimuli upon positive conditioned reflexes, and in this manner successfully demonstrated that they had acquired definite inhibitory properties.

Since in order to become sure of the results these tests had to be repeated several times, Dr. Volborth in one group of experiments accompanied only every alternate test by the unconditioned stimulus. This strict alternation of reinforcement with non-reinforcement was adopted in order to prevent the combination of the positive stimulus with the new and hitherto neutral stimulus from acquiring a pre-dominance of positive or negative properties in itself. But most convincing of all was another form of the experiment in which the test was always accompanied by the unconditioned stimulus. In spite of repeated tests of this kind the recently acquired inhibitory properties of the hitherto neutral stimuli were still prominently exhibited. The following are some of Dr. Volborth's experiments, in which a " natural " alimentary stimulus was employed.

The alimentary conditioned stimulus after extinction was repeatedly applied in conjunction with the sound of a metronome which had previously been rendered entirely neutral. After this procedure had been continued for some time a combination of the action of the metronome with a positive and non-extinguished alimentary reflex was occasionally tested, and this combination was always reinforced by the unconditioned reflex

Experiment of 5th December, 1911, after ten applications of the metronome with the extinguished conditioned reflex.

Time	Stimulus applied during 30 secs.	Salivary Secretion in drops during 30 seconds
12.54 p.m.	Meat powder at a distance	7
1.8 ,,	Meat powder at a distance + metronome	2

Experiment of 1st December, 1911, after 19 applications of the metronome with the extinguished conditioned reflex.

Time	Stimulus applied during 30 secs.	Salivary Secretion in drops during 30 seconds
11.30 a.m.	Meat powder at a distance	7
11.47 ,,	Meat powder at a distance + metronome	1
11.57 ,,	Meat powder at a distance	3
12.7 p.m.	Meat powder at a distance	8

Experiment of 18th December, 1911, after 26 applications of the metronome with the extinguished conditioned reflex.

Time.	Stimulus applied during 30 sec.	Salivary Secretion in drops during 30 seconds.
10.35 a.m.	Meat powder at a distance	9
10.47 ,,	Meat powder at a distance + metronome	1
11.0 ,,	Meat powder at a distance	12

It is obvious that the sound of the metronome which was formerly entirely neutral has acquired inhibitory properties as a result of repeated applications with the extinguished conditioned reflex.

This new inhibitory stimulus of the second order proves itself in every respect similar in properties to those inhibitory stimuli which have been considered already in connection with experimental extinction, conditioned inhibition and delay. For example, a new inhibitory stimulus of the second order which is developed with the help of one definite conditioned reflex can exert an inhibitory effect upon other conditioned reflexes as well. This is shown in the following experiment of 15th March, 1911, in which a different dog is employed.

The sound of a metronome was made always to coincide with an extinguished " natural " conditioned alimentary reflex ; subsequently the effect of the metronome was tested upon an artificial alimentary conditioned reflex to odour of camphor.

Time.	Stimulus applied during 30 secs.	Salivary Secretion in drops during 30 secs.
3.8 p.m.	Camphor	5
3.21 ,,	Camphor	4
3.40 ,,	Camphor + metronome	1
3.55 ,,	Camphor	1
4.18 ,,	Camphor	5

It can be seen also in the above experiment that the effect of the conditioned inhibitory stimulus of the second order is not limited to the time of its actual administration, but reveals itself also in a definite inhibitory after-effect which is subject to summation. Furthermore, conditioned inhibitory stimuli of the second order are, equally with the primary ones, subject to dis-inhibition by agencies belonging to the group of external inhibitors. We thus come to the following conclusion : when perfectly neutral stimuli fall upon the hemispheres at a time when there prevails a state of inhibition they acquire an inhibitory function of their own, so that when they act subsequently upon any region of the brain which is in a state of excitation they produce inhibition.

A point to which further reference will be made should be mentioned here, namely, that every extraneous stimulus which falls upon the hemispheres and remains without any further consequence to the animal, if repeated causes the spontaneous development of a cortical inhibition. Therefore, in the type of experiments just described, it is always necessary to ascertain the extent to which the acquisition of inhibitory properties by hitherto neutral stimuli depends on their simultaneous application with inhibitory stimuli, and to what extent these inhibitory properties have developed independently.

LECTURE VII

The analysing and synthesizing activity of the cerebral hemispheres : (a) The initial generalization of conditioned stimuli. (b) Differential inhibition.

STIMULI which evoke conditioned reflexes are perpetually acting as signals of those agencies in the environment which are in themselves immediately favourable or immediately destructive for the organism. Such signals are drawn sometimes from only one elementary property of the environing agencies, sometimes from a whole complex of these properties. This is possible only because the nervous system possesses on the one hand a definite analysing mechanism, by means of which it selects out of the whole complexity of the environment those units which are of significance, and, on the other hand, a synthesizing mechanism by means of which individual units can be integrated into an excitatory complex. Thus in studying the nervous activity of the cerebral cortex it is necessary to deal with two further and distinct phenomena, one involving a neuro-analysis and the other involving a neuro-synthesis. The analysing and synthesizing functions of the nervous system constantly superimpose themselves upon and interact with one another.

Every type of nervous system presents a more or less complex analysing apparatus which readily admits of subdivision into what we may term the **nervous analysers.** For example, the visual analyser selects the vibrations of light, the acoustic analyser selects the vibrations of sound, and so on. Furthermore, each analyser differentiates its own selective medium of the environment into a very large number of elementary physiological stimuli. With regard to the structure of the analysers, each includes, on the one hand, the peripheral receptor with all its afferent nerves, and, on the other hand, the nerve cells which lie at the central termination of the nerve fibres. The peripheral receptors can be regarded as " transformers," which, in the case of any single analyser, are capable of accepting only one definite form of energy as an adequate stimulus for the initiation of a nerve impulse. It is obvious that both the peripheral receptors and the central nervous elements are involved in the analysing function of the nervous system. Inferior analysing qualities are of course manifested by lower parts of the nervous system, and even by the crudely differentiated nervous substance in those animals which lack a nervous system proper. An organism deprived of its cerebral hemispheres still responds in a great variety of ways to stimuli applied to its receptor surfaces, according to the site of application, the intensity and the quality of the stimuli. However, the highest and most subtle analysing activity of which an animal is capable can be obtained only with the help of the cerebral cortex. It is evident also that only with the progressive development of the analysing activity of the nervous system is the organism enabled to multiply the complexity of its contacts with the external world and to achieve a more and more varied and exact adaptation to external conditions. In contemporary research the study of the analysing function forms a very important section of the so-called physiology of the sense organs. This section has reached a very high state of development in the hands of some of the greatest physiologists, especially Helmholtz, and presents an abundant wealth of data concerning the activities of the peripheral structures of the different analysers and of their cerebral terminations. A good deal is known also about the limits of the analysing functions in man. But while the study of the physiology of the special sense organs suggests explanations of many complicated cases of the analysing function, and enunciates many fundamental laws to which this activity conforms, the greater part of the material which has been gathered is of a subjective character, being based on our psychical apperceptions which are the most elementary subjective indications of the objective correlations between organism and environment. This fact constitutes the greatest defect of this section of physiology, since it excludes the study of the analysing function in animals outside man, and therewith all the advantages of animal experimentation. The method of conditioned reflexes, however, gives over the study of the whole of this most important function of nervous analysis into the hands of the purely experimental physiologist. With the help of conditioned reflexes the scope and limits of the analysing functions in different animals can be exactly determined, and the laws regulating this function made clear. Although the study of the physiology of analysers has been as yet but little developed, research upon the new lines is making rapid progress and may be expected to add largely to our knowledge of the mechanism by which the exact correspondence between the organism and its environment is maintained.

The first step was to find a method by which the activities of the analysers could be objectively studied in animals by means of visible outward reactions. As was mentioned before, even insignificant changes in the external environment call forth if not a special inborn or acquired reflex activity, then a reaction of orientation (the " investigatory reflex "). It is obvious that the investigatory reflex can be used to determine the degree to which the nervous system of a given animal is capable of discriminating between various stimuli. If, for example, among the different environing agencies there is present a definite musical tone, any, even slight, alteration of its pitch will suffice to evoke an investigatory reflex in the form of a definite orientation of the ears and maybe of the whole body of the animal in relation to the tone. The same is true even of slight changes in various other elementary or compound stimuli. The investigatory reflex, of course, takes place only provided that the structure of the analysing apparatus is sufficiently delicate to register the change in the environment. This reflex can be used for the purpose of our investigation by itself, or, much better, through its inhibitory or dis-inhibitory effects upon conditioned reflexes, since these are the most delicate nervous reactions of which the animal is capable. However in spite of the high degree of sensitivity mani- fested by the investigatory reflex this reaction is in many respects unsuitable as a basis for the study of the analysing activity of the nervous system. One of its chief defects is that in the case of certain weak stimuli the reaction is only transient and cannot be repeated, and it is therefore useless for the purpose of exact experi- mentation. The detailed investigation of a conditioned reflex reaction, on the contrary, provides an eminently suitable method for an exact experimental research into the analysing function. A definite external agent is made, for example, to acquire by our usual technique the properties of a definite conditioned stimulus. By repeated reinforcement this particular stimulus is strengthened in its new properties, while the stimulus nearest to it in intensity, position or quality is always contrasted by being left without reinforcement, with the result that it becomes readily and exactly differentiated from the established positive conditioned stimulus.

The successful development of analysis of external agencies by means of conditioned reflexes is always preceded by what we call a

" period of generalization " (which may possibly be regarded as some form of synthesizing activity).

For instance, if a tone of 1000 d.v. is established as a conditioned stimulus, many other tones spontaneously acquire similar properties, such properties diminishing proportionally to the intervals of these tones from the one of 1000 d.v. Similarly, if a tactile stimulation of a definite circumscribed area of skin is made into a conditioned stimulus, tactile stimulation of other skin areas will also elicit some conditioned reaction, the effect diminishing with increasing distance of these areas from the one for which the conditioned reflex was originally established. The same is observed with stimulation of other receptor organs. This spontaneous development of accessory reflexes, or, as we have termed it, generalization of stimuli, can be interpreted from a biological point of view by reference to the fact that natural stimuli are in most cases not rigidly constant but range around a particular strength and quality of stimulus in a common group. For example, the hostile sound of any beast of prey serves as a conditioned stimulus to a defence reflex in the animals which it hunts. The defence reflex is brought about independently of variations in pitch, strength and timbre of the sound produced by the animal according to its distance, the tension of its vocal cords and similar factors.

Besides this we have encountered in conditioned reflexes another form of generalization, the vital importance of which is not so immediately apparent. So far we have been dealing with a temporary form of generalization within a single analyser in the case of simultaneous and delayed reflexes. In the case of conditioned long-trace reflexes, with a pause of 1-3 minutes, the generalization becomes permanent and of a wider scope. Trace reflexes, like all delayed reflexes, present two phases—an initial, inactive phase based on internal inhibition, and a second, active phase based on nervous excitation. All that has been said about the effect of extra stimuli upon these two phases in the case of delayed reflexes is true also for the two phases in trace reflexes. The trace reflexes, however, have another characteristic of their own, namely, that they exhibit a permanent and universal generalization, involving all the analysers. For example, if we establish a long-trace conditioned reflex to a tactile cutaneous stimulus, it is found that stimuli which belong to other analysers and which have never been connected with the given reflex begin to act as conditioned stimuli to the same trace reflex.

We shall deal with this phenomenon at some length, since the investigation presents some special points of interest.

The following experiments bearing upon this question are taken from a research by Dr. Grossman :

A tactile stimulation of the skin is used as the conditioned stimulus for a long-trace reflex to acid, the interval between the end of the conditioned stimulus and the beginning of the unconditioned being one minute. The experiments show the effect of a thermal stimulus at 0°C. and of a given musical tone, both applied for the very first time.

Time	Stimulus applied during one minute	Salivary Secretion in drops during successive minutes from the beginning of the conditioned stimulus	Remarks
	Experiment of 6th February, 1909.		
11.39 a.m.	Tactile	0, 3	⎫ Reinforced by in-
11.55 ,,	Tactile	0, 7	⎬ troduction of
			⎭ acid.
12.6 p.m.	Thermal at 0°C.	1, 4, 7, 7	⎰ Not reinforced by ⎱ acid.
12.22 ,,	Tactile	0, 4	Reinforced.
	Experiment of 7th February, 1909.		
2.36 p.m.	Tactile	0, 9	⎫ Reinforced by in-
2.45 ,,	Tactile	0, 15	⎬ troduction of
			⎭ acid.
2.54 ,,	Tone	0, 3, 4, 6, 2, 0	Not reinforced.
3.2 ,,	Tactile	0, 0	⎫ Reinforced by in-
3.10 ,,	Tactile	0, 1	⎬ troduction of
3.22 ,,	Tactile	0, 6	⎭ acid.

It is thus seen that stimuli which had previously never been connected with the reflex to acid have now acquired the property to excite this reflex. Furthermore, the stimuli, although applied for the very first time, act in the same manner as the stimulus used to establish the trace reflex, their effect being manifested not at the time of their application, but chiefly or exclusively after they have been discontinued. This similarity made us inclined to regard them as being due to a generalization of the original trace reflex. Of course, the evidence from a few isolated experiments of this type was not sufficiently strong to establish this conclusion beyond doubt, and in view of the intrinsic interest of this phenomenon it was subjected to rigid investigation.

On the experimental evidence available concerning conditioned reflexes only two further possible explanations of this phenomenon suggested themselves. In the first place a long-trace reflex is always formed slowly and with difficulty, and it was observed in our earlier experiments that before the formation of the trace reflex other conditioned reflexes were very easily established to any chance stimuli which happened to coincide with the actual administration of the unconditioned stimulus and of which the experimenter himself was often the cause. In the case we are speaking of at present the danger of interference by extraneous stimuli was therefore considerable, and these experiments had to be repeated in our new laboratory so as to make sure that any possible accidental influence of the experimenter upon the animal was excluded. Under these conditions the generalized character of the long-trace reflex was still found to persist.

The second explanation which suggested itself was as follows : When conditioned reflexes are being established in dogs for the first time, it is found that the whole experimental environment, beginning with the introduction of the animal into the experimental room, acquires at first conditioned properties. This initial reflex could be called, therefore, a conditioned reflex to the environment. But later on, when the special reflex to a single definite and constant stimulus has appeared, all the other elements of the environment gradually lose their special conditioned significance, most probably on account of a gradual development of internal inhibition. However, this inhibition is at first very easily dis-inhibited by any extra stimulus. The following is a striking example of such a case which was very common, when, as formerly, the experimenter remained in the room with the dog. The reflex to environment had in the given experiments just come to an end, the glands being now in a resting state except when the special positive conditioned stimulus was applied. As soon, however, as I myself entered the room, in order for the first time to watch the experiments, a copious secretion of saliva was produced by the dog, which persisted as long as I remained in the room. I myself presented in this case the extra stimulus disinhibiting the reflex to environment which had only just recently undergone extinction. Now it occurred to us that the phenomenon of the universal generalization of the long-trace reflexes might really be nothing but a dis-inhibition of the reflex to environment. However, after a thorough examination, this explanation had to be discarded. In the first place, a considerable generalization of long-trace reflexes could easily be observed even in dogs in which the reflex to environment had been deeply inhibited so long ago that it was now almost impossible to dis-inhibit it. In the second place, the supposition of dis-inhibition when followed up necessitated a further assumption which was easily disproved. It has been seen already that dis-inhibition of the inactive phase in delay was obtained immediately on application of the extra stimulus, *i.e.* without any such latent period as is observed for trace reflexes. If the generalized character of trace reflexes was in reality nothing but dis-inhibition, we should expect all the different stimuli also to act immediately, but as we have seen they act only after their termination and after about the same latent period as the initially established trace reflex. If it is still assumed that the effect is due to dis-inhibition of the reflex to environment, then in the case of trace reflexes all the different stimuli must act for some reason as very powerful extra stimuli which do not dis-inhibit the reflex to environment, but temporarily abolish all conditioned activity by producing a very powerful inhibition (as is also the case with very powerful extra stimuli in delay), and the ensuing dis-inhibition must be brought about by their traces which represent weaker stimuli. This assumption, however, is contradicted by the following facts. It is known that repeated application of the same powerful extra stimulus is followed by a gradual diminution of its inhibitory effect, which gives place, as was seen with delay, to dis-inhibition. But in the case of the generalized stimuli in long-trace reflexes the latent period does not diminish in spite of repeated applications. This shows that the reflex activity is due to a genuine generalization of the trace reflex and not to dis-inhibition. Finally, there is this striking fact, that in the case of trace reflexes following the application of various stimuli, which of course are never reinforced, the effect of the special conditioned stimulus to which the trace reflex was experimentally established also becomes temporarily diminished, and the secretion may fall to zero, a fact which cannot be reconciled with any supposition that we are dealing with a dis-inhibition of the reflex to environment. Indeed, there is no doubt that this weakening of the effect of the special conditioned stimulus represents a simple instance of extinction, as the result of non-reinforcement, of a reflex which has become generalized within the hemispheres.

Thus it is seen that in the course of the establishment of simultaneous and delayed reflexes a temporary generalization develops in the form of a number of accessory conditioned reflexes to associated stimuli. Generalization of the reflexes can be effected also through the whole environment acting on the organism by the sum total of its individual units and leading to the formation of what we may call a synthetic environmental reflex. In other cases, namely, in long-trace reflexes, it is effected in virtue of the intrinsic properties of the nervous system itself, which give a more or less generalized character to the individual external stimuli in their capacity as conditioned stimuli. In many instances, some of which we have referred to above, it is obvious that this fact of generalization of stimuli has a definite importance in the natural correlation between the animal and its environment, but in other cases the generalization can have only a limited or temporary significance. In the latter cases the approximate, general, and under some conditions useful connection with the environment as a whole is replaced by a precise and definitely specialized connection with a definite stimulatory unit.

The question can now be discussed as to how the specialization of the conditioned reflex, or, in other words, the discrimination of external agencies, arises. Formerly we were inclined to think that this effect could be obtained by two different methods : the first method consisted in repeating the definite conditioned stimulus a great number of times always accompanied by reinforcement, and the second method consisted in contrasting the single definite conditioned stimulus, which was always accompanied by reinforcement, with different neighbouring stimuli which were never reinforced. At present, however, we are more inclined to regard this second method as more probably the only efficacious one, since it was observed that no absolute differentiation was ever obtained by the use of the first method, even though the stimulus was repeated with reinforcement over a thousand times. On the other hand, it was found that contrast by even a single unreinforced application of an allied stimulus, or by a number of single unreinforced applications of different members of a series of allied stimuli at infrequent intervals of days or weeks, led to a rapid development of differentiation. The method of contrast is now always employed in our experiments, as leading to a differentiation of external agencies in an incomparably quicker time.

We can now follow out the development of differentiation between external stimuli in the conditioned reflexes in greater detail. In the first place an interesting observation which remained for a long time without explanation may be considered : It was noticed that when, after a conditioned reflex to a definite stimulus (*e.g.* a definite musical tone) had been firmly established, the effect of another closely allied stimulus (a neighbouring musical tone) was tried for the first time, the conditioned reflex which resulted from the new stimulus was frequently much weaker than that obtained with the original conditioned stimulus. On repetition of the stimulus of the neighbouring tone, always, of course, without reinforcement, the secretory effect increased until it became equal to that given by the originally established stimulus, but subsequently on further repetition began to diminish, falling finally to a permanent zero. Thus it appeared that at first the two closely allied stimuli were discriminated straight away, but that later this discrimination for some reason disappeared, only gradually to re-establish itself and finally to become absolute. To provide an explanation of this phenomenon we can revert to an interpretation which was advanced previously for similar events occurring in the process of development of conditioned inhibition. It will be remembered that when, in the formation of conditioned inhibition, a conditioned stimulus was accompanied for the first time by the new stimulus which later acquired the properties of a conditioned inhibitor, the combination produced either a very small positive effect or else remained totally ineffective. Later, although the inhibitory combination was never reinforced by the unconditioned stimulus, it produced again a reflex of full strength, which, however, after further repetitions gradually fell to a permanent zero. The explanation given in the case of conditioned inhibition, and fully borne out by experimental evidence, was that the additional stimulus elicited on its first application an investigatory reflex which immediately produced an external inhibition of the conditioned reflex ; on repetition the strength of the investigatory reflex rapidly diminished and the positive effect of the conditioned stimulus was temporarily restored, being later gradually suppressed by the development of internal inhibition. Similarly, in the case of differentiation it is possible to regard stimuli neighbouring on the definite positive conditioned stimulus as bearing two aspects, one of similarity to, and the other of difference from, the positive conditioned stimulus. On account of the element which is in common, these neighbouring stimuli can act similarly to the positive conditioned one ; it is the presence of the second factor, of difference, which determines a temporary investigatory reflex, bringing about external inhibition of the excitatory effect, but later serving as foundation for the development of a permanent and final differentiation of allied stimuli.

Time	Stimulus applied during 30 secs.	Salivary Secretion recorded by divisions of scale (5 div. = 0·1 c.c.) during 30 secs.	Remarks

Experiment of 15th February, 1917.

| 3.13 p.m. | Object rotating clockwise | 27 | Reinforced. |
| 3.25 ,, | Object rotating anti-clockwise | 7 | Not reinforced. |

Experiment of 16th February, 1917.

1.4 p.m.	Object rotating clockwise	24	Reinforced.
1.14 ,,	,, ,, ,,	26	,,
1.25 ,,	,, ,, ,,	27	,,
1.34 ,,	Object rotating anti-clockwise	10	Not reinforced.

Experiment of 17th February, 1917.

| 2.45 p.m. | Object rotating anti-clockwise | 12 | Not reinforced. |

Experiment of 18th February, 1917.

| 2.48 p.m. | Object rotating clockwise | 19 | Reinforced. |
| 3.33 ,, | Object rotating anti-clockwise | 34 | Not reinforced. |

Experiment of 20th February, 1917.

| 3.7 p.m. | Object rotating anti-clockwise | 26 | Not reinforced. |
| 3.28 ,, | Object rotating clockwise | 26 | Reinforced. |

Experiment of 21st February, 1917.

| 3.0 p.m. | Object rotating anti-clockwise | 12 | Not reinforced. |

The strength of the reflex which is undergoing differential inhibition now diminishes progressively with small fluctuations until it reaches a permanent zero.

The correctness of this interpretation is borne out by the striking similarity in detail in the development of differentiation and of conditioned inhibition. The same variations occur in both cases. The initial diminution in the strength of the reflex during the first few applications of the new stimulus is sometimes succeeded by a transitory increase in strength as compared with the normal, and after this the reflex diminishes steadily below its normal value until it finally attains a permanent zero ; in most cases, however, the initial diminution is succeeded by a phase of increase to the normal level, after which the reflex again falls steadily to zero with the development of the final differentiation ; it rarely happens that a development of differentiation is established without such fluctuations, or that a gradual diminution of the reflex follows directly upon the sudden initial drop. While, in describing the formation of conditioned inhibition, the fluctuations received a considerable share of attention, no records of experiments were given. A presentation of the analogous experiments on the establishment of differential inhibition will make the matter clear.

In the first series of experiments (see p. 119), which were conducted by Dr. Gubergritz, an object rotating in a clockwise direction served as the positive conditioned stimulus, while the same object rotating in the opposite direction served as the stimulus undergoing differentiation.

Time	Stimulus applied during 30 secs.	Amount of Saliva recorded by divisions of scale (5 div. = 0·1 c.c.) during 30 secs.	Remarks

Experiment of 12th October, 1917.

Time	Stimulus	Amount	Remarks
12.28 p.m.	Tone	30	Reinforced.
1.0 ,,	Tone	35	Reinforced.
1.10 ,,	Semitone	9	Not reinforced.

Experiment of 13th October, 1917.

Time	Stimulus	Amount	Remarks
12.54 p.m.	Tone	36	Reinforced.
1.5 ,,	Tone	36	Reinforced.
1.12 ,,	Semitone	32	Not reinforced.
2.1 ,,	Semitone	16	Not reinforced.
2.18 ,,	Tone	29	Reinforced.

The reflex to the semitone continues to fluctuate, gradually diminishing in strength until at the thirteenth repetition it has fallen to zero.

The above experiments were conducted on another dog, a musical tone serving as a conditioned alimentary stimulus and its semitone as the stimulus undergoing differentiation.

The dog employed in the next series of experiments is the same as was used in the first series. A luminous circle was used for a conditioned alimentary stimulus, and a luminous square of equal surface and equal brightness for the stimulus undergoing differentiation.

Time	Stimulus applied during 30 secs.	Amount of Saliva recorded by divisions of scale (5 div. = 0·1 c.c.) during 30 secs.	Remarks

Experiment of 28*th December*, 1917.

| 1.20 p.m. | Circle | 14 | Reinforced. |
| 1.53 ,, | Square | 3 | Not reinforced. |

Experiment of 29*th December*, 1917.

| 2.44 p.m. | Circle | 16 | Reinforced. |
| 3.0 ,, | Square | 7 | Not reinforced. |

Experiment of 30*th December*, 1917.

| 1.24 p.m. | Circle | 15 | Reinforced. |
| 1.32 ,, | Square | 10 | Not reinforced. |

Then with small fluctuations the reflex diminishes progressively, until after the eleventh repetition the square becomes permanently ineffective.

Some other interesting points besides those connected with the interference of the investigatory reflex have also come to light in recent experiments. In the first place it has been shown that the development of a differentiation of two very closely allied stimuli may be attempted directly, or, on the other hand, the same differentiation may be effected in stages, leading up through the differentiation of more remote stimuli. There is a considerable difference between the rates of development of a precise differentiation by these two methods. For example, if we begin with the first method we generally find that

the differentiation does not become established even after a considerable number of contrasts of the two very closely allied stimuli ;
but if we proceed to establish a differentiation of a remoter stimulus,
working up gradually through finer differentiations until the very
closely allied stimulus is again reached, it is found that this differentiation is now very rapidly established. The following experiments
of Dr. Gubergritz serve to illustrate these relations :

A circle of white paper provided a conditioned alimentary stimulus
from which it was required to differentiate a circle of grey paper of
similar size made of No. 10 in Zimmermann's scale (50 shades from
white to black). Seventy-five applications of the grey circle No. 10
without reinforcement, contrasted with frequent applications of the
white circle which always remained reinforced, failed to produce the
slightest sign of differentiation. A much darker circle No. 35 was
now contrasted with the white, and a differentiation was quickly
established. Differentiation was now carried out for grey circles
Nos. 25 and 15, after which the attempt to differentiate circle No. 10
was made again, with the result that complete differentiation was
established after a total of only 20 applications, in all, of the four
different circles.

A similar experiment, also with a visual stimulus, but in a modified
form, was carried out on another dog. In this case the conditioned
alimentary stimulus was again a circle, while the stimulus to be
differentiated from it was an ellipse cut from the same paper and of
equal surface, with the semi-axes in the ratio of 8 : 9. Although at
the beginning 70 applications of the ellipse were made with the method
of contrast, no differentiation was obtained. Successive differentiations were now obtained in stages for ellipses with ratio of the
semi-axes 4 : 5, 5 : 6, 7 : 8, and finally with the ellipse of the ratio
8 : 9. A precise differentiation of the latter was finally established
after a total of only 18 applications, in all, of the four ellipses.

In building up a differentiation by stages, beginning with a
remote stimulus, the development of the first crude differentiation
takes place comparatively slowly, especially if it is desired to obtain
an absolute differentiation giving a permanent zero. When, however,
an absolute, or almost absolute, differentiation has been obtained,
the succeeding stages of progress towards the finer differentiation
are passed through with increasing rapidity, becoming, however,
somewhat retarded as the limit of the analysing activity is
approached. One example may be given in illustration :

A white circle of a given surface area was used for a conditioned stimulus, while ellipses of the same area and whiteness but with different ratios of semi-axes provided the stimuli undergoing differentiation. In order to obtain a pronounced differentiation of the first ellipse, in which the ratio of the semi-axes was 4 : 5, twenty-four applications were required, with, of course, frequent contrastings by the circle. At this stage the circle elicited a secretion of 34 divisions of the scale in 30 seconds, whereas the effect of the ellipse was measured by only four divisions. The next ellipse, with a ratio of 5 : 6, required only 3 applications in contrast to the circle before it became fully differentiated. Three repetitions were required also for the next ellipse, in which the semi-axes were in the ratio 6 : 7.

It should be noted that irregularities in the curve of development of differentiation do not depend always on the disturbing influence of the investigatory reflex due to external stimuli ; in all probability they are sometimes caused by variations in the intensity of the underlying nervous activity.

The stability of differentiation of a given stimulus can be measured by the length of time reckoned from the last application of the positive stimulus during which differentiation is fully maintained. When differentiation has only recently been established, the length of time during which the differentiated stimulus without intermediate practice will yet give a full zero on its next application is short ; this length of time increases, however, as the differentiation becomes more firmly established. For practical purposes we take a differentiation as being fully established when it is maintained for not less than 24 hours, still giving a zero reflex when applied as the very first stimulus in an experiment.

Our repeated experiments have demonstrated that the same precision of differentiation of various stimuli can be obtained whether they are used in the form of negative or positive conditioned stimuli. This holds good in the case of conditioned trace reflexes also. The following experiment from a paper by Dr. Frolov gives an illustration of the differentiation of a trace stimulus :

A rate of 104 beats per minute of a metronome was established as a conditioned alimentary stimulus. The conditioned trace inhibitor undergoing differentiation was given by a definite tone of an organ pipe (No. 16) which was sounded for 15 seconds and followed after a pause of one minute by the stimulus of the metronome which remained in this case without reinforcement. A combination of the metronome with a trace of the tone of the next organ pipe (No. 15, an interval of one tone from the first) was contrasted with the first, being reinforced so that it became an excitatory stimulus. The differentiation of the trace inhibition is illustrated in the following experiment:

Experiment of 25th April, 1922.

Time	Stimulus	Duration of Stimulus	Salivary Secretion in divisions of the scale during successive periods of 15 seconds
1.34 p.m.	Tone of organ pipe No. 16	15 seconds	0.
	Interval	60 ,,	0, 0, 0, 0.
	Metronome	30 ,,	15, 40,* not reinforced.
1.40 ,,	Tone of organ pipe No. 16	15 ,,	0.
	Interval	60 ,,	0, 0, 0, 0.
	Metronome	30 ,,	0, 15, not reinforced.
1.48 ,,	Tone of organ pipe No. 15	15 ,,	0.
	Interval	60 ,,	0, 0, 0, 0.
	Metronome	30 ,,	25, 65, reinforced.

It should be added that the above differentiation was obtained by passing through a long series of crude differentiations, beginning with traces measured by seconds, and with wider intervals of tones; but once developed the differentiation could be repeated from day to day.

With regard to the nature of the nervous process by which the initially generalized conditioned stimulus comes to assume an extremely specialized form, we have abundant experimental evidence

* Differentiations of trace-conditioned inhibitors are very easily subjected to dis-inhibition and are very unstable. It can be noticed in the above experiment that the first application of the organ pipe No. 16, the after-effect of which should have inhibited the secretory action of the metronome, failed to do so, when applied, as in this experiment, as the first stimulus after an interval of 24 hours from the preceding experiment. The second application of the organ pipe No. 16 exerted a powerful inhibitory after-effect, giving a secretion of only 15 divisions with a latent period of over 15 seconds as compared with a secretion of 90 divisions with a very short latent period with the use of organ pipe No. 15.

that it is based upon internal inhibition ; in other words, we may say that the excitatory process which is originally widely spread in the cerebral part of the analyser is gradually overcome by internal inhibition, excepting only the minutest part of it which corresponds to the given conditioned stimulus. This interpretation of differentiation as based upon internal inhibition rests upon evidence to be described now.

A differentiation is established between two closely allied stimuli, so that one of them which is reinforced gives a constant positive conditioned effect, while the other, which remains unreinforced, gives no secretory effect. If, however, the positive stimulus is applied a short time after the differentiated one, there is found to be a considerable diminution of its secretory effect. An illustration of such an experiment can be given from a research by Dr. Beliakov :

A definite tone of an organ-pipe has been given properties of an alimentary conditioned stimulus, and an interval of $\frac{1}{8}$th lower has been firmly differentiated from it by the usual method of contrast.

Experiment of 14*th February*, 1911.

Time	Stimulus applied during 30 secs.	Salivary Secretion in drops during 30 secs.	Remarks
12.10 p.m.	Tone	5	Reinforced.
12.25 ,,	Tone $\frac{1}{8}$ lower	0	Not reinforced.
12.26 ,,	Tone	0·5	Reinforced.
12.56 ,,	Tone	4	Reinforced.

It follows that after application of the differentiated tone there remains in the nervous system a state of inhibition which is for some time sufficiently powerful to weaken the excitatory process set up by the application of the positive stimulus.

The inhibition which is exhibited in differentiation must be recognized as constituting the fourth type of internal inhibition, which may be called **differential inhibition.**

It would to our mind be quite appropriate to bring conditioned inhibition also under the heading of differential inhibition, since in both cases we deal with a removal by means of internal inhibition of an excitatory effect of simple or complex stimuli which acquired their excitatory properties spontaneously in virtue of their partial resemblance to the original positive conditioned stimulus.

The inhibitory after-effect in differential inhibition corresponds exactly with the inhibitory after-effect in conditioned inhibition, both becoming shortened by repetition. At the beginning they may persist upwards of an hour, but they become restricted finally to a matter of a few seconds.

It is necessary to emphasize in this place the fact that the finer the degree of differentiation the greater is the intensity of the inhibitory after effect. The following experiments of Dr. Beliakov serve to illustrate this point :

A definite tone represents the conditioned stimulus in an alimentary reflex ; intervals of one-half and one-eighth were used for differentiation.

Time	Stimulus applied during 30 seconds	Salivary Secretion in drops during 30 seconds	Remarks

Experiment of 19*th March,* 1911.

12.17 p.m.	Semitone	0	Not reinforced.
12.37 ,,	Tone	4	Reinforced.
1.7 ,,	Tone	4	Reinforced.

Experiment of 29*th March,* 1911.

3.55 p.m.	One-eighth	0	Not reinforced.
4.15 ,,	Tone	1·5	Reinforced.
4.30 ,,	Tone	4	Reinforced.

Apart from the close connection already mentioned between conditioned inhibition and differential inhibition, the latter provides a close parallel in all other respects to the three types of internal inhibition which have been dealt with in previous lectures. Thus the inhibitory after-effect in differential inhibition, similarly to other forms of internal inhibition, undergoes summation on repetition of the stimulus. The following experiments are again taken from the researches by Dr. Beliakov :

Another dog is taken in which a conditioned alimentary reflex is established to a definite musical tone, while a semitone lower is firmly differentiated as an inhibitory stimulus.

Time	Stimulus applied during 30 seconds	Salivary Secretion in drops during 30 secs.	Remarks
Experiment of 8th June, 1911.			
2.5 p.m.	Tone	10	Reinforced.
2.35 ,,	Semitone	0	Not reinforced.
2.38 ,,	Semitone	0	Not reinforced.
2.39 ,,	Tone	7	Reinforced.
2.50 ,,	Tone	12	Reinforced.
Experiment of 14th June, 1911.			
1.45 p.m.	Tone	12	Reinforced.
2.0 ,,	Semitone	0	Not reinforced.
2.2 ,,	Semitone	0	Not reinforced.
2.4 ,,	Semitone	0	Not reinforced.
2.6 ,,	Semitone	0	Not reinforced.
2.7 ,,	Tone	1·5	Reinforced.
2.30 ,,	Tone	13	Reinforced.

In differentiation as in the other types of internal inhibition the intensity of inhibition stands in direct relation to the strength of the excitatory process on the basis of which it was established, and can therefore be disturbed by any increase in the intensity of the stimulus which developed the inhibitory properties, or by any change in the general or local excitability of the central nervous system. To illustrate this last condition we may take instances of differential inhibitions established on the basis of an alimentary reflex. If, for example, the dog has been kept entirely without food for a much longer period than usual before the experiment is conducted, the increase in excitability of the whole alimentary nervous mechanism renders the previously established differential inhibition wholly inadequate. Again, if the general excitability of the central nervous system has been increased, for example by an injection of caffeine, the previously established differentiation similarly becomes disturbed. This effect of an alteration of the general nervous excitability is fully illustrated by an experiment of Dr. Nikiforovsky :

A tactile stimulation of the fore-paw serves as a positive conditioned alimentary stimulus, while a tactile stimulation of the back is completely differentiated from it.

Time	Stimulus applied during 1 minute	Salivary Secretion in drops during successive minutes from the beginning of the conditioned stimulus	Remarks
12.52 p.m.	Tactile stimulation of back	0, 0, 0	Not reinforced.
1.5 ,,	Tactile stimulation of fore-paw	5	Reinforced.
	Subcutaneous injection of 5 c.c. of 1% solution of caffeine	—	—
1.18 ,,	Tactile stimulation of fore-paw	4	Reinforced.
1.33 ,,	Tactile stimulation of back	3, 3, 2	Not reinforced.
1.45 ,,	Tactile stimulation of fore-paw.	7	Reinforced.

Lastly, in common with the other three groups of internal inhibition, differential inhibition is subject to dis-inhibition, becoming temporarily removed under the influence of mild extra stimuli belonging to the group of external inhibitors, so as to reveal the underlying excitatory process. Two experiments by Dr. Beliakov carried out on the same animal are given in illustration :

A tone of 800 d.v. served as a conditioned alimentary stimulus, and an interval of one-eighth (812 d.v.) was thoroughly differentiated from it. A sound of bubbling water and an odour of amyl acetate served as mild extra stimuli which by themselves did not evoke any secretory effect.

Time	Stimulus applied during 30 seconds	Salivary Secretion in drops per 30 seconds	Remarks
	Experiment of 18th June, 1911.		
12.30 p.m.	800 d.v.	3·5, —	Reinforced.
1.0 ,,	812 d.v.	0, 0	Not reinforced.
1.20 ,,	800 d.v.	3, —	Reinforced.
1.35 ,,	812 d.v. + odour of amyl acetate	2, 2	Not reinforced.

Time	Stimulus applied during 30 seconds.	Salivary Secretion in drops per 30 seconds.	Remarks
	Experiment of 23rd June, 1911.		
11.55 a.m.	800 d.v.	4, —	Reinforced.
12.10 p.m.	812 d.v. + bubbling water	2, 1	Not reinforced.
12.30 ,,	800 d.v.	3, —	Reinforced.
12.40 ,,	800 d.v.	3, —	Reinforced.

It is interesting to note that dis-inhibition can also be obtained when mild extra stimuli influence the hemispheres while the after-effect of differential inhibition is still persisting. The following is an experiment carried out by Dr. Beliakov on the same animal. The extra stimulus is given by the sound of a metronome which by itself produced no secretion.

Time	Stimulus during 30 seconds	Secretion of Saliva in drops	Remarks
	Experiment of 17th May, 1911.		
11.10 a.m.	Tone	4·5 during 30 secs.	Reinforced.
11.30 ,,	Tone	4 ,, ,,	Not reinforced.
11.40 ,,	Tone $\frac{1}{8}$ lower	0 ,, ,,	,, ,,
11.44 ,,	Tone $\frac{1}{8}$ lower	0 ,, ,,	,, ,,
11.44$\frac{1}{2}$,,	Metronome during 1 minute	1$\frac{1}{2}$ during 1 minute	,, ,,

Among the extra stimuli which have been employed there were some which evoked, not an ordinary investigatory reaction, but specific reflexes of greater intensity and complexity ; in these cases the dis-inhibitory after-effect was very much prolonged. An example of the use of such an extra stimulus can again be taken from an experiment by Dr. Beliakov performed on the same animal as before.

A strong extra stimulus was provided by the blare of a toy trumpet which produced voluminous and exceedingly discordant noises. The dog reacted by barking wildly, trembling and trying to break away from the stand.

Time	Stimulus applied during 30 seconds	Salivary Secretion in successive periods of 30 seconds	
10.58 a.m.	Trumpet	0	
10.58½ ,,	Inhibitory tone (812 d.v.)	6, 3, 2	
11.3 ,,	,, ,, ,,	3, 1, 1	Stimuli
11.7 ,,	,, ,, ,,	1, 1, 1	not
11.11 ,,	,, ,, ,,	1·5, 1·5, 0	reinforced.
11.15 ,,	,, ,, ,,	Traces	

The experimental evidence advanced in this lecture leaves us in no doubt but that the establishment of differentiation is based upon the development of internal inhibition in respect to the differentiated agent.

On the evidence of our experiments we are also forced to the conclusion that there is an important difference between the cruder form of differentiation depending upon external inhibition, and the finer form of differentiation depending upon internal inhibition. The former and more generalized inhibition is brought about by the intervention of an excitatory process, in most cases in the form of an investigatory reflex, and this has only a secondary inhibiting or dis-inhibiting effect upon the conditioned reflexes ; the latter is brought about by a primary development of an inhibitory process, resulting, so to speak, from a conflict between excitation and inhibition. This supremacy of the inhibitory process is sometimes gained only with considerable difficulty, and in some cases it is even beyond the power of the nervous system to resolve the conflict in favour of either process. In the latter case the antagonism between the excitatory and inhibitory processes may not always bring about a full utilization of the results of analysis of external stimuli for the general benefit of the organism. This being so the study of the analysing activity of the nervous system by the method of conditioned reflexes will also have its limitations—a fact which in itself presents a problem of considerable interest.

LECTURE VIII

The analysing and synthesizing activity of the cerebral hemispheres (continued) :
(c) Examples of the analysis of stimuli. (d) Synthesis and analysis of compound
simultaneous stimuli. (e) Synthesis and analysis of compound successive
stimuli.

It was shown in the preceding lecture that the animal at first general-
izes any definite individual stimulus of the outer world, but that
with repetition the stimulus becomes more and more specialized as a
result of the development of an inhibitory process (differentiation).
In this final form conditioned reflexes provide a reliable method
for an experimental study of the scope and limits of the activity of
the different cortical analysers. Our knowledge of the different
analysers in the dog has recently been considerably advanced through
the study of conditioned reflexes,—a fact which affords a striking
example of the practical utility of this method of research. It should,
moreover, be mentioned with regard to these particular experiments,
that while considerable difficulties were sometimes encountered in
the course of the work, these did not arise in the physiological part
of the technique, but derived from instrumental limitations, since
in many cases it has been exceedingly difficult to obtain or construct
suitable physical apparatus. The main requirement is for instruments which are capable of producing a perfectly isolated and
unvarying elementary stimulus of a definite degree of intensity.
This, however, is very often a practical impossibility. For example,
it is exceedingly difficult to find an apparatus for tactile stimulation
of the skin which will not produce some slight sound during its
application. It is also not easy to obtain an alteration in the pitch
of a tone without simultaneously affecting its strength. Indeed, it
seems to me that future experimentation upon the analysers of
animals will exhibit an interesting competition between the delicacy
of the nervous analyser and the skill of the instrument maker.

We shall turn now to a consideration of the experiments at our
disposal, taking first those dealing with the visual analyser of the
dog. In respect of discrimination of luminosity this analyser was

found to be greatly superior to that of man. Thus, for example, a conditioned reflex was established in a dog to the presentation of a black screen prefectly uniform in shading, without any traces of graining or spots. A white screen of identical shape and size, and also of uniform luminosity, was differentiated from the black screen by the usual method of contrast. The experimenter was provided with a number of screens of different shades (50 numbers of Zimmermann's collection) ranging from white through different shades of grey to black. After the differentiation of white had been firmly established the same method of contrast was used to obtain finer degrees of differentiation of grey screens approximating more and more nearly to black. It was found in this way that the visual analyser of the dog was capable of distinguishing between the neighbouring shades Nos. 49 and 50, while to the human eye there appeared not the slightest difference between them, whether they were examined successively at different intervals of time or simultaneously. This was also true for several other shades separated further from one another on the scale, which could not be discriminated by the human eye but which the dog differentiated perfectly. The following experiment shows an evident, though not absolute, differentiation of the screens Nos. 49 and 50 [experiments by Dr. Frolov] :

Time	Conditioned Stimulus applied during 30 seconds	Secretion of Saliva in drops during 30 seconds	Remarks
3.13 p.m.	Screen No. 50	10	Reinforced.
4.1 ,,	,, ,,	12	
4.9 ,,	Screen No. 49	6	Not reinforced.

It thus becomes evident that as regards the analysis of intensity of illumination the visual analyser of the dog is so highly developed that we were unable to determine the limit to which this activity extends.

In the case of analysis of various colours the results obtained were quite different. Dr. Orbeli in a first series of experiments was unable to detect any differentiation of colours on the part of his dogs. In a second series of experiments, however, positive results were obtained in one dog, but only with great difficulty, and even in this case the experiments were still open to criticism. The results obtained by other investigators, both Russian and foreign, lead to the conclusion that colour vision in dogs, if present, is only of a very rudimentary form, and that in most dogs it cannot be detected at all.

Dr. Orbeli studied also the differentiation of figures. Examples of figures for which an absolute differentiation was obtained, are given in Fig. 6.

Experiments with regard to differentiation of shapes were continued by Dr. Shenger-Krestovnikova. An alimentary conditioned reflex was established in a dog to a luminous circle which was projected on to a screen placed in front of the dog. After the reflex had attained a constant strength the animal was made to differentiate from the circle a number of ellipses of equal surface and luminosity. In the first of the ellipses the ratio of the semi-axes was 2 : 1, and differentiation was established with ease. This was followed up by a series of ellipses which gradually approximated to the circle in shape, and so required a finer and finer differentiation. The ellipse with ratio of the semi-axes 9 : 8 proved to be the limit at which differentiation just failed. Some indication of differentiation appeared at first, but on repetition it gradually disappeared, and with it disappeared also all the previously established coarser differentiations. To renew these it was necessary to work up carefully from the very beginning, starting with the first ellipse with a ratio of the semi-axes 2 : 1. When all the coarser discriminations had again been obtained, the ellipse with the ratio 9 : 8 was tried once more. Its first application showed a complete discrimination, giving a zero secretion of saliva. Further tests, however, led to the same results as before. Not only was it impossible to obtain the differentiation again (if the first trial can be regarded as a real differentiation at all), but all the earlier, coarser differentiations disappeared as well. In this phenomenon we have a clear reproduction of the case referred to at the end of the preceding lecture. When the stage of minute differences between stimuli is reached, analysis of itself appears still feasible, but the relations existing between the excitatory and the inhibitory processes seem to present an insurmountable obstacle to its continued and permanent utilization by the animal for an appropriate responsive activity.

The differentiation of direction of motion of figures and points was also investigated in our laboratories, but the limit of discrimination was not determined in these cases.

The analysing activity of the acoustic apparatus in the dog was

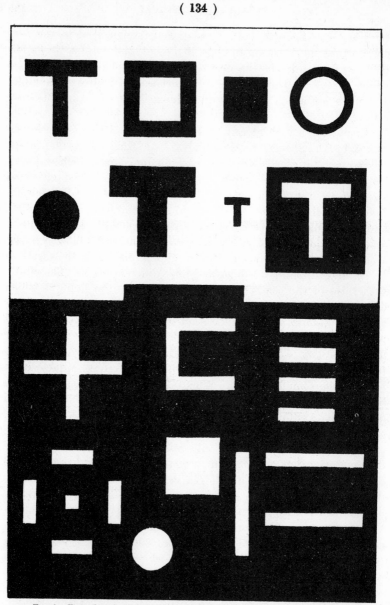

FIG. 6.—Examples of different figures which were successfully differentiated in experiments by Dr. Orbeli. The letter ⊤, shown in the upper left-hand corner of the figure, served for the positive stimulus; the other black figures and the white letter ⊤ where differentiated from the positive stimulus.

In another dog the white cross was the positive stimulus from which the other white figures were differentiated.

investigated in especial detail and in various directions. In the first place we shall consider the analysis of different intensities of the same sound. It was found that any definite degree of intensity of a sound could easily be made into a stable conditioned stimulus and could be differentiated from slightly higher or slightly lower intensities of the same sound [experiments of Dr. Tichomirov]. A tone of 1740 d.v. was sounded by an organ pipe into which air was blown at a constant pressure of 3·6-3·8 cms. of water by means of a spirometer. The organ-pipe was fitted in the centre of a wooden board covered by a thick layer of cotton wool. Above this board and over the pipe was suspended a wooden box, open below and also coated inside with cotton wool. By raising or lowering this box to different heights over the pipe definite dampings of the sound were obtained. The limit of differentiation to the intensities of a given sound could now be determined for the dog and compared roughly with that of human beings. Thus it was found that an intensity very closely approaching the one employed as a positive conditioned stimulus could be differentiated by the dog with an absolute precision even when a pause of 17 hours was made between the two stimuli. The experimenter found himself able to detect a difference between these two intensities of the sound only when they succeeded each other immediately. The following is an example taken from these experiments :

Time	Conditioned Stimulus	Secretion of Saliva in drops during 30 seconds	Remarks
4.28 p.m.	Usual intensity of tone	6	Reinforced.
4.43 ,,	Same tone but of slightly different intensity	0	Not reinforced.
4.49 ,,	Usual intensity of tone	3	Reinforced.

In the continuation of these experiments the intensity of the inhibitory tone was brought still nearer to the intensity used for the positive conditioned stimulus, and an absolute differentiation was obtained even after a pause of three hours between the stimuli. Unfortunately these experiments were conducted in our old laboratory where the effect of the inhibitory stimulus was easily disturbed, and it must be left to the future to repeat these experiments under more perfect conditions in our new laboratory.

A great number of experiments have also been carried out on the differentiation of pitch. To produce tones of different pitch wind instruments were chiefly employed, and the limit to which we were able to carry our tests was an interval of one-eighth of a tone (800 and 812 d.v.). This interval, as has already been shown in the previous lectures (p. 125), was differentiated with perfect accuracy by the acoustic analyser of the dog. It was not possible to carry our determination of the physiological limit of differentiation of pitch any further, since we could not be sure that our apparatus would accurately reproduce smaller intervals than one-eighth. The repetition of these experiments with the use of pure tones, produced by telephones with resonators, showed that this differentiation could still be obtained as easily as with the richer tones of wind instruments [experiments of Drs. Anrep and Manuilov].

The upper limit of the auditory range of the dog was demonstrated by Dr. Bourmakin with the use of a Galton's whistle, and by Dr. Andréev with the use of an apparatus producing pure tones, to be very much higher than in man. Conditioned reflexes were successfully established to tones of such high pitch as to be quite inaudible to man. It was indeed interesting to observe how sharply and precisely the dog reacted to sounds which were non-existent to the human ear.

The differentiation of timbre and the differentiation of direction of sounds were also submitted to investigation, but no exact limits of differentiation were determined in the cases of these special qualities.

While discussing the functional capacity of the acoustic analyser we may refer to those experiments in which differentiation was based not upon the differences in the properties of the sounds but upon differences in the rhythm of successive applications of one and the same single sound. The sound in this case was produced by a metronome beating regularly, but at different rates in the various experiments. Differentiations of this type were quite easily obtained, but the main interest of these investigations lay in the determination of the limit of differentiation, which for the dog was found to be far more subtle than the discrimination which could be recognized in man. The dog was capable of a very precise differentiation between such rates as 100 and 96 beats per minute even when applied at a very long interval after one another (i.e. a discrimination of 0·024 seconds).

A few experiments have been conducted with the analysers for tactile and thermal cutaneous stimuli. Differentiation could easily be established for the site of stimulation, and was found to be very precise, but no determination was made as to the actual limit.

Differentiations were obtained also for different types of tactile stimulation, namely pressure by smooth and rough surfaces, pressure by blunt points arranged in various patterns, and by scratchings in various directions with a small brush. Furthermore, differentiations were also obtained for different degrees of temperature.

The most perfect analyser in the dog is the chemical analyser of smell, but our information concerning it is scanty, mainly on account of instrumental difficulties. It has been exceedingly difficult, if not impossible up to the present, to obtain the same accuracy in graduation of olfactory stimuli as of any other stimuli. It is impossible also to limit the action of olfactory stimuli to any exact length of time. Furthermore, we do not know of any subjective or objective criterion by which small variations in intensity of odours can be determined. On this account only a small number of experiments could be conducted. Differentiations were obtained for various odours— camphor, vanillin and many others. Some of these were made into positive conditioned alimentary stimuli or positive conditioned stimuli for acid, while others were given the corresponding inhibitory properties. Experiments upon differentiation were also conducted with mixtures of odours, into which some new odour could be introduced.

Lastly, some experimental data have been obtained concerning the chemical analyser of taste. In this case matters were more complicated, because the unconditioned stimuli which were usually employed in the experiments (food and rejectable substances), both act on this analyser. In order to study the analyser of taste in a manner similar to that employed for other analysers, it would be necessary to employ an unconditioned reflex belonging to some other analyser and to use various taste stimuli for establishing the corresponding positive and negative conditioned reflexes. Experiments of this kind have not been performed. We adopted, however, another method in which a number of conditioned reflexes were established each associated with a different nutritive or rejectable substance (meat powder, bread crumbs, sugar, cheese, acid, soda, etc.), and their interaction and mutual inhibition were then observed. The following is an example of such an experiment by Dr. Egorov :

A tactile stimulation of the skin presented a conditioned stimulus to the consumption of a mixture of meat powder with bread crumbs ;

a rotating object was used as a conditioned stimulus to the consumption of Dutch cheese.

Time	Conditioned Stimulus	Secretion of Saliva in drops during 30 secs.	Remarks
3.12 p.m.	Tactile	5	
3.29 ,,	,,	5	All reflexes rein-
3.50 ,,	Rotating object	8	forced by their re-
3.57 ,,	Tactile	0·5	spective uncondi-
4.4 ,,	,,	2·5	tioned stimuli.
4.11 ,,	,,	5	

Since the conditioned stimulus of the rotating object (3.50 p.m.) was reinforced by administration of cheese, the above form of the experiment does not tell us whether the subsequent diminution in the conditioned reflex to the tactile stimulus (*i.e.* the conditioned stimulus for meat and bread) was due to the conditioned stimulus of the rotating object or to its reinforcing agent (*i.e.* cheese). To determine this point similar experiments were conducted with the use of the conditioned stimuli applied without reinforcement. The following is an example of such an experiment.

Tactile stimulation of the skin usually resulted in this dog in a conditioned secretion varying from 5 to 6 drops of saliva during 30 seconds. The stimulus of the rotating object which is given prior to the application of the tactile stimulus remains unreinforced.

Time	Conditioned Stimulus	Salivary Secretion in drops during 30 seconds	Remarks
3.12 p.m.	Rotating object	8	Not reinforced.
3.20 ,,	Tactile	2	Reinforced after 30 secs.
3.35 ,,	,,	1	Reinforced after 30 secs.
3.45 ,,	,,	—	Reinforced simul- taneously with the
4.0 ,,	,,	—	beginning of the tactile stimulus.
4.17 ,,	,,	2·5	Reinforced after 30 secs.
4.38 ,,	,,	2	Reinforced after 30 secs.

The very considerable and protracted diminution in the reflex to the tactile stimulus shows that it is the analysing activity of the cerebral part of the chemical analyser of taste which is involved in this case, since the conditioned stimulus to cheese was in itself sufficient without reinforcement to bring about a profound diminution in the reflex to the tactile stimulus.

Another set of experiments was performed [by Dr. Savich] in which "natural" conditioned reflexes to the appearance of meat powder and to the appearance of granulated sugar were employed. The dog's usual diet outside the experiment consisted of oatmeal porridge with meat and bread. Later on meat and bread were excluded from the meal, but a large amount of sugar was added to the porridge. After this diet had been maintained for some time the conditioned reflex to the appearance of meat powder was found to be considerably increased, while the reflex to the appearance of sugar had disappeared almost entirely.

Similar experiments, but with greater precision of detail, were carried out by Dr. Hasen with conditioned reflexes to rejectable substances. He took advantage of two facts which had previously been noticed in reflexes to acid, viz., that in most of the cases the magnitude both of conditioned and of unconditioned reflexes gradually rises towards the end of an experimental day, and that the magnitude of the reflexes also rises, up to a certain maximum, in the course of a series of experiments conducted on successive days. Dr. Hasen modified his experiments in the following manner. After the first application of the conditioned stimulus, which was reinforced, acid was introduced several times in succession without the conditioned stimulus, and finally the conditioned stimulus was again applied. The effect of the conditioned stimulus on this last application was found always to be increased as compared with the effect on its first application. At a later stage in the experiments, which were performed on two dogs, the daily routine was interrupted by three intervals, of five days each in one series of experiments, and of three days each in another. During the first interval the one dog received in the form of an enema, and the other dog received through a stomach tube, a considerable amount of dilute acid. During the second interval a solution of sodium carbonate was given in a similar manner, and during the third interval the dogs received no injections at all. The conditioned reflexes and the unconditioned reflexes were tested after each of these intervals. It was found that after the interval in which acid was introduced the magnitude of the reflexes remained the same or was but slightly diminished as compared with the experiments preceding the pause ; after the interval in which nothing was administered the magnitude of the reflexes fell considerably ; and after introduction of soda the reflexes diminished still more. In the course of daily experiments a definite amount of acid introduced into the mouth of one of these dogs produced from the submaxillary gland on an average a salivary secretion of 5·1 c.c., while the conditioned stimulus elicited a secretion of 4 drops during 30 seconds. After the interval during which nothing was administered the figures were 3·8 c.c. and 2 drops respectively; after the interval in which sodium carbonate was introduced 3·7 c.c. and a secretion of zero were respectively produced ; finally, after the interval in which acid was administered, the secretions obtained amounted to 4·5 c.c. and 3 drops respectively. Thus it is evident that the variations in the chemical composition of the blood which resulted from excess of acid or alkali were differentiated by the cerebral termination of the chemical analyser, being manifested by an increase or a decrease in the excitability of the central part of the analyser. When the animal absorbed an excess of acid the excitability of the " acid " part of the chemical analyser increased, with the result that on encountering acid from the outer world the organism responded by more vigorous motor and secretory reflexes directed towards the exclusion of the further introduction of acid. The same, of course, takes place in the case of nutritive substances, a corresponding increase or decrease being observed in the positive or negative reactions to different substances or different quantities of them. It is thus seen that the chemical analyser of taste in its central part forms a connecting link between the internal and external media of the organism, and by regulating their relations one to the other secures a certain constancy of the internal medium.

The experiments which have just been described, and which, unfortunately, were not subsequently repeated, belong to the earlier period of our work, when the novelty and complexity of the subject afforded numerous sources of error. Nevertheless, even so, they show definitely that the study of the chemical analyser of taste, though complex, can be conducted successfully by the use of conditioned reflexes.

With regard to the synthesizing activity of the nervous system, as compared with its analysing activity, little is known up to the present. It would, indeed, be futile for us to attempt to discuss the nature of its intimate mechanism : it can only be suggested that, in the future, synthesizing activity will be referred to the physico-chemical properties of synaptic membranes or anastomosing neuro-fibrils. Our immediate task must consist in accumulating experimental material concerning the synthesizing activity.

In addition to the formation of the conditioned reflex itself—which is, of course, primarily an expression of the synthesizing activity, and which has constantly formed the starting-point of our investigations—we have also examined the properties of compound conditioned stimuli. Compound stimuli were used with either simultaneous or successive action of their component parts.

In the case of compound simultaneous stimuli the following important relations have been observed :

When the stimuli making up the compound act upon different analysers, the effect of one of them when tested singly was found very commonly to overshadow the effect of the others almost completely, and this independently of the number of reinforcements of the compound stimulus. For example, a tactile component of a stimulatory compound was usually found to obscure a thermal component, an auditory component to obscure a visual component, and so on. Thus, in the following experiment by Dr. Palladin a conditioned reflex to acid was established to a simultaneous application of a thermal stimulus of 0° C. and a tactile stimulation of the skin. Tests were made both of the compound stimulus and of its individual components applied singly.

Time	Conditioned Stimulus	Salivary Secretion in c.cs. during 1 minute
11.15 a.m.	Tactile	0·8 c.c.
12.45 p.m.	Thermal	0·0 c.c.
1.10 p.m.	Tactile + thermal	0·7 c.c.

Another example may be taken from an experiment by Dr. Zeliony. A conditioned alimentary reflex was established to the simultaneous application of the tone of a pneumatic tuning-fork, which was considerably damped by being placed within a wooden box coated with wool, and of a visual stimulus of three electric lamps placed in front of the dog in the slightly shaded room.

Time	Conditioned Stimulus	Secretion of Saliva in drops during 30 seconds
3.37 p.m.	Tone + lamps	8
3.49 ,,	Lamps	0

In the above experiments the action of the thermal and visual components by themselves was ineffective, being completely over-shadowed by the other respective components. It is obvious, however, that the ineffective components in the stimulatory compounds could easily be made to acquire powerful conditioned properties by independent reinforcement outside the combination. The true interpretation of the phenomenon which has just been described is revealed by experiments in which both components of a stimulus belong to one and the same analyser. For example, in one experiment there were used as components in a stimulatory compound two different tones, which appeared to the human ear to be of equal intensity. When the conditioned reflex to the compound became fully established, the tones sounded separately were found to produce an equal effect. In another experiment, a conditioned reflex was formed to a compound in which the two individual tones were of very different intensities. The effect of the tone of weaker intensity when tested singly was now very small or absent altogether. Such a case is illustrated in the following experiment by Dr. Zeliony. An alimentary reflex was established in a dog to a compound stimulus made up of the sound of a whistle and the sound of the tone d' sharp of a pneumatic tuning-fork. Both these sounds appeared to the human ear to be of equal intensity, and both when tested separately elicited a secretion of 19 drops of saliva during one minute. In addition to this, another compound stimulus was established, made up of the same sound of the whistle plus the tone a' of a tuning-fork of weaker intensity. When tested separately the whistle in this case elicited a secretion of seven drops of saliva during thirty seconds, and the tone only one drop.

It is evident from the above experiments that the obscuring of one stimulus by another belonging to the same analyser is determined by differences in their strength, and it is natural to assume that this explanation can be applied also to compound stimuli, the components of which belong to different analysers. On this assumption tactile cutaneous stimuli in our experiments should be regarded as being relatively stronger than thermal cutaneous stimuli, and auditory stimuli should be regarded as being relatively stronger than visual stimuli. The natural deductions from such an assumption are far-reaching, and it will be necessary at some future date to test its validity by the use of stimuli compounded from different analysers and varying as much as possible in their intensities, a very weak auditory stimulus being combined with a very strong visual one, and so on.

The phenomenon in which one stimulus is obscured by another in a simultaneous stimulatory compound, when the two stimuli belong to different analysers, presents several interesting features. The effect of the compound stimulus is found nearly always to be equal to that of the stronger component used singly, the weaker stimulus appearing therefore to be completely overshadowed by the stronger one. If, however, the stronger stimulus is even at long intervals of time, repeated singly without reinforcement by the unconditioned reflex, while the compound stimulus is constantly reinforced, the stronger stimulus by itself becomes completely ineffective, whereas in the stimulatory compound there is no diminution in its effect. It is evident, therefore, that although the effect of the weaker stimulus when tested singly is invisible, it nevertheless plays an important part in the stimulatory compound [experiments by Dr. Palladin].

Another feature of interest has been already described in the fourth lecture [experiments of Dr. Perelzweig, page 56]. If the weak component, which may be even quite ineffective when applied alone, is repeated at short intervals without reinforcement—*i.e.* is extinguished below zero—then both the compound and the stronger component undergo secondary extinction. In this experiment, therefore, the component which is normally of itself apparently ineffective becomes temporarily transformed by the process of experimental extinction into a strong inhibitory stimulus.

The following was observed in a single, but so far as the experimental conditions were concerned a perfect, experiment. When two stimuli belonging to different analysers were first separately made into conditioned stimuli, and only afterwards applied simultaneously to form a compound stimulus, which was repeatedly reinforced, the overshadowing of the one component by the other did not occur. From this it may be concluded that in the usual case where two hitherto neutral stimuli are used to form a compound stimulus, the stronger stimulus at once prevents the weaker from forming a corresponding connection with the centre for the unconditioned reflex. If, however, this connection has been established already, it is not disturbed during the subsequent establishment of the reflex to the compound stimulus. The mechanism on which the predominance of one component of a stimulatory compound over another depends is most probably a form of inhibition. This matter will be examined in detail in a subsequent lecture.

The cases mentioned above show that a definite interaction takes place between different cells of the cortex, resulting in a fusion or synthesis of their physiological activities on simultaneous excitation. In the case of a compound simultaneous stimulus made up of components of unequal strength belonging to the same analyser this synthesis is not so obvious. However, it comes out very clearly that even in these cases there is no summation of the individual reflex effect of each single component, the effect of the stronger component applied singly being equal to that of the compound stimulus.

The phenomenon of synthesis of stimuli belonging to the same analyser is much more evident in a modification of the experimental conditions which was first used in Dr. Zeliony's experiments, then again by Drs. Manuilov and Krylov, and has since been widely practised. It was noticed that if a conditioned reflex to a compound stimulus was established as described above, it was easy to maintain it in full strength and at the same time to convert its individual components, which gave a positive effect when tested singly, into negative or inhibitory stimuli. This result is obtained by constant reinforcement of the compound stimulus, while its components, on the frequent occasions when they are applied singly, remain without reinforcement. The experiment can be made with equal success in the reverse direction, making the stimulatory compound into a negative or inhibitory stimulus, while its components applied singly maintain their positive effect. We leave the discussion of this phenomenon to Lecture XVI, and shall pass on to consider the second type of stimulatory compounds, namely, compound successive stimuli.

In this second type of stimulus, in which the component stimuli are applied not simultaneously but in succession, the synthesizing function of the nervous system is still more obvious. The compound stimuli employed were of many different kinds. In some cases the compound was made up of successive repetitions of one and the same stimulus. For example, a definite tone was repeated three times for one second with an interval of two seconds between the first and second applications, and an interval of one second between the second and third ; this rhythm was repeated after a pause of five seconds, and was now accompanied by the unconditioned stimulus. In other experiments the stimulatory compound was made up of three or four different stimuli all belonging to one analyser ; the stimuli were made to succeed one another in a definite order, being each of equal duration, and with equal pauses between them. There were used, for example, in one case the four tones C, D, E, F of one octave ; and in another case the four stimuli were made up of a noise, two different tones and the sound of a bell. Finally, in other experiments there was employed a stimulatory compound composed of three or four stimuli belonging to different analysers, each stimulus being of equal duration, the pauses between them being also equal. Conditioned reflexes were readily obtained to all these different compound stimuli, and after a certain amount of practice of the reflexes all the individual components when tested singly were found to exhibit a positive conditioned effect, which varied in magnitude according to the quality and relative strength of the individual stimuli.

The next step was the introduction of different modifications of these compound stimuli. In the first case the order of the two pauses between the repetitions of the tone was reversed, the longer pause being now made between the second and third applications instead of between the first and second. In the remaining cases the order in which the different stimuli were applied was changed, either completely by reversing it, or in the case of the compound consisting of four component stimuli by reversing the order of the two middle ones. These modified compounds were repeatedly applied without reinforcement, but when the stimuli were applied in their original order the compound was always reinforced, with the result that ultimately the original compounds became differentiated from their modifications, which latter finally lost their positive conditioned effect and acquired an inhibitory one [experiments by Drs. Babkin, Stroganov, Grigorovich, Ivanov-Smolensky and Eurman].

The following is an example of the different permutations of four tones (1, 2, 3, 4) which were successfully differentiated by the dog in experiments by Dr. Babkin, the sequence 1234 being the positive stimulus and the sequence 4321 the first stimulus to be differentiated ; this was followed by development of an absolute differentiation of all the remaining sequences. The vibration frequencies of the four tones employed were 290, 325, 370 and 413 d.v. respectively.

1234	2134	3124	4123
1324	2314	3214	4213
1342	2341	3241	4231
1243	2143	3142	4132
1423	2413	3412	4312
1432	2431	3421	4321

In the following experiment [by Dr. Eurman] the positive alimentary conditioned stimulus was made up of the flash of an electric lamp (L), a tactile cutaneous stimulation (C), and a sound of bubbling water (S), applied in that order, namely, L-C-S. The inhibitory compound was made up in the reverse order, namely, S-C-L.

Time	Conditioned Stimulus	Secretion of Saliva in drops during 30 seconds	Remarks
11.38 a.m.	L-C-S	10	⎫ Reinforced.
11.45 ,,	,,	11	⎭
11.57 ,,	S-C-L	0	Not reinforced.
12.13 p.m.	L-C-S	7	Reinforced.
12.22 ,,	S-C-L	0	Not reinforecd.
12.32 ,,	L-C-S	5	⎫ Reinforced.
12.45 ,,	,,	7	⎭

The following is an experiment by Dr. Ivanov-Smolensky. The positive conditioned alimentary stimulus was made up of a hissing sound (H), a high tone (hT), a low tone (lT), and the sound of a buzzer (B), applied in that order, namely H-hT-lT-B. The inhibitory stimulus was made up with the order of the two middle components reversed, namely H-lT-hT-B.

Time	Conditioned Stimulus	Secretion of Saliva in drops during 30 seconds	Remarks
3.10 p.m.	H-hT-lT-B	4	Reinforced.
3.17 ,,	H-lT-hT-B	0	Not reinforced.
3.27 ,,	H-hT-lT-B	3	} Reinforced.
3.32 ,,	,, ,,	4	
3.38 ,,	H-lT-hT-B	0	Not reinforced.
3.46 ,,	H-hT-lT-B	2	Reinforced.

The formation of these inhibitory reflexes usually required a great deal of time : although a relative differentiation could sometimes be observed quite early, absolute differentiation was obtained in extreme cases only after more than one hundred repetitions without reinforcement. Indeed, in order to obtain a complete differentiation it was sometimes necessary to proceed by gradual stages, commencing with differentiation of comparatively simple compound stimuli. It was especially difficult to obtain a differentiation of the stimulatory compound of sound, low tone, high tone and buzzer from the compound in which the tones were reversed. All the differentiations, and especially those exceptionally difficult of formation, proved very unstable. On the one hand they suffered considerably from frequent repetition (see Lecture XIV), and on the other hand any interruption in the work caused them to weaken or to disappear for a time altogether. So soon as complete differentiation between such compound stimuli had been established, the individual components when tested singly were found to have lost all their initial positive conditioned effect.

From a purely physiological point of view, the study of differentiation between a compound stimulus and its modification, which both contain the same elements but in a different order of succession, is of considerable interest. The experiments show that a compound stimulus the component units of which remain in themselves unaltered, and consequently most probably affect the same cells of the cerebral cortex, behaves in different modifications as a different stimulus, evoking in these cells now an excitatory process and now an inhibitory one. Plainly the experiments reveal the great importance of the synthesizing activity of the cortical cells which are undergoing excitation. These cells must form, under the conditions of a given experiment, a very complicated excitatory unit, which is functionally identical with the simple excitatory units existing in the case of more elementary conditioned reflexes. Such active cortical cells must necessarily influence one another and interact with one another, as has clearly been demonstrated in the case of compound simultaneous stimuli. The mutual interaction between the excited or inhibited cortical elements in the case of compound successive stimuli is more complicated ; the effect of an active cortical cell upon the one next excited varies according to the influence to which it was itself subjected by the cell last stimulated. In this way it is seen that the order in which a given group of stimuli taking part in a stimulatory compound are arranged, and the pauses between them are the factors which determine the final result of the stimulation, and therefore most probably the form of the reaction, and we know already that different intensities of the same stimulus can be differentiated very accurately, one definite intensity being connected with excitation and another with inhibition.

It is evident from the description given in the present lecture that we must distinguish in animals an elementary, from a higher, type of analysis and synthesis. The former, and especially the elementary type of analysis, is based principally upon the properties and activity of the peripheral receptors of the analysers, while the latter is based principally upon those of the central ends of the analysers. Conditioned reflexes afford the means of investigating experimentally the functions both of the peripheral and of the central parts of the analysers, and such investigations have been conducted in our laboratories. The examples to be given during the remainder of this lecture will illustrate the scope of this field of animal experimentation.

In the first example I shall describe, it was sought to obtain by means of conditioned reflexes experimental data regarding the resonance theory of Helmholtz. We conceived that by partial destruction of the organ of Corti the disappearance of conditioned reflexes to certain tones would possibly be obtained. The following experiment was conducted by Dr. Andréev, who is still working on this subject. Pure tones were employed, being produced by two sets of apparatus, one giving tones from 100 to 3,000 and the other from 3,000 to 26,000 double vibrations per second. Various conditioned alimentary reflexes were established in the dog, namely, to tactile stimuli, visual stimuli, and different auditory stimuli (sound of a buzzer, metronome, a noise, and numerous pure tones). The cochlea was first completely destroyed on one side. When tested for the first time, six days after the operation, all the auditory conditioned reflexes were found to be present. A second operation (10th March, 1923) was now performed on the cochlea of the other side with the object of excluding only the lower part of the tonic scale. The osseous part of the cochlea was opened at the junction of its middle and upper thirds, and the exposed part of the membranous cochlea with the organ of Corti was injured with a fine needle. Already on the tenth day after the operation all the auditory stimuli, excepting tones of 600 double vibrations per second and lower, were found to be fully effective. In the course of three months following the operation, however, the effect of tones from 600 to 300 double vibrations became gradually restored. From numerous tests carried out from this period up to two years after the operation, the upper limit of the tones that had disappeared was fixed as somewhere between 309 and 317 double vibrations per second. The lower limit could not be determined, since we had no pure tones below 100 double vibrations per second at our disposal.

The following two tables are taken from the final period of the investigation :

Time	Conditioned Stimulus	Secretion of Saliva in drops during 30 seconds	Remarks

Experiment of 17th March, 1924.

6.8 p.m.	Metronome	13	⎫ Alimentary motor
6.19 ,,	Tone of 390 d.v.	8	⎬ reaction.
6.25 ,,	,, ,,	8	⎭

Experiment of 19th March, 1924.

5.35 p.m.	Metronome	7	⎫ Alimentary motor
5.39 ,,	,,	9	⎭ reaction.
5.45 ,,	Tone of 315 d.v.	0	No motor reaction.
6.17 ,,	Metronome	5	Alimentary motor reaction.
6.24 ,,	Tone of 315 d.v.	0	No motor reaction.
6.32 ,,	Metronome	8	Alimentary motor reaction.

All reflexes are reinforced.

A histological examination of the cochlea has not yet been carried out, the dog still being used for experiments. It is evident, however, that the positive results of our experiments successfully replace the negative results obtained by Kalischer [1] with regard to this question.

Another problem which engaged our attention was whether the participation of both hemispheres was necessary for differentiation of sounds by their direction. This question was solved by the experiments of Dr. Bikov. The corpus callosum was severed in a dog, and after the animal had recovered from the operation the establishment of new conditioned alimentary reflexes was begun. Their formation presented no special difficulties, and proceeded at the same rate as in normal animals. One of the reflexes was established to the sound of a whistle, 1,500 double vibrations per second. The whistle, which was placed in a cardboard case, was supported on the wall on a level with the left ear and at a definite distance from the dog. The reflex appeared at the eighth repetition, and attained a maximum and permanent strength after 70 repetitions. The whistle was then transferred to the right side of the dog, and in this position was not reinforced by the unconditioned reflex. By repeatedly contrasting the sound from the left with that from the right, a differentiation of the direction of the sound was attempted. There was, however, not the slightest sign of any differentiation, even after 115 applications of the non-reinforced stimulus from the right, and we considered it futile to continue beyond this number of repetitions. It was concluded that a differentiation of the direction of a sound required a united activity of both hemispheres. The following is one of the most recent experiments :

Time	Conditioned Stimulus	Secretion of Saliva in drops during 30 seconds	Remarks
3.40 p.m.	Whistle on left side	9	} Reinforced.
4.0 ,,	,, ,,	14	
4.20 ,,	Whistle on right side (112th application)	14	Not reinforced.
4.35 ,,	Whistle on left side	12	} Reinforced.
4.46 ,,	,, ,,	13	

[1] O. Kalischer. " Weitere Mitteilung über die Ergebnisse der Dressur als physiol. Untersuchungsmethode auf den Gebieten des Gehör-, Geruchs- und Farbensinns." *Archiv f. Anatomie und Physiologie, Physiologische Abteilung,* p. 303, 1909.

Other differentiations were obtained in this dog easily and rapidly, but never one involving localization of the source of a sound. In normal dogs the differentiation of sounds by their direction presents no more difficulty than any other differentiation, and is capable of great precision.

The experiments described in this and the preceding lectures leave no doubt in my mind that all the questions which have hitherto been considered as belonging to the domain of the so-called physiology of the organs of special sense can actually be investigated objectively by the method of conditioned reflexes. Are not Helmholtz's famous " unconscious conclusions "—in his *Physiological Optics*—in reality conditioned reflexes ? We may take as an example the case of a drawing imitating the visual character of a relief. In actual experience, of course, the tactile and muscular stimuli proceeding from a relief represent the initial and fundamental stimuli : the visual stimuli provided by its areas of light and shade form the signalling conditioned stimuli, which only subsequently obtain a vital significance by being constantly reinforced by the tactile and muscular stimuli. In the further course of our lectures we shall refer to other examples which can be studied objectively in dogs, and which correspond fully with phenomena usually described only in connection with the physiology of the organs of special sense.

LECTURE IX

The irradiation and concentration of nervous processes in the cerebral cortex :
(a) The irradiation and concentration of inhibition within a single analyser.

UP to the present we have been concerned chiefly with what may be called the external aspect of the cortical activity. We have studied the general laws governing the establishment of the most complicated and delicate correlations between the organism and its environment. It was shown that in response to an unlimited number of stimuli there can be brought about in the cerebral hemispheres an activity which serves to signal the approach of the comparatively small number of agencies which are of vital importance to the organism either in a favourable or in an injurious sense. It is through the hemispheres that corresponding reactions are brought about, thus anticipating the actual contact or clash of the organism with those agencies. The conditioned significance of stimuli is constantly corrected or changed by the hemispheres, so that when a given stimulus no longer corresponds to the correlations existing at a given time between the organism and its environment such a stimulus may be rendered temporarily or permanently ineffective. Finally, we have seen that in harmony with the perpetual and varied fluctuation of nature the hemispheres may invest with a rôle of conditioned significance on the one hand the minutest elements of the environment individually (" analysis "), and on the other hand various complexes compounded of these elements (" synthesis ").

The present and the following lectures will be devoted to the study of the internal aspect of the cortical activity, and we shall consider first the part played in it by the fundamental nervous processes of excitation and inhibition.

The first point which must receive our attention is the irradiation and concentration of these two processes.

It frequently happens in physiological investigation that where a broad group of phenomena is to be examined, the investigation of one of the members of this group may be more convenient than that of others. A detailed investigation of this aspect of internal inhibition proved, in the present case, to be the most advantageous. At the same time this investigation provided a striking illustration of the numerous advantages presented by the cutaneous analyser with its extensive and easily accessible receptor surface.

The experiment which revealed this new and important chapter in the physiology of the cerebral hemispheres was conducted by Dr. Krasnogorsky, to whom we owe several of the succeeding experiments.

Five small apparatuses for tactile stimulation of the skin were arranged along the hind leg of the dog. The first was fixed over the paw, and the remaining four were spaced out up the leg at distances of 3, 9, 15 and 22 cms. respectively from the first. Stimulation over the paw was given the properties of an inhibitory stimulus, while stimulations at the four upper places were given positive conditioned properties. This effect was obtained by the usual method of experimental differentiation. That is to say, a positive conditioned alimentary stimulus was established first of all to a tactile stimulation of one of the four upper places ; on account of the initial generalisation of the reflex, all the other places as well became spontaneously more or less effective upon stimulation. The positive conditioned effect of stimulation of the four upper places on the animal's leg was equalized by reinforcement with food, while by the method of contrast the stimulation over the paw, which was given always without reinforcement, lost all its positive conditioned properties and acquired inhibitory ones. In the experiments given below the conditioned stimulus was applied in every case during 30 seconds. The place on the skin which was stimulated is indicated by a number : 0 represents the inhibitory place ; 1, 2, 3, 4 represent the positive places taken in order. The number of the positive place is accompanied by a figure giving its distance from the inhibitory place.

It is seen from the table (p. 154) that stimulation of each of the three places 4, 3, and 1 produced in the beginning identical positive conditioned effects, measured by 5 drops of salivary secretion during 30 seconds. The four places 1, 2, 3 and 4 were now separately tested at an interval of exactly one minute after the last of three successive applications of the inhibitory stimulus. The stimulation of place 1, nearest to the inhibitory place, was at the first test absolutely ineffective, and at the second test its effect was barely distinguishable (less than one drop). The stimulation of place 2, next in distance from the inhibitory place, gave only half its normal positive conditioned effect, but the stimulation of the remaining places (3 and 4) gave a full or even an increased positive effect. The significance of this experiment is clear. The different sensory places on the skin must be regarded as projecting themselves upon

Time-interval between separate stimuli	Place of stimulation	Secretion of Saliva in drops during 30 seconds
—	4 (22 cms.)	5
10 minutes	3 (15 cms)	5
10 ,,	1 (3 cms.)	5
10 ,,	0	0
1 ,,	0	0
1 ,,	0	0
1 ,,	1 (3 cms.)	0
10 ,,	0	0
1 ,,	0	0
1 ,,	0	0
1 ,,	2 (9 cms.)	3
10 ,,	0	0
1 ,,	0	0
1 ,,	0	0
1 ,,	3 (15 cms.)	6
10 ,,	0	Trace
1 ,,	0	0
1 ,,	0	0
1 ,,	4 (22 cms.)	7
10 ,,	0	0
1 ,,	0	0
1 ,,	0	0
1 ,,	1 (3 cms.)	Trace
10 ,,	0	0
1 ,,	0	0
1 ,,	0	0
1 ,,	2 (9 cms.)	3
10 ,,	0	0
1 ,,	0	0
1 ,,	0	0
1 ,,	4 (22 cms.)	5

corresponding areas in the cortex of the hemispheres. Therefore it is reasonable to suppose that the inhibitory process initiated in a definite point of the cortex by the tactile stimulation of the inhibitory place irradiates into the surrounding region, giving a smaller inhibitory effect with increase of distance from the inhibitory point and becoming indistinguishable at the more distant points.

A different intensity of the inhibitory process can be produced, either by varying the number of successive applications of the inhibitory stimulus, of which the after-effects are summated, or by varying the interval between the last inhibitory stimulus and the application of the positive stimulus.   In either case different figures are obtained for the salivary reflex, but their general significance remains the same.   This is shown in the following experiment :

Interval of time between separate stimuli	Place of stimulation	Secretion of Saliva in drops during 30 seconds
—	1 (3 cms)	7
10 minutes	4 (22 cms.)	6
10 ,,	2 (9 cms.)	6
10 ,,	0	1
$\frac{1}{4}$ minute	0	0
$\frac{1}{4}$,,	0	1
$\frac{1}{4}$,,	0	0
$\frac{1}{4}$,,	4 (22 cms.)	3

The inhibitory after-effect was tested in this experiment after a shorter time ($\frac{1}{4}$ minute), and after four applications of the inhibitory stimulus instead of three ; under these conditions a considerable inhibitory influence was exerted even upon the positive place 4, which in the previous experiment when tested one minute after three successive applications of the inhibitory stimulus gave a full reflex.

If the various positive stimuli are applied in one and the same experiment at different times after the last inhibitory stimulus, it can clearly be brought out how the initially widely irradiated inhibition gradually frees from its after-effect first the remoter areas, and subsequently those areas nearer to the cortical point in which the inhibition arose primarily.   An example of such an experiment is given in the table shown on p. 156.

It is thus seen that the furthest place (4) was free of inhibition after half a minute, place 2 after five minutes, and place 1 after ten minutes.

The more frequently the differentiation is exercised in the course of days or weeks, the more rapidly are the more remote places freed from the inhibitory after-effect, a fact which is sometimes exhibited in the course of a single experiment after the positive and negative stimuli have been repeated several times.

It is worthy of note that experiments upon the irradiation of inhibition have been successfully demonstrated on numerous occasions without serious interference by the presence of a stranger with the experimenter in the animal's room, and have even been carried out successfully at crowded meetings of the Petrograd Medical Society.

Interval of time between separate stimuli in minutes	Place of stimulation	Secretion of Saliva in drops during 30 seconds
—	1 (3 cms.)	7
10	0	0
1	0	0
$\frac{1}{4}$	4 (22 cms.)	4
10	0	0
1	0	0
$\frac{1}{2}$	4 (22 cms.)	8
10	0	0
1	0	0
1	1 (3 cms.)	2
10	0	0
1	0	0
5	1 (3 cms.)	3
10	0	0
1	0	0
10	1 (3 cms.)	8
10	0	0
1	0	0
1	2 (9 cms.)	3
10	0	0
1	0	0
5	2 (9 cms.)	8

We have now to inquire into the nature of the recession of inhibition from those cortical points into which it was irradiated. Does this represent a destruction or waning of the inhibition in these places, or is it some kind of return or active concentration of the inhibition to its starting-point due to some antagonistic process ? In face of the constant fact that strengthening of differentiation by repeated contrasts is accompanied by a corresponding shortening of the duration and extent of irradiation of the inhibitory after-effect, we are naturally more inclined to accept the second hypothesis, namely, that we deal with the reverse of irradiation, *i.e.* " concentration " of the inhibition toward its initial point of origin in the cortex. A number of important facts in support of this conclusion will be adduced later. Meanwhile, it may be noted that in Dr. Krasnogorsky's experiments the waning of the inhibition occupied several minutes. The actual spread of inhibition, however, proceeded with such rapidity in these experiments that Dr. Krasnogorsky was unable to follow it.

The preliminary observations upon the antagonistic processes of irradiation and concentration seemed to us of such fundamental importance as to demand a thorough investigation by modifying and controlling the experiments in all possible ways. Our attention, therefore, was next directed to that form of internal inhibition which has been discussed under the name of experimental extinction, and these experiments were also conducted with the use of tactile cutaneous stimuli [experiments of Dr. Kogan]. As a preliminary a conditioned reflex to acid was established for a tactile stimulation of some place on the skin. While it was still in its initial, generalized phase the reflex was equalized as far as possible in strength for stimulation of any place on the skin along the whole of the surface of one side of the body before the experiments were proceeded with. A definite place was then selected to which the stimulus was applied for a minute, without reinforcement, and repeated every two minutes until the first zero was obtained. At different intervals of time, following the first zero of extinction at the given place, tactile stimulations were tried at various other places of the skin and the resulting secretory effect was compared with their usual one. These other places were found also to suffer inhibition temporarily to a greater or less extent. The place subjected to experimental extinction is termed the *place of primary extinction*, and the places which become involved in the inhibitory after-effect are termed *places of secondary extinction*. We are familiar with this terminology from our discussion of the phenomenon of experimental extinction in the fourth lecture, where it was made quite clear that the extinctive inhibition does not confine itself to the actual point in the cortex which was called into activity by the specific external stimulus, but irradiates over a wide area. We have, in other words, a phenomenon similar to that which has already been discussed in connection with differential inhibition.

It was essential in these experiments to vary the place subjected to the primary extinction. Otherwise, instead of the extinctive inhibition—from which the primarily extinguished reflex frees itself in a few minutes, or at the most 1-2 hours—there would have developed a differentiation with its very stable and lasting form of internal inhibition.

An example of an experiment such as has just been described is given in the following table :

Date	Place to which conditioned stimulus was applied	Interval of time between zero of extinction and stimulation of new place	Secretion of Saliva in drops during 1st, 2nd, and 3rd minutes	Percentage of inhibition
		Dog No. 1.		
10th Nov. 1913	Left shoulder (place primarily extinguished)		9, 2, 1 2, 0, 1 5, 1, 0 1, 0, 0 0	
11th Nov. 1913	Left side of chest Left shoulder (place primarily extinguished)	1 minute	**1**, – – 9, 1, 0 3, 0, 1 2, 0, 0 1, 0, 0 0	84
	Left thigh	1 minute	**8**, – –	12
		Dog No. 2.		
17th Oct. 1913	Left side of neck (place primarily extinguished)		10, 2, 0 3, 0, 0 2, 0, 0 1, 0, 0 0	
18th Oct. 1913	Left shoulder Left side of neck (place primarily extinguished)	3 minutes	**0**, – – 9, 3, 1 4, 1, 0 1, 0, 0 0	100
	Left thigh	3 minutes	**5**, – –	45

It is plain that, the further away on the skin the secondarily inhibited place is from the place which undergoes the primary inhibition, the weaker is the irradiated inhibitory after-effect.

If the stimulation is applied to one definite place at different intervals of time after the reflex has been extinguished to zero at another place, the greater this interval the weaker is the inhibition in the secondarily extinguished place. This is borne out by the following experiments.

Date	Place to which conditioned stimulus was applied	Interval of time between zero of extinction and stimulation of new place	Secretion of Saliva in drops during 1st, 2nd, and 3rd minutes	Percentage of inhibition
	Dog No. 1.			
18th Nov. 1913	Left fore limb (place primarily extinguished)		9, 2, 0 3, 0, 1 1, 0, 0 0	
21st Nov. 1913	Left side of abdomen Left fore limb (place primarily extinguished)	60 seconds	**8**, – – 9, 2, 1 3, 0, 1 3, 0, 0 1, 0, 0 0	12
20th Nov. 1913	Left side of abdomen Left fore limb (place primarily extinguished)	30 seconds	**4**, – – 10, 2, 1 4, 0, 1 3, 0, 1 0	56
	Left side of abdomen	15 seconds	**2**, – –	80
	Dog No. 2.			
28th Nov. 1913	Left thigh (place primarily extinguished)		10, 4, 1 4, 1, 0 1, 0, 0 0	
29th Nov. 1913	Left scapula Left thigh (place primarily extinguished)	15 minutes	**9**, – – 9, 2, 0 2, 0, 0 1, 1, 0 0	10
30th Nov. 1913	Left scapula Left thigh (place primarily extinguished)	7 minutes	**4**, – – 8, 1, 0 2, 0, 0 2, 0, 0 0	56
	Left scapula	2 minutes	**0**, – –	100

It is obvious that in this experiment we deal again with the concentration of inhibition, the inhibition being gradually withdrawn from the periphery of its irradiation and concentrated at its initial point. Further, it becomes evident that the rate at which the inhibition is withdrawn from the places undergoing secondary inhibition varies very considerably with individual dogs, so that, for example, a process which occupies only one minute in dog No. 1 requires fifteen minutes in dog No. 2. This, of course, is a fact of considerable importance, since it gives a numerical expression to one of the most intimate sides of the highest nervous activity. That these individual differences in the three animals were not accidental is shown by the fact that they remained constant during many months in which the experiments proceeded.

In the experiments of Dr. Kogan it was possible to observe also the progress of the spreading of the inhibitory after-effect. I shall give the actual experiments in which the degree of secondary inhibition corresponding to the different places of the skin was determined *immediately* after complete primary extinction had been obtained :

Dog No. 2.

Date	Place at which conditioned stimulus was applied	Secretion of Saliva in drops during 1st, 2nd, and 3rd minutes	Percentage of inhibition
25th Jan. 1914	Right side of chest	12, 1, $\frac{1}{2}$ 2, 0, 0 0	
25th Jan. 1914	Right hind paw Right side of chest	**$11\frac{1}{2}$**, – – $13\frac{1}{2}$, $1\frac{1}{2}$, $\frac{1}{2}$ 0	4
26th Jan. 1914	Adjacent place Right side of chest	**0**, – – 12, $1\frac{1}{2}$, $\frac{1}{2}$ 0	100
26th Jan. 1914	At a distance of 1 cm. Right side of chest	**0**, – – 14, 2, $2\frac{1}{2}$ 6, 2, $\frac{1}{2}$ 0	100
4th Feb. 1914	Right hind paw Left side of chest	**13**, – – 12, 2, 0 0	7
5th Feb. 1914	Left front paw Left side of chest	**$11\frac{1}{2}$**, – – $9\frac{1}{2}$, 1, 0 0	4
	Left scapula	**$3\frac{1}{2}$**, – –	64

A comparison of these results with those of the preceding experiment on the same dog shows clearly that immediately after the full development of inhibition for the primarily extinguished place, a complete secondary inhibition is obtained only for adjacent places, the inhibitory after-effect being absent or hardly distinguishable for places more remote.

It is interesting to note that in the three dogs employed in these experiments the effect of stimulating the remoter places immediately after the primary inhibition had been produced varied considerably. In dog No. 1 not only was the reflex to stimulation of the remoter place not inhibited, but it even produced a considerably enhanced positive effect, whereas dog No. 3 under similar conditions revealed a considerable degree of secondary inhibition. This fact, which was frequently observed in the experiments both of Dr. Krasnogorsky and Dr. Kogan, and which will form the subject of more detailed discussion in the eleventh lecture, is well illustrated in the following experiments :

Date	Place at which conditioned stimulus was applied	Secretion of Saliva in drops during 1st, 2nd, and 3rd minutes	Change in strength of reflex
	Dog No. 1.		
28th Jan. 1914	Left side of chest	$8\frac{1}{2}$, $1\frac{1}{2}$, $\frac{1}{2}$ 0	
6th Feb. 1914	At a distance of 3 cm. Right shank	$\frac{3}{4}$, – – 9, $\frac{1}{2}$, 1 $3\frac{1}{2}$, 1, 0 0	−92%
	Right shoulder	$14\frac{1}{2}$, – –	+60%
	Dog No. 3.		
5th Feb. 1914	Left hind paw	$10\frac{1}{2}$, 2, $\frac{1}{2}$ 0	
11th Feb. 1914	Left fore leg Left shank	6, – – $10\frac{1}{2}$, 2, 0 0	−43%
	Left thigh	0, – –	−100%

In addition to the foregoing, Dr. Kogan made a considerable number of observations which illustrate in detail the length of time occupied in his three dogs by the phases of irradiation and concentration of inhibition in the tactile cutaneous analyser. These observations show that in the case of dog No. 1 the phase of irradiation of inhibition occupied about twenty seconds, while the concentration of inhibition occupied about seventy-five seconds. In dog No. 2 the irradiation was complete after three minutes, while the whole inhibitory process in both its phases occupied fifteen minutes. In dog No. 3 the corresponding figures were four to five minutes for the irradiation and twenty minutes for the two phases taken together. It is seen, therefore, that although the duration of the inhibitory after-effect differed considerably in the three dogs, the time ratio between the phases of irradiation and concentration of the inhibition remained almost constant, the phase of concentration taking four or five times as long as the phase of irradiation. It must be admitted, however, that the data relating to the experiments upon extinction cannot be regarded as absolutely faultless, since the original magnitude of the conditioned reflexes sometimes varied considerably in different experiments, and in some cases the causes of these variations could not be definitely determined.

An experimental investigation upon the irradiation of conditioned inhibition was carried out by Dr. Anrep, who also made use of the cutaneous analyser. A generalized tactile cutaneous reflex was first established, and its strength was equalized so that the stimulation of any place resulted in the same intensity of reflex response. The tactile stimulation of one definite place was now repeatedly combined with a stimulus for another analyser (the sound of a buzzer), and in this combination the stimulus remained without reinforcement by the unconditioned reflex. The result was that the stimulus became negative or inhibitory when applied in the combination, although it retained its full positive effect when applied singly. The places on the skin which were stimulated are indicated by numbers : 0, between the neck and chest, in combination with the buzzer, represented the area subjected to the conditioned inhibition. On the left side the following places were used for positive tactile conditioned reflexes : 1, on the fore limb ; 2, on the fore paw ; 3, on the middle of the chest ; 4, on the pelvis ; 5, on the thigh ; and 6, on the hind paw. The experiments were conducted in the following manner. In a given experiment one positive place was first tested, in order to determine the normal magnitude of the conditioned reflex response. The inhibitory combination was now applied, and then the positive place was tested again at different intervals of time. This procedure was performed in separate experiments for all the remaining positive places. The positive and the negative conditioned stimuli were allowed to act in every case during 30 seconds. The following table summarizes the series of experiments on this animal:

Number of the place stimulated	Percentage of inhibition observed at different intervals of time						
	0″	15″	30″	45″	60″	120″	180″
2	30		54		29	19	10
1	45		66		39	22	13
0 (place primarily inhibited)	91		75		50	37	17
3	52	58	69	57	45	34	13
4	37		65		39	22	13
5	27		57		23	17	11
6	19	26	31	22	20	10	7

The first vertical column gives the number of the places stimulated ; the succeeding vertical columns indicate the magnitude of inhibitory after-effect corresponding to these places. The upper horizontal row gives the length of the interval from the end of the inhibitory stimulus to the beginning of the stimulation of any given place.

It is thus seen that in the case of conditioned inhibition the inhibitory process initiated at a definite point spreads over the whole analyser, diminishing in intensity with distance from the primarily inhibited place, and reaching its maximum strength for the whole analyser only by the end of a period of 30 seconds ; after this the inhibitory process undergoes a gradual diminution—again simultaneously over the whole analyser. The only exception which must be made to this general rule is that at the place which is subjected to the primary inhibition the intensity of the inhibitory after-effect does not increase gradually, but is maximal from the start.

Of course, in these experiments also it was essential to take most rigid precautions to avoid casual extraneous stimuli, since these would invariably exert a disturbing influence causing sometimes inhibition of the positive reflexes and sometimes dis-inhibition. Dr. Anrep's experiments were, however, performed in our special laboratory.

The three series of experiments, upon the movement of differential inhibition, experimental extinction and conditioned inhibition, all clearly demonstrate that the inhibition first spreads from its point of initiation over the whole analyser and then gradually recedes. The details of this process, however, are seen to differ considerably according to the type of internal inhibition. In Dr.

Krasnogorsky's experiments on differential inhibition the irradiation of inhibition occurs instantaneously, and the inhibitory after-effect attains its maximum after a zero interval : it is only the concentration of inhibition in this case which proceeds in a measurable interval of time.   In Dr. Kogan's experiments with extinctive inhibition the irradiation of inhibition was progressive, and the nearer places underwent the maximum secondary inhibition much sooner than the more remote places.   The phase of concentration in the extinctive inhibition, however, was four to five times longer in duration than the phase of irradiation.   It is possible that this difference of rate between the irradiation of these two forms of inhibition depends upon the intensity of inhibition developed.   Dr. Krasnogorsky usually repeated the primary inhibitory stimulus several times, regardless of the fact that it produced its full effect at once, while Dr. Kogan confined himself to the first zero.   The differences in the case of conditioned inhibition are much more complicated and important.   Dr. Anrep showed that the conditioned inhibition, like the differential inhibition in Dr. Krasnogorsky's experiments, irradiated simultaneously, although in a varying degree, over the entire analyser ;   after this, in contradistinction from Dr. Krasnogorsky's results, the inhibition increased gradually up to a certain maximum strength during a definite period, and at all places simultaneously.   The gradual diminution in intensity of the inhibition also occurred simultaneously over the entire analyser.   Thus conditioned inhibition differs from differential inhibition and from experimental extinction in that the entire analyser simultaneously reveals, though in different degrees, an inhibitory after-effect; an actual progression or regression of the maximum inhibitory after-effect cannot be observed.

The experiments by Dr. Anrep embrace in detail the following phenomenon, already indicated in part by some previous workers. He observed that both positive and negative conditioned reflexes established to tactile stimulation of different places on one side of the body are reproduced spontaneously and with extreme accuracy to tactile stimulation of the corresponding places on the other side.   The irradiation and concentration of the inhibitory after-effect once initiated on one side, correspondingly and equally involves the other side. This interesting fact will be discussed further on in these lectures.

A series of experiments analogous to those carried out on the irradiation of inhibition over the cutaneous analyser were conducted with the acoustic analyser, and these also confirmed the hypothesis that the peripheral end of the analyser can be regarded as projected geometrically upon the cortex of the hemispheres. In these experiments different musical tones, the beat of a metronome, and a hissing sound served as conditioned stimuli [experiments of Drs. Manuilov and Ivanov-Smolensky]. The reflex to one of these conditioned stimuli was subjected to primary experimental extinction, and the effect upon the reflexes to the remaining stimuli was observed. The following is an account of the experiments of Dr. Ivanov-Smolensky on this subject.

Separate conditioned alimentary reflexes were established, and equalized, to four different tones produced by a Max-Kohl's tone-variator. These tones were chosen in two pairs, separated by an interval of approximately three octaves—the lower tones having vibration frequencies of 123 and 132 respectively, and the upper tones of 1036 and 1161 respectively. Similar reflexes were also established to a hissing sound, and to the sound of a metronome beating at a rate of one hundred per minute. In the course of the experiments one of the conditioned reflexes was extinguished to zero, and then all the remaining reflexes were tested in different experiments, either immediately or after intervals of 1, 3, 5, 7, 10, 12 or 15 minutes. All the reflexes were found to undergo secondary inhibition, but in a varying degree. A part of the results of these experiments is given in the table on page 166.

The table shows that on the extinction of one of the tones belonging to the lower pair the reflex to the other tone of the same pair reaches the maximum inhibition somewhat more rapidly, remains at this maximum longer, and recovers from the inhibition more slowly, than the reflexes to either of the higher tones. On the extinction of one of the high tones, the reflex to the other high tone reaches the maximum inhibition more rapidly, remains longer at this level, and recovers from the inhibitory after-effect more slowly than the reflexes to either of the lower tones. On the extinction of any of the tones the secondary inhibition of the reflexes to hissing and to the metronome is in all respects less than that of the reflexes to the tones. On the other hand, after extinction of the reflex to hissing or to the metronome an intense secondary inhibition of all the reflexes to tones is obtained.

It is obvious that only the experiments with extinction of tones can be brought forward as evidence of a definite geometrical projection of the acoustic peripheral receptor upon the cortical part of the analyser.

The fact that extinction of the reflexes to the metronome and to hissing produces intense inhibition of the reflexes to tones, whereas extinction of the reflexes to tones results only in comparatively weak inhibition of the reflexes to the metronome and hissing may perhaps be accounted for by the greater strength and by the more mixed character of the latter stimuli.

Primarily extinguished reflex	Secondarily extinguished reflex	Interval after the beginning of the conditioned inhibition							
		0	1'	3'	5'	7'	10'	12'	15'
		Percentage of inhibition							
Conditioned reflex to 123 d.v.	Conditioned reflex to 132 d.v.	71	95	100	100	—	100	—	65
	Conditioned reflex to 1161 d.v.	57	60	86	94	—	53	—	45
	Conditioned reflex to hissing sound	10	—	50	73	47	—	8	—
Conditioned reflex to 1161 d.v.	Conditioned reflex to 1036 d.v.	75	100	95	100	—	91	—	80
	Conditioned reflex to 123 d.v.	67	80	100	90	—	80	—	46
	Conditioned reflex to metronome	5	—	45	63	42	—	0	—
Conditioned reflex to 123 d.v.	Conditioned reflex to metronome	5	—	93	67	42	—	4	—
Conditioned reflex to metronome	Conditioned reflex to 123 d.v.	73	—	100	100	76	—	65	—

It is highly probable that irradiation and concentration of inhibition, which takes place as described in the cutaneous and acoustic analysers, follow a similar course also in the case of other analysers. However, the experimental determination of the relationships in these cases is at present extremely difficult or even impossible owing to purely technical obstacles. If in the future these obstacles should be overcome and the laws governing the spread of inhibition be determined for all the analysers, an experimental method would be provided for the study of the internal structure of the different analysers.

LECTURE X

Irradiation and concentration of nervous processes in the cerebral hemispheres (continued) : (b) Irradiation and concentration of inhibition over the entire cortex ; (c) Irradiation and concentration of excitation.

IN the last lecture it was shown how internal inhibition, initiated in a single definite point of the cortical part of an analyser, rapidly irradiates over the whole analyser, after which it is slowly concentrated upon its initial point. Furthermore, it was found that the progress of irradiation of internal inhibition can be traced step by step within the analyser.

In the present lecture we shall trace the progress of inhibition from one analyser to another over the whole cerebral cortex. Experiments bearing upon this process have been conducted for all the forms of internal inhibition recognized up to the present.

It was mentioned in the description of differential inhibition that when the inhibition is initiated in one analyser it reveals itself in other analysers as well, in the form of an inhibitory after-effect. In a series of experiments by Dr. Beliakov it was found that differential inhibition of a small intensity does not involve in its after-effects any other analyser than the one in which the inhibition was primarily developed, but that when the intensity of the inhibition is great the inhibitory after-effect involves other analysers as well. However, secondary inhibition of other analysers is in every case much weaker than that of the analyser in which the differentiation was primarily developed. A number of experiments will be described to illustrate these relations :

A conditioned alimentary reflex was established to a tone of 4,000 d.v. produced by a Galton's whistle ; from this a pitch of one semitone lower was differentiated. A second positive conditioned alimentary reflex was established to a noiselessly rotating object. The reflex to the auditory stimulus gave an average secretion of 11-12 drops during 30 seconds, and the reflex to the visual stimulus gave an average of 7-8 drops. The results of a series of experiments

167

upon the irradiation of differential inhibition are illustrated by the following table :

Time	Stimulus applied during 30 seconds	Salivary Secretion in drops during 30 seconds
Experiment of 8th June, 1909.		
2.5 p.m.	Tone of 4000 d.v.	12
2.35 ,,	Semitone lower	0
2.38 ,,	,, ,,	0
2.39 ,,	Tone of 4000 d.v.	5
2.50 ,,	,, ,,	11
3.5 ,,	Semitone lower	0
3.8 ,,	,, ,,	0
3.9 ,,	Rotating object	7
3.20 ,,	,, ,,	7
Experiment of 11th June.		
1.35 p.m.	Tone of 4000 d.v.	12
1.45 ,,	,, ,,	11
2.0 ,,	Semitone lower	0
2.2 ,,	,, ,,	0
2.4 ,,	,, ,,	0
2.6 ,,	,, ,,	0
2.7 ,,	Rotating object	3
2.25 ,,	,, ,,	7
Experiment of 14th June.		
1.45 p.m.	Tone of 4000 d.v.	11
2.0 ,,	Semitone lower	0
2.2 ,,	,, ,,	0
2.4 ,,	,, ,,	0
2.6 ,,	,, ,,	0
2.7 ,,	Tone of 4000 d.v.	1
2.30 ,,	,, ,,	11

The significance of these experiments is obvious. After the inhibitory semitone had been repeated twice with an interval of 3 minutes between the successive repetitions, the positive tone tested half a minute later had lost more than 50% of its effect, while the visual stimulus showed no diminution in its effect at all (experiment of 8th June). After a greater summation of the inhibitory after-effect by four successive repetitions of the semitone with intervals of 2 minutes between them, the reflex to the visual stimulus tested half a minute later (in the experiment of 11th June) showed a diminution of 60%, while the inhibition of the reflex to the auditory stimulus (tested in the experiment of 14th June) was nearly complete.

Similar results are obtained with extinctive inhibition, as shown in a series of experiments by Dr. Gorn. In these experiments, owing to the introduction of certain modifications into the technique, the irradiation of the inhibitory process was even more clearly exhibited, especially as regards the earlier removal of its after-effect from the secondarily involved analysers. The following are some of the experiments :

Separate conditioned alimentary reflexes were established in a dog to the tone c′ sharp of a pneumatic tuning-fork and to flashes of three electric lamps, each of 16 candle-power.

Time	Stimulus applied during 30 seconds	Salivary Secretion in drops during 30 seconds	

Experiment of 15th December, 1911.

Time	Stimulus	Drops	
1.55 p.m.	Light	9	
1.58 ,,	,,	4½	
2.1 ,,	,,	Trace	Not reinforced
2.4 ,,	,,	0	
2.7 ,,	,,	0	
2.31 ,,	,,	Trace	

Experiment of 26th January, 1912.

Time	Stimulus	Drops	
2.17 p.m.	Tone	10	Reinforced
2.32 ,,	Light	8	
2.35 ,,	,,	3½	
2.43 ,,	,,	4	Not reinforced
2.46 ,,	,,	1	
2.49 ,,	,,	0	
2.52 ,,	,,	0	
2.52½ ,,	Tone	4	Reinforced

Experiment of 27th October, 1911.

Time	Stimulus	Drops	
1.25 p.m.	Tone	12	Reinforced
1.37 ,,	Light	11	
1.40 ,,	,,	10	Not reinforced
1.43 ,,	,,	½	
1.46 ,,	,,	0	
1.49 ,,	,,	0	
1.52 ,,	Tone	12	Reinforced

The conditioned reflex to light was in these experiments subjected to extinction, and the inhibitory after-effect was tested upon the reflex to the auditory stimulus. The reflex to the visual stimulus itself, after extinction up to the point of two consecutive zeros, showed the first signs of spontaneous recovery only after an interval of $23\frac{1}{2}$ minutes (15th December, 2.31 p.m.). The reflex to the auditory stimulus, on the other hand, when tested immediately after a similar extinction of the visual reflex was diminished in strength by only 60% (26th January, 1912, 2.52$\frac{1}{2}$ p.m.), and when tested in the third experiment after a pause of $2\frac{1}{2}$ minutes it was quite free of any inhibitory after-effect (27th October, 1912, 1.52 p.m.). It is thus seen that the inhibition irradiated from the visual to the acoustic analyser—never, however, producing a full inhibitory after-effect, and quickly retreating from it. That the rapid removal of the inhibitory after-effect from the acoustic analyser in these experiments was not due to a smaller intensity of the primary inhibition within the visual analyser is proved by the following details. In the case of the visual stimulus the interval between the repetitions ($2\frac{1}{2}$ minutes) led to a progressive diminution of the reflex through all the stages of extinction, whereas in the acoustic analyser an identical interval sufficed for a complete restoration of the reflex. Moreover, when in the second experiment the extinction of the visual reflex had led to a reduction of the secretion to $3\frac{1}{2}$ drops as against the usual 8 drops, a prolongation of the interval on purpose to $7\frac{1}{2}$ minutes served only to check the progress of the diminution in the strength of the reflex, and did not result in any appreciable restoration (2.43 p.m.), while the acoustic analyser was after that interval already completely free from any inhibitory after-effect. Neither was the difference between the restoration of the primarily and the secondarily extinguished reflexes due to any peculiarities of the cortical elements of the visual and auditory cells, as was proved by experiments in which the tone was subjected to the primary extinction, and the effect of secondary inhibition was observed on the visual analyser. The relations between the rates of recovery from the inhibition in the primarily and secondarily extinguished analysers in these experiments were exactly the same as before, and there is no need, therefore, to give separate tables. It can now reasonably be assumed that in the secondarily extinguished analyser we deal with the periphery of the irradiated inhibition, and that its recessional movement begins at the periphery and proceeds towards the point of initiation of the inhibition exactly in the same manner as within the single cutaneous analyser (concentration of inhibition).

Experiments on irradiation of extinctive inhibition over the entire cortex of the hemispheres were performed with a great number of variations. For example, two conditioned reflexes were developed in the analyser which was subjected to primary extinction (*e.g.* visual analyser), and the inhibitory effect of experimental extinction of one of these reflexes was observed upon both of them and also upon reflexes belonging to other analysers. Recovery from the inhibitory after-effect was found first of all in secondarily extinguished reflexes belonging to other analysers. Shortly afterwards recovery occurred in the secondarily extinguished reflex belonging to the visual analyser itself, and finally, but after a much longer time, the reflex which underwent the primary extinction became freed from the inhibitory after-effect. The difference in the length of time necessary for the recovery of the two reflexes belonging to the primarily inhibited visual analyser clearly points to a regional localization of reflexes within the analysers, such as was already suggested in the preceding lecture.

Experiments performed with irradiation of conditioned inhibition gave, on the whole, very similar results. One definite additional stimulus was used as a common conditioned inhibitor for conditioned reflexes belonging to different analysers, each of the conditioned stimuli in turn being repeated with the additional stimulus and remaining in the compound always without reinforcement, so that the compound conditioned stimulus developed inhibitory properties. The actual experiments were conducted as follows. First one of the conditioned stimuli was applied, and its secretory effect recorded. Next the conditioned inhibitor was applied in combination with the same or another conditioned stimulus, and the combination was repeated several times in succession. Finally, the effect of the first conditioned stimulus applied singly was again tested at different intervals of time after the last application of the inhibitory combination. When the positive reflex tested was the one employed in the inhibitory combination, it was found to be considerably inhibited, and was only slowly freed from the inhibitory after-effect ; when, however, the inhibitory combination was made with a stimulus from another analyser, the stimulus undergoing the test was only slightly inhibited, and rapidly recovered its original strength. It is thus seen that the inhibitory after-effect was very powerful and prolonged in the analyser of the reflex subjected to the primary conditioned inhibition, but was only weak and of short duration in other analysers.

In a series of experiments conducted by Dr. Degtiareva separate conditioned alimentary reflexes were established to a metronome (M) and to flashes of electric lamps (L). A noiselessly rotating object (R) was used as a conditioned inhibitor common to both positive stimuli. The application of the conditioned stimuli both singly and in the inhibitory combination was always continued during one minute, and the amount of saliva secreted during this time was recorded. The following experiments give the final result of the determination of the minimal interval which was necessary for complete recovery of the conditioned reflexes from their secondary inhibition.

Time	Stimulus	Salivary Secretion in drops during one minute
Experiment of 13th May.		
4.20 p.m.	M	11
4.26 ,,	M + R	3
4.29 ,,	,,	0
4.32 ,,	,,	0
4.35 ,,	,,	0
4.38 ,,	,,	0
4.46 ,,	M	12
Experiment of 16th May.		
4.16 p.m.	M	12
4.22 ,,	L + R	4
4.25 ,,	,,	0
4.28 ,,	,,	0
4.31 ,,	,,	0
4.34 ,,	,,	0
4.35$\frac{1}{4}$,,	M	11

These experiments show that after five repetitions of the inhibitory combination of which the metronome formed part, the minimum period necessary for the complete recovery of the positive reflex to the metronome was 7 minutes (experiment of 13th May, 4.46 p.m.). On the other hand, the minimum period required for the complete restoration of the reflex to the metronome after five repetitions of the inhibitory combination of rotating object plus visual stimulus was only 15 seconds (experiment of 15th May, 4.35¼ p.m.).

Finally, we have studied the irradiation of that form of internal inhibition which develops during the first phase of reflexes with a long delay. Owing to the peculiar character of this type of internal inhibition, occurring as part of a diphasic phenomenon, it might naturally be expected to exhibit peculiarities with regard to its after-effect, and such was actually found to be the case. The results obtained in experiments with different dogs varied considerably, and only in a certain number of cases could the irradiation of the inhibition easily be followed over the entire cortex. The experiments were performed in the following manner. The stimulus for the delayed reflex was continued only during the first part of the inhibitory phase of the delayed reflex, and was then followed either immediately or after some interval of time by a conditioned stimulus from another analyser ; the strength of this stimulus had previously been determined, and was now again tested to find the magnitude of the inhibitory after-effect. Some of these experiments are given below.

Two conditioned reflexes delayed for 30 seconds were established, the conditioned stimulus being in the first case flashes of electric lamps, and in the second tactile stimulation of the skin ; a third conditioned reflex to a metronome was delayed for 3 minutes; the inhibitory phase of this reflex was equal to 1½-2 minutes : all three reflexes were established with the help of acid.

Time	Stimulus	Salivary Secretion in drops
Experiment of 26th January.		
3.24 p.m.	Tactile stimulation	During 30″, 9
3.41 ,,	Metronome (applied during only one minute)	During 1st 30″, 0 ; 2nd 30″, 1
3.42 ,,	Tactile stimulation	During 30″, **4**
Experiment of 28th January.		
3.20 p.m.	Flashes of lamp	During 30″, 7
3.36 ,,	Metronome (applied during only one minute)	During 1st 30″, 0 ; 2nd 30″, 1
3.37 ,,	Flashes of lamp	During 30″, **2**

The result is quite definite. The inhibition evoked by the metronome in the first stage of its action has irradiated from the acoustic analyser into both the visual and tactile cutaneous analysers, diminishing their reflexes by 60-70%.

In another dog the results were almost completely reversed. The conditioned stimuli applied immediately after the inhibitory phase of the delayed reflex produced an increased positive effect. The reason of this difference was found without difficulty. In the first dog, when an interval of 2 minutes was introduced between the isolated action of the metronome and the application of the succeeding conditioned stimulus, the excitation phase of the delayed reflex never appeared during these 2 minutes. In other words, the inhibitory phase of the delayed reflex in this dog was effectively isolated from the excitatory phase. On this account, under the conditions of the experiments, the inhibition became obvious in its after-effect upon both the visual and tactile stimuli. In the second dog, on the other hand, when the same interval was introduced between the isolated action of the metronome and the application of the succeeding conditioned stimulus, the active phase of the reflex to the metronome became revealed during the interval. In this dog, therefore, under the conditions of the experiment, the effect of the positive conditioned stimuli falling within the positive phase of the delayed reflex was not diminished but considerably increased on account of summation of the two reflexes. In this second dog the excitatory process appeared earlier and was more powerful ; in other words, the separation of the inhibitory phase of the delayed reflex from the excitatory phase was not complete. It is interesting to note in this connection that in the first dog the inhibitory process in general predominated over the excitatory one.

In this and the preceding lecture I have adduced numerous experiments illustrating the spread of the inhibitory after-effect over the cerebral cortex, and it may be that to some readers I have seemed to over-stress this point. However, such multiplication of experiments was necessary in order to emphasize sufficiently how often this phenomenon occurs in simple and pure forms. The facts hitherto considered present only the fundamental interrelations between the inhibitory and excitatory processes revealed by special methods of experimentation, and often merely owing to special individual peculiarities of the animal. In many cases these fundamental interrelations are obscured by various accessory elements which render the whole process much more complex.

At the very beginning of our investigation of the irradiation of internal inhibition we were struck by the paradoxical and un-expected results of certain experiments [Dr. Krasnogorsky]. Dr. Krasnogorsky's experiments on the irradiation and concentration of differential inhibition within the cutaneous analyser were described in the preceding lecture (page 153). The preliminary test of a con-ditioned reflex to tactile stimulation of the skin at a place situated at a distance of 22 cm. from the place primarily inhibited elicited 8 drops of salivary secretion during 30 seconds, while a visual reflex gave a secretion of 5 drops. One minute after the last of three successive stimulations of the inhibitory place the visual reflex was found to be reduced to zero ; in other words, the inhibitory after-effect spreading from the tactile into the visual analyser had com-pletely overshadowed the excitatory effect of the visual stimulus. After ten minutes' interval the inhibitory place was again stimulated, now four times in succession, and on testing the tactile reflex at the place 22 cms. away, one minute after the last inhibitory stimulus, it was found to be completely free from inhibition.

Similar phenomena have been recorded in experiments on con-ditioned inhibition conducted by Dr. Chebotareva. Several con-ditioned reflexes were established in a dog to stimuli belonging to different analysers. A conditioned reflex to a metronome, when applied in conjunction with a conditioned inhibitor in the form of a visual stimulus, failed to elicit a single drop of saliva. A minute or two later the metronome applied singly (when, of course, it was reinforced) produced its full secretory effect. Conditioned reflexes to a tactile stimulus and to an odour of camphor, however, when tested shortly afterwards were still found to be considerably inhibited.

It appears, therefore, from these experiments that, contrary to our expectation, the reflexes recovered from the inhibitory after-effect in the primarily inhibited analyser sooner than in any other. However, on careful consideration of the records of the development of the various reflexes in the animals, it became obvious that these apparently anomalous results were obtained only in cases when the secondarily inhibited reflexes belonging to other analysers were but recently established or, in the case of old reflexes, when they had not been exercised for a considerable time or were weak through having been established with the help of stimuli of small intensity. Hence it follows that if a certain area which was originally under the influence of inhibition has become free from the inhibitory after-effect, it does not necessarily mean that the inhibition is also with-drawn from the regions surrounding this area : under certain definite conditions the process of excitation in some areas of the cortex may prevail over the co-existing and somewhat weakened inhibition of the surrounding areas. It is, indeed, our experience that conditioned reflexes in which the phase of initial generalization has not been succeeded by sufficient specialization, as well as reflexes of small intensity of excitation, become very easily disturbed, both by external and by internal inhibition. Those strong conditioned reflexes in which the specialization has been carried to a high degree, on the other hand, are not so easily influenced by external or internal inhibition. The question of stability and of resistance of strong and well-developed positive and negative conditioned reflexes will be considered in the thirteenth lecture.

In order to elucidate these exceptional phenomena, which appeared to contradict the more general rule for the irradiation and concentration of inhibition, the following experiments were specially conducted by Dr. Pavlova.

Conditioned reflexes were established to several stimuli belonging to different analysers, particular attention being directed to main-taining an equal number of repetitions of all the various stimuli, always, of course, with their reinforcement. After the maximum intensity of every one of the reflexes had been reached, a conditioned inhibition was developed for one of the reflexes by the usual method of non-reinforcement of the corresponding stimulus when applied in combination with the conditioned inhibitor. The strengthening of the conditioned inhibition was carried to the point when the inhibitory after-effect as tested by the application of the correspond-ing stimulus became limited to two minutes. Of course, during the period of development of the conditioned inhibition all the positive reflexes continued to be reinforced an equal number of times. At this stage of the experiment all the other stimuli, which up till then had not been combined with the conditioned inhibitor, were now for the first time tested in company with the inhibitor. It was found that these reflexes also, with only one exception, became free of inhibitory after-effect two minutes after initiation of the con-ditioned inhibition. The exception in question was a weak conditioned reflex to the appearance of a somewhat dim light, which was found to be still inhibited for some time after the recovery of the others. From these experiments it becomes clear that one and the same intensity of inhibition, when it had ceased to produce any diminution of the stronger reflexes, nevertheless exercised a definite action upon the weaker ones.

This dependence of the inhibitory after-effect upon the intensity of the secondarily inhibited reflexes is only one of several factors complicating the otherwise smooth progress of irradiation and concentration of inhibition. In the next lecture we shall describe another factor of much greater importance, producing a more profound disturbance in the progress of irradiation and concentration.

We shall turn now to a discussion of the experimental evidence with regard to the after-effect of the excitatory process ; this has not, however, yet been studied to so great an extent as the after-effect of the inhibitory process.

The first experiments upon the after-effect of excitation were conducted by Dr. M. Petrova on similar lines to the early experiments on the irradiation and concentration of inhibition. Five separate apparatuses for tactile stimulation of the skin were arranged at equal distances apart along the hind limb of a dog, the first of the series being placed over the paw and the fifth over the pelvis. In one animal the tactile stimulation of the paw (No. 1) served to evoke a conditioned reflex to acid, while in another animal it served to evoke a conditioned alimentary reflex. Owing to initial generalization of the reflex, the stimulation of the remaining places (Nos. 2, 3, 4 and 5) also evoked at first positive alimentary reflexes or defence reflexes to acid. These places, however, rapidly became differentiated by the method of contrast, giving finally a zero effect, so that only the stimulation of the paw remained positive. At the beginning of each experiment the tactile stimulation of the paw (the positive stimulus) was applied during 30 seconds, and the amount of salivary secretion was recorded during the first half and during the second half of the period of stimulation. After 30 seconds of stimulation the reflex was reinforced. Then, after some interval of time, the paw was again stimulated, but now the stimulation was continued during only the first 15 seconds, and was followed immediately by stimulation of one or another of the inhibitory places during the second 15 seconds. Results were obtained as follows. On changing the stimulus from the positive place (No. 1) to the nearest inhibitory place (No. 2) the salivary secretion during the second period of 15 seconds was diminished only slightly, or even not at all, as compared with the secretion observed during the first period of 15 seconds (action of apparatus No. 1). But when the remotest apparatus (No. 5) acted during the second period of 15 seconds, the salivary secretion was considerably diminished. Stimulation of the places Nos. 3 and 4 under identical conditions gave rise to a secretion intermediate between that evoked at places Nos. 2 and 5, the secretory effect at place No. 3 exceeding that at place No. 4.

In further experiments not only was the salivary secretion during the 15 seconds of the actual stimulation of the inhibitory places recorded, but also the entire secretory after-effect. In these experiments the difference in the effect of the nearer and the more remote stimuli was exhibited almost without exception and with great distinctness. For example, stimulation of the nearest place (No. 2) evoked a far more prolonged and greater secretion than did stimulation of the remotest place (No. 5). The following experiments illustrate this case. The dog used in these experiments had its tactile conditioned reflexes established with the use of acid.

Time	Stimulus	Salivary Secretion in drops during successive periods of 15 seconds, starting with the preliminary application of the positive conditioned stimulus No. 1		Remarks
		Period of stimulation	Secretory after-effect	

Experiment of 14th November, 1913.

2.0 p.m.	No. 1	8, 7		⎫ Reinforced
2.10 ,,	,,	7, 11		⎬
2.23 ,,	No. 1 followed by No. 2	7, **5**	**5, 3, 1, 1**	Not reinforced
2.40 ,,	No. 1	4, 9		Reinforced

Experiment of 16th November, 1913.

1.45 p.m.	No. 1	5, 9		⎫ Reinforced
2.0 ,,	,,	3, 7		⎬
2.10 ,,	No. 1 followed by No. 5	6, **2**	**1, 0, 0, 0**	Not reinforced
2.26 ,,	No. 1	2, 8		Reinforced

Time	Stimulus	Salivary Secretion in drops during successive periods of 15 seconds, starting with the preliminary application of the positive conditioned stimulus No. 1		Remarks
		Period of stimulation	Secretory after-effect	

Experiment of 19th November, 1913.

Time	Stimulus	Period of stimulation	Secretory after-effect	Remarks
1.45 p.m.	No. 1	4, 8		⎫ Reinforced
2.45 ,,	,,	6, 7		⎭
3.10 ,,	No. 1 followed by No. 2	7, 5	3, 2, 1, 0	Not reinforced
3.25 ,,	No. 1	2, 8		Reinforced
3.37 ,,	No. 5	0, 0	0, 0, 0, 0	Not reinforced

Experiment of 21st November, 1913.

Time	Stimulus	Period of stimulation	Secretory after-effect	Remarks
1.32 p.m.	No. 1	6, 12		⎫
2.32 ,,	,,	9, 15		⎬ Reinforced
3.10 ,,	,,	10, 13		⎭
3.22 ,,	No. 1 followed by No. 5	8, 4	2, 0, 0, 0	Not reinforced
3.35 ,,	No. 1	7, 11		Reinforced

Experiment of 23rd November, 1913.

Time	Stimulus	Period of stimulation	Secretory after-effect	Remarks
12.40 p.m.	No. 1	7, 11		⎫
1.0 ,,	,,	9, 13		⎬ Reinforced
1.10 ,,	,,	10, 12		⎭
1.22 ,,	No. 1 followed by No. 2	12, 8	4, 3, 1, 0	Not reinforced
1.36 ,,	No. 1	3, 9		Reinforced

Experiment of 28th November, 1913.

Time	Stimulus	Period of stimulation	Secretory after-effect	Remarks
1.30 p.m.	No. 1	7, 8		⎫ Reinforced
1.43 ,,	,,	6, 10		⎭
1.59 ,,	No. 1 followed by No. 5	8, 5	1, 0, 0, 0	⎫ Not
2.5 ,,	No. 2	0, 0	0, 0, 0, 0	⎬ reinforced
2.18 ,,	No. 1	2, 10		Reinforced

The results of these experiments are very definite. In the cases when the positive stimulus, No. 1, was succeeded by the nearest inhibitory one, No. 2, the amount of salivary secretion recorded during the first 15 seconds (action of No. 1) was in the three different experiments 7, 7, 12 drops respectively, while the secretion during the remaining period (action of No. 2 plus the secretory after-effect) was 15, 11 and 16 drops respectively. In the cases when the positive stimulus, No. 1, was succeeded by the remotest stimulus, No. 5, the secretion during the first 15 seconds amounted to 6, 8 and 8 drops respectively, while the secretion during the action of the remotest stimulus, No. 5, plus the secretion during the period of the excitatory after-effect amounted to only 3, 6 and 6 drops respectively. The total secretion subsequently to the first 15 seconds was, therefore, in the first case (with stimulus No. 2) definitely greater than during the 15 seconds' action of the positive stimulus No. 1, and in the second case (with No. 5) definitely smaller. On changing from the positive stimulus, No. 1, to the nearest inhibitory stimulus, No. 2, the secretory after-effect persisted during 45-60 seconds, while on changing to the remotest stimulus, No. 5, the secretory after-effect persisted during only 15 seconds. These results assume a still greater significance when it is remembered that the inhibitory properties of the nearest stimulus, No. 2, ought to be greater than those of the remotest stimulus, No. 5, since, as we have learned already, the more delicate the differentiation the more intense is the underlying inhibitory process. That this actually was the case was definitely established by special experiments, in which the inhibitory after-effects from Nos. 2 and 5 were tested upon the positive reflex from No. 1 and upon some conditioned stimuli from other analysers. The following is an example of the inhibitory after-effect upon the positive reflex from the place No. 1, as tested $4\frac{1}{2}$ minutes after the use of the inhibitory stimuli Nos. 2 and 5 respectively. The experiments were carried out on the same dog as before.

Time	Conditioned stimulus applied during 30 seconds	Salivary Secretion in drops during 30 seconds
3.45 p.m.	No. 1	12
3.55 ,,	,,	18
4.10 ,,	No. 2	0
4.15 ,,	No. 1	4
4.20 ,,	,,	15
4.35 ,,	No. 5	0
4.40 ,,	No. 1	12
4.45 ,,	,,	15
4.50 ,,	,,	12

The inhibitory after-effect following stimulation of place No. 2 was still very powerful after an interval of $4\frac{1}{2}$ minutes, whereas the inhibitory after-effect following stimulation of place No. 5 was negligible.

In view of the results of these further experiments, there seems to be no reason to doubt that the excitation evoked by the positive stimulus in the previous experiments exerted a greater effect on the place nearest to it than on the place most remote. The whole phenomenon must, therefore, be regarded as a result of an irradiation of excitation.

Some experiments upon the irradiation of excitation have recently been repeated by Dr. Podkopaev. The places for tactile stimulation were taken on the skin of one side of the body, the first apparatus being arranged over the fore paw and the remaining apparatuses being placed at equal distances apart along the trunk and hind limb of the dog, the last being arranged over the hind paw. Stimulation of the area over the fore paw was given the properties of a positive alimentary conditioned stimulus, while stimulations of the remaining areas were given the properties of negative stimuli. The salivary secretion was recorded during successive periods of five seconds. Usually the positive conditioned stimulus was continued during 30 seconds and was then immediately reinforced, but for the purpose of the tests the stimulus was occasionally allowed to act during only 15 seconds, and was followed by a pause of 15 seconds before the reinforcement. In this manner it was possible to follow the course of the secretion during 30 seconds when the stimulus was acting throughout, and also during 30 seconds when the stimulus was abbreviated to the first 15 seconds. With the longer stimulation the ratio of the secretion during the first 15 seconds to that during the second 15 seconds came out as $1 : 2\cdot4$; in the case of the abbreviated stimulation it came out as $1 : 1\cdot25$. In the next stage of the experiments the positive stimulus after acting during the first 15 seconds was followed immediately by an inhibitory stimulus which acted during the succeeding period of 15 seconds, and this stimulus was given by stimulation of a nearer or a remoter place. The ratio of the amount of secretion during the first 15 seconds to that during the second 15 seconds came out in the former case as $1 : 1\cdot35$, and in the latter case as $1 : 0\cdot53$. It is obvious, therefore, that in this case, as in the previous experiments, the excitatory after-effect of the positive stimulus was strong in places nearest to it and negligible in the remoter places.

Neither this last nor the preceding series of experiments permits us to determine with which phase of the movement of excitation we have to deal, whether the phase of irradiation or the phase of concentration. Experiments are at present being conducted in which the inhibitory stimuli are applied, not immediately on cessation of the positive stimulus, but after a short pause of varying length. Unfortunately, the direct experimental data concerning irradiation and concentration of excitation at our disposal are limited to the facts described above. There are, however, a number of isolated observations which have some bearing upon this subject, and these will now be described.

One of our animals—a sheep-dog—had a very exaggerated form of what might be called " the warding reflex." The experimenter [Dr. Besbokaya], who always worked with the dog in a separate room, used to prepare it for the experiment without the slightest difficulty, placing it in the stand and adjusting the various apparatuses for recording and for stimulation. Under Dr. Besbokaya's control the experiments on conditioned reflexes proceeded quite smoothly, but the moment a stranger appeared in the experimenting room the dog always developed a powerful aggressive reaction, especially if the stranger (in that case myself) took the place of the experimenter. Applying the established conditioned alimentary stimulus under these circumstances, I always obtained a secretory reflex considerably above normal, the dog consuming its food with obviously exaggerated muscular effort. This aggressive reaction evoked by my presence became diminished in intensity when I intentionally kept quite still : the only part of the reflex still remaining was the gaze of the animal, which was kept fixed on me. The conditioned alimentary stimulus now produced a much smaller salivary secretion than the normal, and sometimes even no secretion at all. As soon, however, as I relaxed my attitude, and especially if I moved about, the aggressive reaction returned in full vigour, and the salivary and motor reactions in response to the conditioned alimentary stimulus became considerably increased in their intensity. It is interesting to note that although this dog grew calm in the presence of a stranger who kept quite still, the aggressive reaction returned after each reinforcement after the end of the conditioned stimulus, the reaction continuing for some time, even though the stranger remained motionless. There appears to be only one possible explanation of this phenomenon. The powerful excitatory effect of the intruder and his movements must have irradiated over the hemispheres, and increased amongst others the excitability of that area which is related to alimentary functions. When, however, this excitation diminished on account of weakening and concentrating of the external stimulus the reverse took place, and the excitability of remoter areas became diminished as compared with the normal (effect of external inhibition). In a similar manner the eating of food temporarily heightened the excitability of the centre for the aggressive reaction.

A similar phenomenon was observed in experiments conducted [by Dr. Prorokov] with another exceptional dog. In this dog tactile stimulation of the skin evoked a peculiar and very definite motor reaction, akin to a reaction to tickling, and possibly of a sexual character. It elicited also a conditioned alimentary reflex which was abnormally powerful, exceeding any of the other conditioned alimentary reflexes to non-tactile stimuli. As a rule, tactile stimulation of the skin evoked first of all its own special motor reaction, and was then succeeded after 10-15 seconds by an exceedingly powerful alimentary motor reflex. When the special motor reaction was overcome by the use of a technique which will be discussed in the last lecture, the conditioned alimentary reflex to the tactile stimulus became reduced to a normal level, and became less powerful, for example, than homogeneous reflexes to auditory stimuli. This phenomenon must unquestionably be regarded as a further example of irradiation of excitation.

We are inclined to give a similar interpretation also to the following fact. In the case of interaction of conditioned reflexes based upon the use of different alimentary substances, the inhibition of some of them by others does not develop immediately, but only after an interval of some minutes. It is quite conceivable that at first an irradiation of excitation is initiated from the cortical point corresponding to some definite alimentary substance. The excitability of neighbouring points thereby becomes temporarily increased, and it is only afterwards, when the excitation gets weakened and concentrated, that the inhibition reveals itself [experiments of Dr. Savitch].

A similar argument can be advanced in explanation of some unexpected results obtained by Dr. Vassiliev in the course of formation of heterogeneous conditioned reflexes to thermal stimuli. A conditioned reflex to acid was established by the application of a thermal stimulus of 0° C. to the skin of the animal, and a conditioned alimentary reflex by means of a thermal stimulus of 47° C. The development of these reflexes required a considerable time, and when finally established they were found to show the following extremely interesting peculiarity. If the conditioned reflex to cold (based on acid) was repeated with reinforcement several times in succession, the alimentary conditioned reflex to heat when evoked directly afterwards became transformed into a defence reflex to acid similar to that obtained with the stimulus of cold. Reversely, cold applied after several reinforcements of the conditioned alimentary reflex to heat brought about an alimentary reaction instead of the customary reaction to acid. The fact of this transformation was quite distinct and beyond doubt, since the nature of the reflex could easily be established by, for example, observing the motor reactions of the animal, which differ considerably for the two reflexes. In the case of the alimentary reflex the dog turned towards the experimenter, dividing its gaze between him and the source of food and smacking its lips ; in the case of the reflex to acid the dog turned away from the experimenter, snorting and whining, shaking its head and making ejective movements with its tongue. Moreover, the reflexes could easily be distinguished by the composition of the saliva from the submaxillary salivary gland, which in the case of the alimentary reflex was thick and mucous, and in the case of the reflex to acid, fluid or watery. These points of difference were established in the given case with especial care. The persistent and prolonged transformation of one reflex into the other was the more strange and unexpected, since such a confusion of heterogeneous reflexes never occurs in other analysers ; for example, in the acoustic analyser, even if the two stimuli to heterogeneous reflexes differ by less than a tone no transformation occurs, although it might be thought that the difference between two neighbouring tones was of much smaller vital significance than the difference between heat and cold.

The explanation turns on a certain peculiarity in the relations of the analysers for heat and cold. As is well known the peripheral ends of these analysers are interspersed with one another over the surface of the skin. Now it has been proved experimentally by Dr. Shishlo that the cortical ends of the two analysers overlap and it is tempting, therefore, to conjecture that the cortical ends are interspersed similarly to the peripheral ends. In that case irradiation from the one analyser to the other would be facilitated and such a confusion between the reflexes as is illustrated in the above experiments can be accounted for.

I shall now return to a further consideration of a phenomenon which was referred to in the preceding lecture in connection with the analysing activity of the cortex, but which, from the point of view of its intimate mechanism, has to be dealt with in this section. This concerns the initial generalization of any recently established conditioned stimulus, representing an apparently spontaneous positive activity of stimuli which had never previously been applied, but which constitute an allied group with the stimulus which had acquired conditioned properties on account of reinforcement. As an example we may take a series of experiments on the cutaneous analyser conducted by Dr. Anrep. Six apparatuses for tactile stimulation of the skin were arranged at definite places along one side of the body. The action of apparatus No. 0 at a place on the thigh was given positive alimentary conditioned properties in a short trace reflex. The remaining places were distributed as follows :

No. 1 on the hind paw, No. 2 on the pelvis, No. 3 on the middle of the trunk, No. 4 on the shoulder, No. 5 on the fore leg, No. 6 on the front paw. Stimulation of any of the latter places produced a spontaneous conditioned secretory effect, although none of them had been combined with food ; the intensity of their secretory effect decreased very gradually with the distance from the place on the thigh, No. 0. The table gives the average figures obtained with one of the three dogs employed for these experiments. The amount of saliva is expressed in drops, each equal to 0·01 c.c. The secretion was recorded for the 30 seconds during which the stimulation lasted.

Number of place stimulated -	1	0	2	3	4	5	6
Secretion - - - -	33	53	45	39	23	21	19

The stability of generalization varies considerably in different dogs, and it is not always easy to keep it on a definite level during a series of experiments. If the stimuli were applied to new places, and reinforced every time, the reflexes would become completely generalized. On the other hand, if these stimuli remained without reinforcement an opportunity would be provided for the development of a differential inhibition. In view of this, and in order to secure more or less exact and comparable results which could be verified by repetition, the stimuli were alternately applied with and without reinforcement, or else the applications were repeated at long intervals of time (2-3 weeks).

It remains now to inquire into the intimate mechanism of generalization, and the following interpretation seems best to agree with our present knowledge. It may be assumed that each element of the receptor apparatus gains representation in the cortex of the hemispheres through its own proper central neurone, and the peripheral grouping of the receptor organs may be regarded as projecting itself in a definite grouping of nervous elements in the cortex. A nervous impulse reaching the cortex from a definite point of the peripheral receptor does not give rise to an excitation which is limited within the corresponding cortical element, but the excitation irradiates from its point of origin over the cortex, diminishing in intensity the further it spreads from the centre of excitation, exactly as we have seen in the case of inhibition. Just as the initial point of cortical excitation becomes connected with the centre of the unconditioned reflex, so also do the secondary points of cortical excitation, and this leads to the formation of many accessory reflexes. These reflexes decrease progressively in strength with increasing distance of the secondarily excited areas from the point of primary cortical excitation, since the magnitude of the conditioned reflex is rigidly determined by the intensity of excitation. This interpretation agrees with Dr. Koupalov's observation that an experimental generalization of a localized tactile reflex develops gradually and progressively, and that complete equalization of the effect of stimulating any place of the skin is only reached after a considerable time. This, of course, is only natural, since conditioned reflexes from points further removed from the primary excitation appear considerably later, the accessory tactile reflexes being much weaker to start with at the remoter places.

The explanation advanced as regards the initial generalization of simultaneous conditioned reflexes within a single analyser can be effectively applied to the type of universal generalization which is observed in long-trace reflexes (Lecture VII). In the case of the long pause between the conditioned and the unconditioned stimulus, the excitation initiated by the conditioned stimulus has time to spread over the entire cortex, and in this manner all the individual cortical points can now link up with the centre for the unconditioned reflex as soon as this becomes excited.   In the case of a short pause between the two stimuli the centre for the unconditioned reflex determines a concentration of the conditioned excitation towards itself, thus limiting any extensive irradiation over the general mass of the hemispheres.

LECTURE XI

Mutual induction of excitation and inhibition : (a) *Positive induction.* (b) *Negative induction.*

THE first aspect of the intimate nature of the cortical activity which came into our field of investigation concerned the irradiation and concentration of excitation and inhibition. Only considerably later was a second aspect of this activity discovered and also subjected to a rigorous analysis. This second aspect concerned the reinforcing effect exerted by the one process upon the other, both in respect to the cortical points directly excited or inhibited and those into which the excitation or inhibition has irradiated.

This effect will be referred to as *induction*—a term introduced by E. Hering and C. S. Sherrington. Induction is mutual, or reciprocal, excitation leading to increased inhibition and inhibition leading to increased excitation. The former is referred to as " the phase of negative induction," and the latter as " the phase of positive induction," or, briefly, " negative " and " positive " induction respectively.

The phenomenon of induction was observed many years ago, but, as so frequently happens in scientific research, its full significance was for a long time obscured in our minds by the idea of a smoothness of propagation of nervous processes, and those irregularities which are now known to be the result of induction, were always attributed to various casual disturbing influences, the danger of which is so great in our investigations. The first indication of induction was found in the experiments of Dr. Kogan, in which, as was shown in the ninth lecture (page 161), the stimulation of a place on the skin following *immediately* upon the complete extinction of another definite place much further removed revealed almost invariably a state of *increased* excitability. No systematic investigation of this phenomenon was, however, attempted, until recently some experiments of Dr. Foursikov focused attention upon the matter and led to its energetic investigation. The following is one of the earlier experiments of Dr. Foursikov.

A conditioned alimentary reflex was established to tactile stimulation of the front paw. A similar tactile stimulation of the hind paw was differentiated, the inhibition being complete, so that not a single drop of saliva appeared in response to stimulation of the inhibitory place.

Time	Conditioned stimulus applied during 30 seconds	Salivary Secretion in drops during 30 seconds	Latent period of the salivary reaction in seconds
4.20 p.m.	Front paw	8	3
4.36 ,,	,,	7·5	3
4.45 ,,	Hind paw	0	–
4.45½ ,,	Front paw	12	2
4.58 ,,	,,	5	8
5.10 ,,	,,	6·5	5

It is seen that the secretory effect was increased almost 50% when the positive conditioned stimulus was applied immediately after the termination of the inhibitory stimulus, and that the latent period of the reflex was definitely shortened. Moreover, the intensity of the motor alimentary reaction of the animal was also considerably increased. Evidently, under the influence of the inhibitory stimulus (hind paw), the corresponding cortical area develops a state of inhibition, which is, as we know, retained for some time after the termination of the inhibitory stimulus. On the other hand, the cortical area corresponding to the positive stimulus (front paw), on termination of the inhibitory stimulus must be temporarily in a state of increased excitation. In this instance the interpretation is helped by the spatial relation of the two points of stimulation. The problem, however, becomes more complicated when both the positive and negative stimuli act upon one and the same cortical point, as, for example, in cases of differentiation of a stimulus according to its intensity or according to its continuous or interrupted character, or as regards the frequency of interruption in one and the same type of stimulus. The phenomenon of induction can, nevertheless, be seen in these cases also. The following is another experiment taken from Dr. Foursikov's research :

A conditioned alimentary reflex is established to a rate of 76 beats per minute of a metronome, and from this a rate of 186 beats per minute is completely differentiated, both with regard to the secretory and motor components of the reflex.

Time	Conditioned stimulus applied during 30 seconds	Salivary Secretion in drops during 30 seconds	Latent period of the salivary reaction in seconds
5.5 p.m.	76 beats	5·5	5
5.15 ,,	,,	6	5
5.24 ,,	186 beats	0	–
5.24½ ,,	76 beats	8	2
5.43 ,,	,,	5·5	5
5.51 ,,	,,	6	5

The positive stimulus tested immediately after the application of the inhibitory stimulus showed an increase of 30% in the secretory reflex; the motor reaction was correspondingly intensified, while the latent period of the secretory reflex was considerably shortened.

Another example of positive induction may be given from a research by Dr. Kalmykov: a positive conditioned alimentary reflex was established to strong light, and from this a reflex to weak light was completely differentiated.

Time	Conditioned stimulus applied during 30 seconds	Salivary Secretion in drops during 30 seconds	Latent period of the Salivary reaction in seconds
1.46 p.m.	Strong light	7	15
1.55 ,,	,,	7	13
2.5 ,,	Weak light	0	—
2.5½ ,,	Strong light	10	4
2.14 ,,	,,	5·5	13
2.24 ,,	,,	4	11

In this experiment also the positive stimulus, tested immediately after the inhibitory stimulus, showed an increase in the secretory reflex of 40%; the latent period was considerably shortened and the alimentary motor reaction was distinctly increased.

It may be questioned, in the light of the foregoing experiments, whether the phenomenon of positive induction does not really represent a form of dis-inhibition. The plausibility of such an interpretation is obvious, since in experiments on positive induction a new condition is introduced in the *immediateness* of the replacement of the negative conditioned stimulus by the positive one. This new condition might play as potent a rôle as any other fresh change in the environment in evoking an investigatory reaction, so producing dis-inhibition. However, apart from the many points of difference in detail between the phenomena of positive induction and dis-inhibition, this explanation is definitely disproved by the character of the motor reaction of the animal. This never at any time, even from the very beginning, manifests itself as a general investigatory reaction, but always as a distinctly specialized reaction corresponding to the definite positive conditioned reflex.

The duration of induction varies from several seconds to one or two minutes. The cause of this variation has not yet been sufficiently investigated.

After this bare statement of facts, we must now proceed to a more detailed study of positive induction, especially as its occurrence was by no means so constant as might be inferred from the above account. The subject is not even yet entirely under our control, but a number of conditions on which induction depends can already be indicated.

The first of these conditions was revealed accidentally. In certain experiments with a conditioned alimentary stimulus of 100 beats of a metronome per minute Dr. Kalmykov regularly observed a positive induction on testing the positive stimulus immediately after the withdrawal of the inhibitory stimulus of 160 beats per minute. However, when Dr. Kalmykov tried to demonstrate the experiment in the presence of several visitors, including myself, the results obtained were quite different : instead of the customary augmentation, the application of the inhibitory stimulus immediately before the positive one now caused a pronounced diminution in the positive reflex. This unexpected deviation was interpreted as follows. Since the dog was not sufficiently isolated from the sounds produced by the experimenter and the visitors, their conversation must have acted as an external inhibitory stimulus weakening the differentiation, and at the beginning even distinctly dis-inhibiting it. Positive induction could not, therefore, be exhibited at any time during the experiment. The record of this experiment is given on p. 192.

Time	Conditioned stimulus applied during 30 seconds	Salivary secretion in drops during 30 seconds	Latent period of the salivary reaction in seconds
1.27 p.m.	100 beats	7·5	9
1.40 ,,	,,	7	16
1.47 ,,	160 beats (inhibitory stimulus)	4	12
1.55 ,,	100 beats	3	21
2.5 ,,	,,	11·5	7
2.15 ,,	160 beats (inhibitory stimulus)	0	—
2.15½ ,,	100 beats	0	—
2.21 ,,	,,	11	6
2.33 ,,	160 beats (inhibitory stimulus)	0	—
2.33½ ,,	100 beats	2	27
2.42 ,,	160 beats (inhibitory stimulus)	0	—
2.42½ ,,	100 beats	2	26
2.50 ,,	,,	10·5	7

It is seen that the differentiation which previously to this experiment was complete became disturbed on its first application in the presence of visitors, 4 drops of salivary secretion being now obtained (1.47 p.m.).   Later, the inhibitory stimulus applied singly gave the usual zero secretion, but throughout the experiment the inhibitory stimulus never exhibited any power of positive induction ;   the positive reflex tested immediately after the withdrawal of the inhibitory stimulus underwent a diminution, and was therefore influenced immediately by an inhibitory after-effect instead of the usual temporary positive induction (2.15½ p.m., 2.33½ p.m., 2.42½ p.m.).

It may be concluded from the foregoing that the weakening of the inhibitory process leads to the disappearance of induction, so that now the inhibitory after-effect begins to develop immediately, without the intervention of a preliminary heightening of excitation. In order further to test this interpretation Dr. Kalmykov reduced the intensity of the differential inhibition by intentionally subjecting it to external inhibition.   For this purpose the experiment was preceded by the introduction of a rejectable substance into the mouth of the dog, when, as in the case just described, no induction could be observed throughout the experiment. It may be concluded, therefore, that the manifestation of positive induction depends upon some definite intensity of inhibition.

The second condition upon which the development of induction depends was also brought out in experiments on the same dog.

Differential inhibition having been established to the metronome beating at a rate of 160 per minute, it was practised for special purposes a great number of times in the course of several months without testing for induction. A more delicate differentiation to a rate of 112 beats per minute was now established (the rate of the positive stimulation being in both cases 100 beats per minute). When this finer discrimination became absolute, tests for induction were performed with the following definite result:

Time	Conditioned stimulus applied during 30 seconds	Salivary Secretion in drops during 30 seconds	Latent period of the salivary reaction in seconds
1.17 p.m.	100 beats	12	19
1.26 ,,	112 beats	0	—
1.26½ ,,	100 beats	21	6
1.36 ,,	,,	7	22

The inductive action of the new and more delicate differentiation resulted in an immediate increase of the positive secretory reflex by 75% and in a considerable shortening of the latent period. When, however, the older and coarser differentiation of 160 beats was now tested, it was surprising to find that no trace of inductive action could be observed. We thought it possible that this result might have been due to interruption in the practice of the coarser differentiation while the new and more delicate differentiation was being established, and therefore we now practised the two differentiations alternately for periods of 10-15 days each. This procedure did not, however, change the course of events, as is shown in the following tables:

Time	Conditioned stimulus applied during 30 seconds	Salivary Secretion in drops during 30 seconds	Latent period of the salivary reaction in seconds
Experiment of 17th April.			
11.11 a.m.	100 beats	16	8
11.19 ,,	112 beats	0	–
11.19½ ,,	100 beats	20	2
11.30 ,,	,,	0	–
11.37 ,,	,,	4	26

Time	Conditioned stimulus applied during 20 seconds	Salivary Secretion in drops during 20 seconds	Latent period of the salivary reaction in seconds
	Experiment of 20th April.		
11.37 a.m.	100 beats	13	9
11.45 ,,	160 beats	0	–
11.45½ ,,	100 beats	5	23
11.55 ,,	,,	6	23
12.2 p.m.	,,	6	17

It is seen that the new and finer differentiation produced a distinct though temporary effect of positive induction (11.19½ a.m.), whereas the older and coarser one was followed directly by an inhibitory after-effect. On continuation of the experiments the effect of positive induction of the finer differentiation also began to weaken.

In similar experiments conducted by Dr. Frolov a modification was introduced by employing an inhibitory stimulus of greater intensity than the stimulus to the positive conditioned reflex. The tone D of Max Kohl's tone variator, damped to different degrees, provided the stimuli in these experiments. Three intensities of the tone were employed. The weakest served for the positive conditioned stimulus, while the remaining intensities of the tone were given inhibitory properties, the strongest tone being the first to be contrasted. When this differentiation became definitely established a test was made of its effect in producing positive induction :

Time	Conditioned stimulus applied during 30 seconds	Salivary Secretion in drops during 30 seconds
1.28 p.m.	Weak tone	12
1.33 ,,	Strong tone	3
1.42 ,,	Weak tone	11
1.56 ,,	,,	11
2.8 ,,	Strong tone	0
2.8½ ,,	Weak tone	17
2.18 ,,	,,	7

On immediate transition from the inhibitory tone to the weak positive one, the effect of the latter was found to be increased by

50% (2.8½ p.m.). The differentiation to the strong tone was now repeatedly practised for over a month. When tested at the end of this period it was found to have lost completely its effect of positive induction :

Time	Conditioned stimulus applied during 30 seconds	Salivary Secretion in drops during 30 seconds
1.41 p.m	Weak tone	8
1.57 ,,	,,	6
2.3 ,,	,,	9
2.11 ,,	Strong tone	0
2.11½ ,,	Weak tone	**6**
2.24 ,,	,,	6·5

The next stage in the experiment was the formation of a differentiation to the tone of intermediate intensity. This finer differentiation was already nearing completion on its nineteenth application. The following table gives the results of a test for positive induction :

Time	Conditioned stimulus applied during 30 seconds	Salivary Secretion in drops during 30 seconds
1.15 p.m.	Weak tone	12·5
1.19 ,,	,,	11
1.29 ,,	Medium tone	0
1.29½ ,,	Weak tone	**17**
1.45 ,,	,,	9

Exactly as in the preceding experiments by Dr. Kalmykov, the older and coarser differentiation had lost its inductive effect after prolonged practice, while the new and more delicate differentiation, so soon as definitely established, exhibited an intense effect of positive induction.

The natural conclusion to be drawn from these observations is that positive induction represents a temporary, phasic phenomenon, which is associated with the period of establishment of new relations in the nervous system ; induction makes its appearance only with the maximal development of a given cortical inhibition, and disappears after the inhibition has become finally stabilized. This general rule, however, is not without exceptions, since in some cases induction is maintained during long periods of time without showing any signs of subsequent diminution. So far as can be judged from the available data, this depends on whether the rapid replacement of the inhibitory, by the excitatory, stimulus affects one and the same cortical area, as in the experiments just described, or whether the two stimuli affect two cortical areas more or less remote, as in the experiments upon the cutaneous analyser. The conditions under which induction assumes a more permanent character can be settled only by further experiments, such as are at present in progress.

It may, however, be added that a considerable number of experiments were conducted with differentiation of the rate of rhythmic tactile stimulation of some definite area of the skin. In these experiments a high rate of stimulation acted as the positive stimulus, while a low rate of stimulation acted as the inhibitory one. So far we have been unable to observe any positive induction with these stimuli, on rapid transition from the inhibitory to the excitatory one. In all cases there was only an immediate development of an inhibitory after-effect.

Negative induction—*i.e.* an intensification of inhibition under the influence of preceding excitation—was also observed several years ago, but was always wrongly interpreted, and it only received adequate recognition in some quite recent experiments. In these experiments, which were carried out by Dr. Stroganov, the phenomenon of negative induction was repeatedly investigated in many dogs, and can now be estimated at its full value.

Negative induction was first met with in investigations on the destruction of internal inhibition. Some experiments of this type conducted by Dr. Krjishkovsky dealt especially with the destruction of conditioned inhibition. A tone employed singly was given the properties of a positive conditioned stimulus to acid, while in combination with a tactile cutaneous stimulus it served as a stimulus in a conditioned inhibition. The destruction of the inhibition was attempted by reversing the process employed in its formation, the application of the inhibitory combination being alternated with applications of the positive conditioned stimulus singly, but both being this time reinforced. The results obtained were quite unexpected. In spite of ten applications of the inhibitory combination with reinforcement by acid in the course of three days, its inhibitory properties remained undisturbed. These experiments are represented in the following tables :

Time	Conditioned stimulus applied during 30 seconds	Salivary Secretion in drops during 30 seconds	

Experiment of 15th *October,* 1907.

10.24 a.m.	Tone	11	
10.38 ,,	Combination	0	
10.59 ,,	Tone	13	
11.11 ,,	Combination	0	Reinforced in
11.27 ,,	Tone	10	all cases by
11.40 ,,	Combination	0	injection of
11.58 ,,	Tone	11	acid into
12.13 p.m.	Combination	0	the mouth.
12.25 ,,	Tone	10	
12.39 ,,	Combination	0	
12.55 ,,	Tone	12	

Experiment of 16th *October,* 1907.

1.34 p.m.	Tone	8	Reinforced in
1.52 ,,	Combination	0	all cases by
2.41 ,,	Tone	9	injection of
2.55 ,,	Combination	0	acid into
3.10 ,,	Tone	7	the mouth.

Experiment of 17th *October,* 1907.

10.55 a.m.	Tone	7	
11.5 ,,	Combination	0	Reinforced in
11.25 ,,	Tone	6	all cases by
11.35 ,,	Combination	0	injection of
11.53 ,,	Tone	8	acid into
12.6 p.m.	Combination	0	the mouth.
12.19 ,,	Tone	9	

Since this method failed to produce a destruction of the conditioned inhibition, another technique was used on the day following the last experiment. The combination, which remained always reinforced, was now repeatedly applied without any intervening applications of the positive conditioned stimulus singly. Destruction of the inhibition was now rapidly obtained.

Experiment of 18*th October*, 1907.

Time	Conditioned stimulus applied during 30 seconds	Salivary Secretion in drops during 30 seconds	
10.42 a.m.	Tone	10	
10.52 ,,	Combination	0	Reinforced in
11.4 ,,	,,	3	all cases by
11.17 ,,	,,	4	injection of
11.30 ,,	,,	6	acid.
11.41 ,,	,,	6	
11.54 ,,	,,	8	

Although the difference between the results of the two methods seemed obvious enough, the suggestion offered itself that the destruction which developed so rapidly with the second method had been facilitated by the previous reinforcements in the earlier period of alternate application. In order to eliminate this possibility, the inhibitory combination was re-established and practised during a period of over one year, when the second method for the destruction was again applied, the result being as follows :

Experiment of 22*nd November*, 1908.

Time	Conditioned stimulus applied during 30 seconds	Salivary Secretion in drops during 30 seconds	
10.43 a.m.	Tone	8	
10.57 ,,	Combination	0	
11.9 ,,	,,	0	Reinforced in
11.23 ,,	,,	1	all cases by
11.35 ,,	,,	3	injection of
11.49 ,,	,,	5	acid.
12.3 p.m.	,,	10	
12.25 ,,	Tone	14	

These experiments clearly demonstrate an essential difference between the two methods, but, as has already been said, the apparent anomaly presented by the first method remained for many years without any satisfactory explanation, until the question was re-investigated by Dr. Stroganov, who worked with differential inhibition. Conditioned alimentary reflexes were established in four dogs, differentiations being established for musical tones of differing pitch and for different rates of metronome beats. A pronounced difference in the rate of destruction of the inhibitory process by the two methods was clearly exhibited in all the dogs, without any exception. In the case of repeated application of the inhibitory stimulus with reinforcement, destruction of the inhibition was obtained after only a few applications ; in the case of regular alternation of the inhibitory stimulus with the positive conditioned stimulus, on the other hand, both being followed by reinforcement, the destruction of inhibition was very much delayed, and appeared only after a great number of applications. In the different animals employed in this research sometimes the one and sometimes the other method of destruction was used first, and in every case the two methods were repeated many times with each animal. The differentiations were, of course, always well re-established before the succeeding experimental destruction. In addition, several important variations in the experiments were made. The first variation consisted in the application of the positive stimulus after the differential inhibition had been almost altogether abolished by the use of the second method of destruction ; it was found that even one single application was sufficient partially or fully to restore the inhibition (12.6 p.m. in the table below).

A rate of 120 beats of the metronome per minute served for a positive conditioned alimentary stimulus. A rate of 60 beats per minute was firmly established as a stimulus to a differential inhibition. During 41 applications within a period of 40 days it did not elicit a single drop of saliva.

Time	Conditioned stimulus applied during 30 seconds	Salivary Secretion in drops during 30 seconds	
11.25 a.m.	60 beats	0	
11.30 ,,	,,	0	All the stimuli
11.42 ,,	,,	3	were accom-
11.49 ,,	,,	4	panied by re-
11.56 ,,	120 beats	8½	inforcement.
12.6 p.m.	60 beats	0	

A second variation of the experiment consisted in making three successive applications of the positive conditioned stimulus just before the destruction of the differential inhibition by the second method was begun. This preliminary administration of the positive stimuli caused an unusual retardation of the destruction, which now required an additional five or six applications of the inhibitory stimulus.

In another dog the same positive and inhibitory conditioned stimuli were employed, and although the differentiation in this dog was less stable and, therefore, subject more easily to dis-inhibition, a similar delay was observed in its destruction.

Time	Conditioned stimulus applied during 30 seconds	Salivary Secretion in drops during 30 seconds	
12.1 p.m.	120 beats	9	
12.10 ,,	,,	11	
12.21 ,,	,,	5	
12.31 ,,	60 beats	0	All the stimuli were accompanied by reinforcement.
12.43 ,,	,,	0	
12.52 ,,	,,	0	
12.56 ,,	,,	0	
1.2 ,,	,,	$2\frac{1}{2}$	
1.9 ,,	,,	$2\frac{1}{2}$	

In a third variation of the experiment, after the destruction had been carried by the method of alternation to such a degree as to be already appreciable, four or five applications of the positive stimulus in succession were sufficient to reverse this effect, re-establishing the inhibition.

Another method of experiment for the demonstration of negative induction was employed by Dr. Prorokov, who made use of an old observation that the positive conditioned reflex response which was evoked second in an experiment frequently showed the greatest secretory effect. This was most probably owing to an increased excitability of the alimentary centre following on the first reinforcement with the unconditioned reflex; on this account a recently established, but not yet quite stable, inhibitory stimulus is frequently disturbed when applied in an experiment immediately after the first application of the unconditioned stimulus, the reflex being partially dis-inhibited. When several positive conditioned alimentary reflexes are present, and only one of them is associated with a differentiation, it can be observed that if one of the independent conditioned reflexes is applied first in a given experiment, the reflex corresponding to the differentiated inhibitory stimulus applied second is frequently considerably dis-inhibited. When, on the other hand, an experiment begins with the application of the positive one of two differentiated stimuli, the effect of the negative stimulus when applied second is but rarely, and then only slightly, disturbed. The actual experiments of Dr. Prorokov were carried out as follows. A rate of 144 beats of a metronome per minute served as a positive conditioned alimentary stimulus, while a frequency of 72 beats per minute was differentiated from it. The sound of a buzzer served as a further positive alimentary stimulus. When the buzzer was applied first in the experiment, and the inhibitory stimulus of the metronome second, the reflex to the metronome was dis-inhibited in 8 cases out of 12, the maximum disinhibition being 72%. When, however, the inhibitory rate of the metronome was applied after a preliminary application of the positive rate, dis-inhibition was obtained in only two cases out of 12, and it never exceeded 20%. The two procedures were always conducted in different experiments alternately, in order to preclude any effect of an increase in the stability of the differential inhibition following on repeated contrasts. The results show that, at any rate in some cases, the effect of negative induction is more especially connected with the positive stimulus to which a differentiation has been established, any other positive conditioned stimulus, even though it belongs to the same analyser, having but a small, or even no, effect of negative induction upon the inhibitory stimulus of the differentiated pair.

The two forms of experiment just described leave no doubt that under certain conditions the generation of an excitation intensifies a succeeding inhibition.

The recognition of the actual existence of negative induction naturally led us to inquire whether the effect which had previously been described under the name of external inhibition was in essence a form of a negative induction, in which the excitation initiated by extra stimuli falling upon the cortex induced a greater or less degree of inhibition in the surrounding points. The investigation is, however, somewhat difficult, since it is necessary to determine whether the external inhibition is a cortical phenomenon, or whether it takes place entirely in the lower centres of the brain, seeing that in the case of external inhibition the centres of two different unconditioned reflexes are involved. From what is known with regard to the functions of the lower parts of the central nervous system, it must undoubtedly be assumed that in the case of external inhibition of conditioned reflexes an interaction of an inhibitory character does occur between the centres of the two unconditioned reflexes. It must be ascertained, however, whether in the case of external inhibition there is not also a similar interaction between the various points of the cortex, and this is where the difficulties appear. An attempt was made to overcome them in experiments by Dr. Foursikov, the actual experiments being performed in the following way. Two conditioned reflexes based on different unconditioned ones were established, the one alimentary and the other a defence reflex to a strong electric stimulation of the skin. The conditioned stimulus to the defence reflex was applied, and as soon as the defence reaction appeared the conditioned defence stimulus was replaced by the conditioned alimentary stimulus. In the majority of cases the conditioned alimentary reflex suffered inhibition in a greater or less degree. Since, however, the defence reaction was present, it must be assumed that the unconditioned centre for the defence reaction was in a state of excitation, and therefore, that the possibility of an interaction of the unconditioned centres was not eliminated in these experiments. Although, however, the experiments in this form were inconclusive, they provided occasion for an observation which justified the assumption that in some cases an interaction in the form of a negative induction must also exist between the cortical points corresponding to the two conditioned reflexes. It was noticed that after the establishment of the conditioned defence reflex, the older conditioned alimentary reflex when it belonged to a different analyser suffered no diminution in intensity. When the conditioned stimuli for the two reflexes were taken from the same analyser, the establishment of the conditioned defence reflex led to a prolonged diminution in the magnitude of the conditioned alimentary reflex. Moreover, when both the alimentary and defence stimuli were related to different points of the cutaneous analyser, it was found that after the establishment of the conditioned defence reflex a diminution in the strength of the conditioned alimentary reflex was found only for those alimentary points nearest to the one which had been given properties as a conditioned stimulus to the defence reflex, the reflexes for more remote alimentary points retaining their full magnitude. Now, if the external inhibition had been confined to the centres of the unconditioned reflexes, such relations would not have been found in the cortical analysers. These observations render it highly probable that external inhibition can take place as a purely cortical phenomenon, of the same nature as negative induction, and that external inhibition can, therefore, be identified with internal inhibition. It may be noted that the nearest point associated with the alimentary reflex did not under these circumstances manifest any properties peculiar to the point for the defence reaction, and no motor defence reaction ever accompanied the alimentary reflex. At present a series of experiments is being conducted with the object of securing more direct evidence on this point.

There can be no doubt that the phenomenon of mutual induction described above provides a physiological basis for the large group of contrast phenomena described in connection with the physiology of the sense organs. Here, therefore, we are confronted with a further illustration of the successful application of the objective method to the study of problems hitherto considered to be exclusively within the domain of subjective investigation.

LECTURE XII

Interaction of irradiation and concentration with induction.

THE last three lectures were devoted to the irradiation of excitation and inhibition in the cerebral cortex and to their mutual induction. Irradiation and concentration on the one hand, and induction on the other, were dealt with separately, as if they were completely independent. In actual fact, however, it is plain that these processes are superimposed on and interact with one another. Cases of the apparently isolated existence of irradiation and concentration of either excitation or inhibition without the simultaneous presence of induction can only be regarded as exceptional, and must be interpreted either as being an expression of some definite phase of the development of these processes, or as an individual peculiarity of the nervous organization of the experimental animal. It is probable, also, that, at least in some cases, the interpretation of experiments upon irradiation and concentration was simplified artificially, since at first the existence of mutual induction was not thought of. Moreover, in the initial phases of our investigation the whole problem presented such overwhelming and chaotic complexity that many sides of the subject were intentionally ignored. We had to disregard many points, and had to obviate specially difficult problems, replacing dogs which for some reason were unsuitable or presented complex relations difficult to trace. At the present time, however, as a result of many years' experience, special attention can be directed to any new fact or any new peculiarity observed in any individual animal, and such peculiarities now raise fresh problems for investigation.

The mutual relations of irradiation and concentration of the two nervous processes with their mutual induction are exceedingly complex, and a complete knowledge of their interrelations has not yet been attained. The data available on this subject at present do not lend themselves to systematic arrangement, but there is sufficient material to merit consideration.

The simplest case, which will be given first, is taken from an experiment by Dr. Kreps, who worked upon the tactile analyser.

Positive conditioned reflexes were established to tactile stimulation of two places on the thigh (1 and 2), one on the abdomen (3), one on the chest (4), and one on the shoulder (5) ; a place on the fore leg of the animal was completely differentiated from the others, and acted, therefore, as an inhibitory stimulus. All the positive stimuli were equalized as regards the magnitude of their effect. The actual experiments were conducted in the following manner. At the beginning of each experiment the normal magnitude of the secretory reaction for a given positive stimulus was determined ; further on in the experiment the effect of the same positive stimulus was tested again, either immediately or at various intervals of time after the termination of the inhibitory stimulus. This process was repeated with all the rest of the positive stimuli, the whole series of experiments taking a period of about five months for completion. The results are summarized in the two following tables, in which the magnitudes of the positive conditioned reflexes for the different places are expressed as percentages of their normal value, as determined in every experiment prior to the use of the inhibitory stimulus.

First Table.

	0	5 sec.	15 sec.	30 sec.	1 min.	2 min.	3 min.	5 min.
Place 1 -	130	—	—	57	68	70	71	100
,, 2 -	125	—	—	48	70	64	73	98
,, 3 -	125	—	—	59	73	84	77	100
,, 4 -	131	—	—	58	60	75	73	100
,, 5 -	126	—	—	56	64	89	86	100
Average -	127	—	—	56	67	76	76	100

Second Table.

	0	5 sec.	15 sec.	30 sec.	1 min.	2 min.	3 min.	5 min.
Place 1 -	138	123	92	53	71	100	85	100
,, 2 -	141	117	92	64	67	110	—	—
,, 3 -	127	—	97	65	98	112	105	98
,, 4 -	145	123	100	77	88	95	81	—
,, 5 -	127	—	90	80	100	105	106	110
Average -	136	121	94	68	85	108	94	102

The first vertical column gives the number of the positive place of stimulation, while the upper horizontal row indicates the interval of time between the end of the inhibitory and the beginning of the positive stimulus. The first table represents the average figures for the total number of experiments during the whole period of investigation ; the second table gives the average figures only for the last month of the investigation, the intervals of 5 and 15 seconds having been employed during the latter period only.

These experiments show that when the positive stimulus is applied immediately after the termination of the inhibitory stimulus its effect is invariably increased, when it is applied after an interval of 15 seconds its effect is below mormal, and when applied towards the end of 30 seconds its effect is minimal ; only towards the end of the 5th minute is complete recovery of its normal effect obtained (first table). Thus the application of the inhibitory stimulus is followed in the first place by an effect of positive induction ; this is succeeded by an irradiation of inhibition, which gradually disappears so that the effect of the positive stimulus returns to normal again. A similar replacement of positive induction by an inhibitory after-effect might also have been noticed by the reader in experiments given in the previous lecture, when the phenomenon of positive induction was first described (see especially experiment on page 193).

Returning to the experiment described above, the following particulars should be noted. While the magnitude of positive induction increased somewhat towards the later period of the investigation (second table), the inhibitory after-effect diminished, both as regards its duration (being now confined within an interval of two minutes), and as regards the extent of the irradiation (being more obvious at the two positive places nearer to the inhibitory one). The latter phenomenon is a repetition of a fact which has already been discussed in the earlier lectures in connection with the after-effect of different types of internal inhibition.

In the lecture on the irradiation of inhibition attention was drawn to an observation made by Dr. Kogan, that in one of his dogs the complete extinction of the tactile conditioned stimulus in one place was always immediately succeeded by an increased excitability—i.e. positive induction—in the place which was furthest away from it. This phenomenon has been studied in greater detail by Dr. Podkopaev in a series of experiments in which the result of a single non-reinforcement (i.e. the first step in extinction) of a conditioned tactile alimentary reflex was investigated. Conditioned alimentary reflexes were established in a dog to tactile stimulation of several places on one side of the body, all of which were spaced out along a line commencing in front at the lower part of the fore limb, extending along the whole length of the trunk, and finishing at the lower part of the hind limb. All the places were equalized as regards the magnitude of the positive conditioned effect. Every experiment commenced by stimulating some definite place, in order to determine the normal magnitude of the reflex. The stimulation of the same or another place (at a distance of 1, 43 or 89 cms.) was now applied without reinforcement ; then the particular place which had been stimulated first in the experiment was tested again at intervals of from 45 secs. to 12 mins. The experiment was concluded by testing any of the remaining places, in order to confirm the normal positive effect for the given day. Experiments were conducted with intervals of 4-5 days, in order to ensure a more or less stationary condition of the inhibition with respect to its after-effect. However, this expectation was not fulfilled, since the inhibition became more and more centred around the cortical point of its origin as the experiments proceeded, and on this account it is necessary to represent the general results in the form of three tables for three consecutive series of experiments. In the dog on which these experiments were carried out, the magnitude of the positive conditioned effect was so constant that it was possible to utilize each separate experiment instead of taking the mean of several experiments. In the tables given on page 208 the magnitude of the reflex is represented in percentages of the normal positive effect for each day. The intervals of 45 secs., 1 and 3 mins. are given only in the third table, since only at this period of the experiments did the flow of saliva after administration of the non-reinforced conditioned stimulus stop in time enough to allow of a determination of the after-effect of extinction at earlier periods.

It is seen from these tables that at the beginning of the experiments (first table) the inhibition spread to the furthermost place and was still obvious 12 minutes after the extinction. Later (second table) the inhibition became limited within a distance of 43 cm., and after 4 minutes was of smaller intensity than the inhibition occurring in the preceding table after so long as 12 minutes. It can further be observed from the second table that at the remoter places there was sometimes, in the later intervals, an increase, instead of a decrease, of the effect as compared with its normal magnitude. Finally, in the last phase (third table), the inhibitory after-effect could be observed only in the primarily extinguished place, and this at variable periods of time, whereas in the remaining places, with the exception during the first minute of the remotest place, there was either an increase above the normal, or a return to the normal magnitude of the positive effect. The increased positive effect was most probably due to positive induction, which could be detected first at the places more remote from the starting-point of the inhibition, but only after a considerable period of time following extinction.

Interval of time	Distance from the place subjected to extinction			
	0 cm.	1 cm.	43 cms.	89 cms.

First Table.

4 mins.	67	$54\frac{1}{2}$	$53\frac{1}{2}$	61
8 ,,	85	80	65	$52\frac{1}{2}$
12 ,,	$77\frac{1}{2}$	$82\frac{1}{2}$	93	83

Second Table.

4 mins.	87	$88\frac{1}{2}$	94	100
8 ,,	100	$90\frac{1}{2}$	111	89
12 ,,	$96\frac{1}{2}$	100	100	118

Third Table.

45 secs.	$51\frac{1}{2}$	112	100	85
1 min.	100	117	112	71
3 mins.	$91\frac{1}{2}$	115	100	$113\frac{1}{2}$
4 ,,	100	100	100	100
8 ,,	74	100	100	100
12 ,,	100	100	100	100

The magnitude of the reflexes is expressed in percentages of the normal value.

However, the effect of positive induction gradually makes itself felt at places nearer to the starting-point of the inhibition, and appears earlier after the incipient extinction. In other words, both as regards time and space, positive induction gradually overcomes and supersedes the inhibitory process.

The experiments just described present some interesting details. Firstly, they demonstrate the extreme sensitivity of the cortical elements : the effect of a single non-reinforcement exercising over a large region of the cortex a profound influence lasting for a considerable time (more than 12 minutes). Secondly, they afford a further example of the extreme delicacy and lability of physiological processes in the cerebral hemispheres : a relatively small influence repeated at intervals so long as 4-5 days causes a profound change in the general course of events (rapid diminution of inhibitory after-effect). Lastly, it can easily be observed that the state of different cortical points manifests a definite rhythmic undulation, both with respect to time and to distribution of inhibition. Thus in the third table the primarily extinguished place was alternately under the influence of, and free from, inhibition during 12 minutes, and a similar rhythmic oscillation was also observed in space, namely, in the distribution of excitation and inhibition in the cerebral cortex at any given moment. This fact, which is of considerable importance, will be referred to frequently in the further course of these lectures. It should be regarded as a natural result of the interaction and mutual adjustment of the two opposite nervous processes of excitation and inhibition— just as the waves of the third degree on a blood pressure curve represent the result of the interaction of pressor and depressor influences.

In some further experiments on the same dog, in which extinction was not restricted to a single non-reinforcement but was carried to the first zero, a similar undulation was observed, but only at the place nearest to the one undergoing extinction. No such undulations were apparent at more remote places. The results of these experiments are presented in the following table :

	Inhibitory after-effect of extinction to the first zero : magnitude of the reflex tested at different time intervals after the last inhibitory stimulus (expressed as percentage of normal response)												
	0″	10″	30″	1′	3′	5′	8′	12′	15′	20′	25′	30′	40′
Place nearest to the one undergoing extinction (distance 1 cm.)	44	12	—	8	41	57	60	16	59	75	88	75	100
Remoter place (89 cm. from the one undergoing extinction)	66½	29	32	40	50	—	73	70	71	100	—	—	—

It is possible that the steady level of the reflex at the remoter place, which remained unaltered for 7 minutes (8th to 15th minutes), could be regarded as some expression of an undulation, especially since it corresponded to the period of a wave of inhibition at the nearest place.

Dr. Andréev has observed similar undulations in another dog. In these experiments four apparatuses for tactile stimulation of the skin were arranged along the hind limb of the animal from the upper part of the thigh to the lower part of the leg. These places are indicated in order from above downwards by the numbers 0, 1, 2 and 3, and were spaced at equal distances of 15 cms. from one another. Stimulation of any one of the three lower places served as a positive conditioned alimentary stimulus, while stimulation of the upper place was differentiated, and acted, therefore, as an inhibitory stimulus. The differentiation, however, in this dog was not very stable. In the general course of the experiments the intervals between successive stimulations were always 7 minutes. Each experiment began with the conditioned stimulus of a buzzer or a metronome. This was followed by two positive tactile stimuli, which were applied to any of the active places, and these were followed by the positive tactile cutaneous stimulation which was being specially tested in the given experiment. All these stimuli were applied with intervals of 7 minutes. The uppermost apparatus evoking inhibition was used next. After this, and this time at different intervals varying in the different experiments from 0 to 10 minutes, the tactile stimulus which immediately preceded the inhibitory stimulus was again applied and the inhibitory after-effect determined. The following table represents the results of these experiments, the magnitude of the reflexes being calculated as a percentage of the normal positive effect, for which the mean value of the three tactile cutaneous reflexes which preceded the inhibitory stimulus was taken. Each figure given in the table is an average of three observations.

Intervals of time :		0″	15″	30″	60″	2′	3′	5′	6′	7′	8′	9′	10′
Magnitude of the reflex in percentage of normal response	Place No. 1	110	77	90	58	82	62	40	105	93	95	95	100
	No. 2	83	62	86	40	—	75	27	89	60	—	—	70
	No. 3	68	24	20	0	25	65	40	50	—	55	—	100

The complex relations occurring in these experiments can be more readily followed on the following chart:

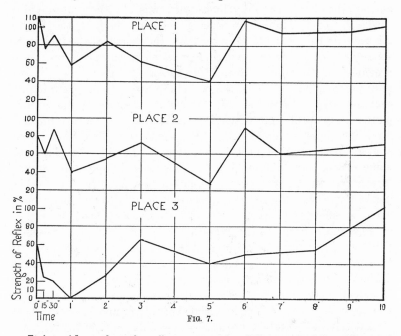

FIG. 7.

It is evident that the effects upon the different positive places of the irradiating inhibition initiated by the stimulation of place No. 0 showed more points of variance than of resemblance. The chief point which they had in common was the following: the inhibitory after-effect in all three places sooner or later reached a maximum and then disappeared. A further point in common was that all three places simultaneously revealed two waves of inhibition, the crest of one occurring at an interval of sixty seconds following the termination of the inhibitory stimulus and the second after an interval of five minutes. Here the resemblance ended; all the other features presented considerable differences. At the place nearest to the inhibitory one there was, immediately on the termination of the inhibitory stimulus, a slight increase of excitability, *i.e.* an effect of positive induction. In the remaining two places the inhibitory after-effect was revealed immediately. The second wave of inhibition at places 1 and 2 was greater than the first, but at place 3 the second wave was expressed only slightly, while during the first wave the inhibition was complete. Moreover, numerous secondary fluctuations were observed at places 1 and 2. At place 3, on the other hand, the only fluctuation was a rather considerable weakening of the inhibition during the first half of the fourth minute. If this had not been present, the course of the inhibitory after-effect would have been as regular as in the cases examined previously in the ninth and tenth lectures. At place 3, again, just as in previous observations, the period of development of the inhibition was several times less than the period of its recession, while at places 1 and 2 the time taken to reach the maximum of inhibition was either equal to, or even less, than the time required for the complete restoration of the normal excitability. Lastly, when the gross value of the total inhibitory after-effect was computed by adding together all the percentages of inhibition calculated from the table, it was found that the inhibition exerted its fullest effect at place 3, a smaller effect at place 2, and the least effect at place 1.

The most natural interpretation of these complex relations between the cortical excitation and the irradiated inhibition is that the induced increase of excitability produced the greatest effect nearest the point primarily inhibited ; for this reason the undulating character of the struggle between the two opposing processes was seen most clearly in the neighbourhood of this cutaneous area. That the underlying excitatory process was actually greatest in this place is obvious from the definite result of positive induction which was observed immediately on the termination of the inhibitory stimulus at this point alone. In remoter places the inhibition was exhibited in a practically unimpeded form, first increasing gradually in strength, and then undergoing a prolonged weakening until the normal positive effect was restored. It must be noted, however, that the individual figures which were averaged exhibited for the first place variations much wider than for the intermediate place, and still wider than those for the remotest place. It is possible that the minor differences between the curves for the different places should to a certain extent be attributed to this. On the other hand, it is possible that the inconstancy in the separate figures was in itself a true expression of the greater fluctuations of the excitability in the nearest place, as compared with the remoter ones.

The following experiments by Dr. Podkopaev, which were performed on a different dog, give another striking illustration of the great complexity of the relations in question. Apparatuses for tactile stimulation of the skin were arranged in linear order along one side of the body of this dog as follows : No. 0 on the front paw, No. 1 on the shoulder, No. 2 on the chest, No. 3 on the abdomen, and No. 4 on the thigh. A positive conditioned alimentary reflex was established by stimulation of the front paw (No. 0) ; the remaining places (Nos. 1, 2, 3 and 4) were rendered inhibitory, and made equal in their action. Immediately after the application of any of the inhibitory stimuli, the place producing a positive reflex was tested, its normal effect having previously been determined at the beginning of the experiment. The experiments to determine the effect of each inhibitory place upon the positive ones were performed without any stereotyped order in the choice, first one and then another being taken. The results cannot, therefore, be attributed to any regular changes in the experimental conditions during the course of the experiments.

The following table contains the data for each of three separate experiments with each inhibitory stimulus, together with the mean figures. The effect of the positive stimulus is expressed as a percentage of its normal magnitude. It should be remembered that the excitatory effect of place No. 0 was in all cases tested *immediately* after applying one or other of the inhibitory stimuli.

Secretory effect of place No. 0 when tested immediately after the stimulation of one or other of the inhibitory places (Nos. 1-4)	After stimulation of place No. 1	133% 128% 125%	Average 128½%
	After stimulation of place No. 2	127% 58% 100%	Average 95%
	After stimulation of place No. 3	100% 100% 100%	Average 100%
	After stimulation of place No. 4	140% 158% 127%	Average 143%

This table demonstrates clearly that the intensity of excitation at the positive place varies considerably, depending on which of the inhibitory stimuli was previously applied. When the nearest or the remotest place was the one previously stimulated, a definite effect of positive induction was readily observed : the secretory activity increased considerably as compared with the normal, the latent period became shorter, and frequently the alimentary motor reaction became increased in intensity. Moreover, the effect of positive induction resulting from stimulation of the remotest place was somewhat greater than that resulting from stimulation of the nearest one. No influence was observed from stimulation of place No. 3, and the effect of stimulation of place No. 2 showed no regularity, being at one test inhibitory, at another test giving rise to positive induction, and at a still further test giving neither effect. The similarity between the figures for the three separate determinations in these experiments (excluding those for place No. 2) was so great that there can be no grounds for doubting the accuracy of the average figures, and the figures relating to place No. 3 can be taken, therefore, as evidence of the existence of an intermediate zone in which neither the inhibitory after-effect nor induction was in the ascendant.

We must now consider what this experiment teaches us with regard to the intimate functional activity of the cortex. If it is assumed that the linear arrangement of the places on the skin corresponds with a similar arrangement of projection points in the cortex, the result obtained above should be regarded as striking evidence of an undulatory distribution of cortical excitability. On this view the cortical area over which a nervous process spreads must be regarded as an alternation of regions with heightened and with diminished excitability, in which now the excitatory and now the inhibitory process predominates. These experiments cannot, however, be regarded otherwise than as suggestive, and the whole hypothesis of the wave-like progression of excitation and inhibition cannot be accepted without further and more direct experimental proof, especially since it involves so many important and far-reaching implications.

The data brought forward in this lecture tend to show that the changes in excitability of different points of the cortex caused by external stimuli, and especially those of an inhibitory character, proceed in a wave-like manner, both in regard to time for a given single place, and in regard to space for different cortical points simultaneously. There is nothing surprising in this phenomenon, considering that the spread of the nervous processes on the one hand and their mutual induction on the other are established facts. Considerable difficulties arise, however, when a general rule governing the interrelations between the two processes is looked for. At present we are still confronted with a series of unrelated facts, which do not explain why in some cases these undulations are present, in others absent ; why in some cases the spreading inhibition is preceded by a positive induction, and why in others the latter is not apparent.   The available experiments, however, indicate that this variability is determined by the co-operation of three factors.   These are, firstly, the functional peculiarities of the central nervous system of the experimental animal employed ;   secondly, the different stages of establishment of new connections in the cortex under the influence of external stimuli ; and thirdly, the form in which such connections are established, since, for example, the different types of internal inhibition are known to differ considerably as regards their intensity and stability.   One of the most important problems in the future complete analysis of the relations in question must be the exact determination of the part played by each of these factors in the cortical activity at any given moment, taking into considera-tion the relative intensities of the nervous processes involved.   Of course, the problem can to some extent be dealt with even at present. In the experiments which were described a tentative approach to a solution of this question could be noticed.   This is even more clearly revealed in experiments which have been recently conducted and are still in progress.   In the last four lectures it could be seen that the inhibition produced by a stimulus applied at a certain point spreads over the analyser, either immediately on the termination of the inhibitory stimulus or after a short preliminary period of positive induction.   For the purpose of determining what happens *during* the actual application of the inhibitory stimulus the following special series of experiments was carried out.   In these experiments other points of the same or of other analysers were tested, not on the termination of the inhibitory stimulation, as was hitherto the practice, but while the inhibitory stimulation was still in progress, *i.e.* the positive stimulus to be tested was, so to speak, superimposed on the background of the inhibitory stimulus.   The investigation was carried out on four different dogs by Dr. Podkopaev.

The experiments with extinctive inhibition will be considered first.   The dog employed was the same which served for the experi-ments upon the irradiation of inhibition after a single non-reinforce-ment of the conditioned stimulus and after extinction to zero.   In the present experiments extinction of the conditioned reflex to tactile stimulation of a definite place of the skin was carried to zero.

The degree of inhibition was tested at two places, one at a distance of 1 cm. and the other at a distance of 89 cm. The positive stimulus was applied at each place at the 30th second of action of the inhibitory stimulus and the combined stimulus was now continued during a further 30 seconds. The stimulation of the nearer place when applied upon the background of the inhibitory stimulus gave $84\frac{1}{2}\%$ of the secretory effect, while that of the distant place gave 88%. In other words, the effect was practically the same at both places. It will be remembered that when the same places were stimulated immediately *after* the termination of the inhibitory stimulus, the nearer point gave 44% and the remoter point $66\frac{1}{2}\%$ (page 209). In order to appreciate these results more fully, it must be noted that in the case of the simultaneous stimulation of the inhibitory, and either of the positive places, the latent period of the reflex was considerably reduced, and the alimentary motor reaction was more sharply expressed than usually. Both these facts are unmistakable evidence of positive induction at all points of the analyser, except the one specially extinguished. The somewhat diminished secretory effect from the other places should undoubtedly be interpreted as the result of an algebraic summation of their effect with the effect of the extinguished place.

In a modification of these experiments another feature of special interest was revealed. The extinction to zero produced at a definite place of the skin was obtained by repeating the conditioned stimulus without reinforcement at intervals of 2 minutes, and the process of extinction was continued to the third zero. At the third zero stimulation of another place of the skin was superimposed on the stimulation of the inhibitory place. The reflex effect obtained from the combined stimulation was in the majority of cases equal to the usual effect of the positive stimulus taken singly. Thus it follows that an intensification of inhibition still further diminished the inhibitory effect upon the surrounding areas during the time the inhibitory stimulus lasted (enhanced induction).

Another point is also clearly brought out in these experiments. As was shown previously (page 209), the reflexes at the two positive places in this dog were still 50% inhibited two minutes after extinction of another place to the first zero. But when the action of one or another of the positive places was superimposed upon the action of the inhibitory stimulus at its third zero, again two minutes after the preceding zero, there was no inhibitory after-effect from the preceding extinction. It must be concluded, therefore, that during the repeated application of the inhibitory stimulus the inhibition again became concentrated at the point at which the inhibitory stimulus was applied. The spread of the inhibitory after-effect has thus to be regarded as proceeding not during, but entirely or mainly after, the termination of the inhibitory stimulus; while during its action the surrounding areas of the cortex are, to all evidence, subjected to positive induction.

Similar results were obtained by Dr. Podkopaev in another dog, in which positive conditioned alimentary reflexes were established to a definite tone and to a metronome beating at a rate of 120 per minute; an inhibitory reflex based upon differentiation was established to a stimulus of 60 beats of the metronome per minute. The tone, when superimposed upon the inhibitory stimulus of the metronome, gave out of nine experiments a slight trace of inhibition once, a normal effect four times, and an effect greater than normal four times.

In further experiments on the same problem two more dogs were employed. In one of these [experiments of Dr. Golovina] positive reflexes were established to a definite tone, to a sound of a whistle, and to a tactile stimulus. Three inhibitory reflexes were also established, all based on differentiation—one to a definite rate of a metronome, another to a tactile stimulus, and the third to flashes of a lamp. When all these reflexes were well established, experiments were performed in which each one of the positive stimuli in turn was applied on the background of one of the inhibitory stimuli. All the tests gave uniform results. A positive stimulus combined in this way gave either a normal or else a somewhat augmented secretion, and the latent period was in most cases reduced.

In the second dog [experiments by Dr. Pavlova] positive conditioned reflexes were established to the sound of a whistle, to a sound of bubbling, and to a tactile stimulus. An inhibitory stimulus based on differentiation was established to a definite rate of a metronome. In these experiments each positive stimulus was applied several times with the inhibitory stimulus. The results were somewhat different from those obtained in the first dog. Although the latent period was in most cases reduced, the positive effect of the combined stimulus was almost constantly, and sometimes considerably, smaller than that obtained with the positive stimulus used singly. In the second dog, therefore, the concentration of the inhibition was not so perfect.

It should be said that the last two dogs possessed functionally different types of nervous system. While in the first dog the differentiations were in general very stable and remained unaffected by the combined stimulation, in the second dog the differentiation was frequently incomplete, and was invariably still further disturbed after the experiments with superimposition.

The series of experiments described in this lecture clearly demonstrate that, on the one hand, the positive induction arising as the result of an inhibitory stimulus applied to a definite place limits the spread of the inhibitory process, and that, on the other hand, the interaction between excitation and inhibition is determined either by the phase of establishing new relations in the cortex [experiments of Dr. Podkopaev] or by the type of nervous system in different animals [experiments by Drs. Golovina and Pavlova].

LECTURE XIII

The cortex as a mosaic of functions : (a) Examples of the mosaic character of the cortex and the more obvious ways in which this character is acquired. (b) Variability of the physiological properties of different points of the cortex in some instances, stability in others.—The cortex as a united complex dynamic system.

IT becomes obvious from all the previous discussion that through the medium of the cerebral cortex a great number of environmental changes establish now positive, now negative, conditioned reflexes, and determine in this manner the different effector activities of the animal organism and its everyday behaviour. All these conditioned reflexes must have definite representation in the cerebral cortex in one or another definite group of cells. One such group of cells must be connected with one definite activity of the organism, another group with another activity : one group may determine a positive activity, while another may inhibit an activity. The cerebral cortex can accordingly be represented as an exceedingly rich mosaic, or as an extremely complicated " switchboard." However, in spite of its extreme complexity as a switchboard, there are always large spaces reserved for the development of new connections. Moreover, points which are already involved in a definite conditioned activity frequently change their physiological rôle and become connected with some other activity of the animal.

The idea of the cerebral cortex as a mosaic of functions is in part indicated in the current anatomical and physiological teaching. The structural complexity of the specific receptor organs of special sense, the rich complexity of the cellular structures of the cortex, and the complexity of their distribution conform quite readily to the idea of the mosaic character of the central nervous system. The rather rough localization of function which has been achieved during the last century of experimental physiology is no less in accord with such a conception. The final resolution of the many delicate problems involved in this conception is, however, a complex and difficult matter ; up to the present it has been possible only to make the very first attempts towards an experimental study of the simplest aspects of the problem, and even these aspects demand the utmost skill and resource of the inquirer.

The existence of a localization of function in the cortex is in some cases sufficiently proved by the evidence of structure alone, definite receptor elements having been shown to stand in connection with definite cortical cells. The study of conditioned reflexes has shown, however, that a conditioned reflex appears at first in a generalized form, *i.e.* that excitation irradiates from its point of initiation to embrace also cells belonging to other receptor elements beyond the boundary of the area of the cortex primarily connected with the stimulated receptor ; the problem becomes still more complicated when we take into account also the subsequent concentration of excitation upon its point of initiation.

Two different problems present themselves for consideration. In the first place the question arises how the functional demarcation of two positive cortical points each connected with a different unconditioned reflex is effected, and in the second place the similar question arises as to the mechanism of the functional demarcation of neighbouring positive and negative cortical points belonging to the same unconditioned reflex. The study of anatomical localization of function is obviously of no assistance in solving these problems. The investigation of the first question is being conducted at the present time, and therefore cannot yet be discussed; our investigations up to the present have been confined almost exclusively to the second problem, since it is the simpler.

We shall commence with a simple and obvious case. A positive conditioned alimentary reflex was established to a tactile stimulation of the skin on the right shoulder, and a negative conditioned reflex to a similar stimulation of the skin on the right thigh. After these reflexes had been thoroughly established, the effect of a tactile stimulation of other places on the skin was tried. The different sites of stimulation were : (1) the front paw 17 cms. below the positive point on the shoulder ; (2) the side of the animal 12 cms. caudally from the positive place on the shoulder ; (3) the side of the animal 15 cms. in front of the negative place on the thigh ; and (4) the hind paw 18 cms. below the negative place on the thigh. The salivary secretion was measured during 30 seconds of isolated stimulation of each of the above places. The results are summarized in the following table :

Conditioned tactile stimulus applied during 30 seconds	Secretion of Saliva in drops during 30 seconds
Front paw	6
Shoulder (the positive place)	8
Point on side nearer to shoulder	7
Point on side nearer to thigh	3
Thigh (the negative place)	0
Hind paw	0

Similar results were obtained in two other dogs [experiments of Dr. Foursikov].

It can be seen that under the influence of two definite external stimuli, which affected the animal under opposite conditions (one reinforced by the unconditioned reflex and the other remaining without reinforcement), two perfectly definite and separate points within the cutaneous analyser were given, the one excitatory, and the other inhibitory, properties. Around each of these points there was established a corresponding region of positive or negative influence, these regions of positive and negative influence extending towards each other, although each maintaining its distinctive properties. The smallness of the positive reflex on stimulating the place on the side of the animal nearer to the thigh, and the absence of positive reflex on stimulating the hind paw, indicate the predominance of inhibitory properties in these respective points. In the absence of a nucleus of inhibition the positive effect due to the initial generalization would have spread over the whole of the analyser in such a manner that the decrement of the positive reflex with increase of distance from its point of initial development would have been gradual, as was shown in the tenth lecture.

The experiments described in this lecture show that external stimuli evoking antagonistic processes provide the first method by which a functional mosaic character of the cortex originates. Many other examples of this can be found in the lecture upon the analysing function of the cortex.

More complicated experiments were conducted upon three more dogs. In two dogs different tones [experiments of Dr. Siriatsky], and in the third dog tactile stimulation of different areas of the skin [experiments of Dr. Koupalov], were used as conditioned stimuli, alternate areas being respectively positive and negative. The object of the experiments was to determine the mode of development of the mosaic character, the stability and the delicacy of its pattern, the interaction of its different points, the effect of stimulation of the spaces intermediate between the positive and negative places, and the effect of development of such a functional mosaic upon the general condition of the animal. Some of the results of these experiments will be given now, others will be described in further lectures, although it should be mentioned that the investigations are still being pursued. In one dog all the tones C of five neighbouring octaves of an organ (64-1024 d.v.) were used as positive conditioned alimentary stimuli, while all the tones F (85$\frac{1}{3}$-1365$\frac{1}{3}$ d.v.) were used as inhibitory conditioned stimuli. In the following tables the respective C's and F's are designated according to Helmholtz's scale. The following experiment illustrates the final result obtained with one dog:

Time	Conditioned stimulus applied during 30 seconds	Salivary Secretion in drops during 30 seconds
11.32 a.m.	c'	9
11.44 ,,	c'''	9$\frac{1}{2}$
11.53 ,,	F (negative)	0
12.1 p.m.	C	10
12.13 ,,	c'''	10$\frac{1}{2}$
12.22 ,,	f'' (negative)	0
12.34 ,,	C	9$\frac{1}{2}$
12.47 ,,	f' (negative)	0
12.59 ,,	C	9

In the second dog different tones from f (170$\frac{2}{3}$ d.v.) to f' sharp (360 d.v.) were used in alternate order as positive and negative conditioned stimuli. e' sharp (335 d.v.) was given the properties of an excitatory stimulus, e' (320 d.v.) properties of an inhibitory stimulus, c' (256 d.v.) excitatory, a (213$\frac{1}{3}$ d.v.) inhibitory, g (192 d.v.) excitatory and f (170$\frac{2}{3}$ d.v.) inhibitory, these tones being enumerated in descending order. As can be seen, the intervals between the respective positive and negative tones were in this dog irregular, and smaller than in the first dog. The final stage of development of the reflex is shown in the following experiment:

Time	Conditioned stimulus applied during 30 seconds	Salivary Secretion in drops during 30 seconds
2.2 p.m.	g (positive)	10
2.9 ,,	f′ sharp (positive)	8
2.16½ ,,	e′ (negative)	0
2.24 ,,	c′ (positive)	7½
2.34 ,,	a (negative)	0
2.43 ,,	g (positive	7
2.51 ,,	f (negative)	0
2.56½ ,,	g (positive)	6

In the third dog the conditioned alimentary reflexes were tactile. The apparatuses used for the stimulation were always arranged in strictly identical positions along a line extending along the left side from the hind leg along the whole length of the body to the left leg, the apparatuses being set at a distance of 12 cms. from each other measured from the centre of one apparatus to the next. The stimulated places are numbered in order from No. 1, the left hind leg, to No. 9, the left fore leg. Stimulations of the places represented by odd numbers were given excitatory properties, and stimulations of the places represented by even numbers inhibitory properties. The following is a typical experiment :

Time	Conditioned stimulation applied during 30 seconds	Salivary Secretion in drops during 30 seconds
12.10 p.m.	Tactile No. 7	9
12.18 ,,	Tactile No. 5	10½
12.30 ,,	Tactile No. 4 (negative)	½
12.34 ,,	Tactile No. 5	4
12.43 ,,	Tactile No. 7	6
12.49 ,,	Tactile No. 3	6½
12.59 ,,	Tactile No. 6 (negative)	0
1.3 ,,	Tactile No. 7	6
1.8 ,,	Tactile No. 7	5½
1.16 ,,	Tactile No. 2 (negative)	½

The development of this functional mosaic of the cortex presented at the beginning some difficulty, but with continuation of the experiments it grew progressively easier. The reflexes were developed not simultaneously but in succession. One of the most interesting points brought out by these experiments was the spontaneous development in the first and third dogs, in the final stages, of some new reflexes, and it is important to note that the new conditioned properties in these cases developed within the region of the antagonistic nervous processes. In the case of the first dog the positive conditioned reflex to c″ was of very long standing. In one experiment this tone c″ evoked a secretion of 8 drops during 30 seconds, while on the contrary f″ even on its first application failed to produce any positive effect. This inclined us to regard f″ as inhibitory from the start, and the truth of such an assumption was definitely proved in an experiment on the following day, when, f″ being used as the first stimulus, it not only remained without any positive effect but also left a considerable inhibitory after-effect, so that the positive reflex to the succeeding stimulus c″ became very much diminished. It is obvious therefore that f″ assumed its inhibitory properties spontaneously, without requiring any contrasting, but to all appearance simply in virtue of its situation in the neighbourhood of the positive cortical point corresponding to c″. The same phenomenon repeated itself with c‴, which when tested for the very first time gave a positive effect apparently in virtue of its proximity to the negative f″.

In the third dog, with tactile conditioned reflexes, the places Nos. 1 and 9 also developed their full positive effect spontaneously without any previous reinforcement, but most probably in virtue of being within the sphere of influence of the previously established negative places Nos. 2 and 8.

Clearly these facts should be interpreted as due to mutual induction initiated by the pre-existing points of excitation and inhibition in regular alternation. These experiments show us why any rhythmic activity is performed more easily and less exhaustingly than an arhythmic one. The experiments on all three dogs showed us that in the case of a regular alternation of positive and inhibitory stimuli all the reflexes were exceedingly precise. In some cases such a regular alternation leads even within one experimental day to a more and more precise functional localization of positive and negative cortical points. This can, of course, most clearly be demonstrated in cases where at the beginning of the experiment the effect of the different points was lacking in precision. The following results were obtained with the dog in which tactile stimuli were employed as the alternating excitatory and inhibitory conditioned stimuli ; the experiment was performed before the negative stimuli became well established :

Time	Conditioned stimulus during 30 seconds	Secretion of Saliva during 30 seconds
1.3 p.m.	Tactile No. 1	$17\frac{1}{2}$
1.12 ,,	Tactile No. 2 (negative)	8
1.19 ,,	Tactile No. 3	14
1.26 ,,	Tactile No. 4 (negative)	4
1.34 ,,	Tactile No. 5	10
1.44 ,,	Tactile No. 6 (negative)	$\frac{1}{2}$
1.53 ,,	Tactile No. 7	$7\frac{1}{2}$
2.7 ,,	Tactile No. 8 (negative)	0
2.23 ,,	Tactile No. 9	6

The following is another example of an experiment on the first dog taken at the time when the reflexes were not yet quite regular :

Time	Conditioned stimulus during 30 seconds		Secretion of Saliva in drops during 30 seconds
10.50 a.m.	c (128 d.v.)		5
10.59 ,,	c (128 d.v.)		7
11.16 ,,	c′ (256 d.v.)	All	3
11.26 ,,	c′ (256 d.v.)	stimuli	7
11.38 ,,	c″ (512 d.v.)	positive	5
11.50 ,,	c″ (512 d.v.)		2
12.1 p.m.	c (128 d.v.)		4

The same dog after 3 days :

Time	Conditioned stimulus during 30 seconds	Secretion of Saliva in drops during 30 seconds
11.50 a.m.	c (128 d.v.)	7
11.59 ,,	F ($85\frac{1}{3}$ d.v.) (negative)	0
12.12 p.m.	c′ (256 d.v.)	6
12.20 ,,	f ($170\frac{2}{3}$ d.v.) (negative)	0
12.31 ,,	c″ (512 d.v.)	6
12.42 ,,	f′ ($341\frac{1}{3}$ d.v.) (negative)	0
12.58 ,,	c (128 d.v.)	6

The above experiments indicate that the mutual induction of the antagonistic nervous processes of excitation and inhibition should be regarded as the second contributing factor to the development of a mosaic of functions in the cerebral cortex.

The same dogs were used to determine the extensity of the excitatory and inhibitory processes around the respective points of stimulation, and to determine also whether there existed any mosaic of neutral territory interwoven with the mosaic of excitation and inhibition. For this purpose, in the dogs in which a mosaic of tones was established, other tones were used intermediate between the tones which had been given positive or negative significance, and the effect produced by these intermediate tones was observed. A positive effect, in the form of a salivary secretion, was a direct evidence of the tone having definite excitatory properties. An absence of secretory effect, on the contrary, gave no special indication whether the tone had any inhibitory conditioned properties or was merely neutral, and special experiments had to be made to test whether such tones left any inhibitory after-effect or exhibited any effect of positive induction. In the following experiment, between the positive tone 256 d.v. and the negative tone 320 d.v. three tones were taken: $266\frac{2}{3}$, 288 and $303\frac{2}{5}$ d.v. respectively.

Time	Conditioned stimulus applied during 30 seconds	Salivary Secretion in drops during 30 seconds
Experiment of 9th October, 1925.		
1.22 p.m.	c' (256 d.v.)	10
1.30 ,,	e' (320 d.v.) (negative)	0
1.40 ,,	c' (256 d.v.)	7
1.50 ,,	d' (288 d.v.)	0
$1.52\frac{1}{2}$,,	Tactile	4
Experiment of 14th October, 1925.		
12.50 p.m.	g (192 d.v.)	10
12.56 ,,	f ($170\frac{2}{3}$ d.v.)	9
1.7 ,,	e' (320 d.v.) (negative)	0
1.15 ,,	c' (256 d.v.)	10
1.25 ,,	c' sharp ($266\frac{2}{3}$ d.v.)	3
Experiment of 20th October, 1925.		
2.14 p.m.	Tactile	4
2.20 ,,	f' sharp (360 d.v.)	13
2.33 ,,	e' (320 d.v.) (negative)	0
2.40 ,,	c' (256 d.v.)	10
2.48 ,,	e' flat ($303\frac{2}{5}$ d.v.)	0
$2.50\frac{1}{2}$,,	Tactile	2

The above experiments show that the tones intermediate between the positive c' and the negative e', namely, the tone d' and the semitones c' sharp and e' flat, assumed a different significance. The semitone c' sharp produced a definite though comparatively small positive effect, *i.e.* it still belonged to the excitatory region of c' ; on the other hand the tone d' and the semitone e' flat at the first glance were equal in their effect, since both gave a zero secretion. It was only by testing their inhibitory after-effect that a difference between these two tones could be revealed. The conditioned tactile stimulus when applied two minutes after the use of the semitone e' flat diminished in its effect by 50%, *i.e.* it was under the influence of the inhibitory after-effect. When, however, tested under precisely the same conditions after the tone d' the tactile stimulus gave a full positive effect. The semitone e' flat, therefore, belonged unquestionably to the region of the inhibitory e' ; the tone d', however, either was entirely neutral or else carried much weaker inhibitory properties, an alternative which can be finally settled only by more delicate experiments. The whole question of the possible existence of completely neutral points in the cortex is being further investigated.

It was mentioned in the first lecture and again in the beginning of the present lecture that additions can always be made in any pattern of the functional mosaic both with respect to its extent and its complexity. Moreover it is subject also to frequent reconstruction, one and the same point changing its physiological significance and becoming connected successively with different physiological activities of the organism. In respect to this we have only one series of experiments, conducted by Dr. Friedman, as follows :

One and the same agent served at first as a conditioned alimentary stimulus, later it was transformed into a conditioned stimulus for acid ; reversely, old conditioned stimuli to acid were transformed into alimentary ones. Two dogs were used for experiments with the first set of transformations, and a third dog was used for the second set. The transformation of conditioned stimuli was effected by the substitution of one unconditioned reflex for the other. The following is the general sequence of events : The conditioned stimulus, on transition from one unconditioned reflex to another very quickly, even within a single experimental day, loses its secretory effect and gives a series of zeros for a comparatively long time ; only after considerable practice with the new unconditioned stimulus does it gradually reassume excitatory properties, and these now belong to a conditioned reflex based on the new unconditioned one, as shown by the very definite change in the composition of the saliva secreted by the submaxillary gland and in the character of the motor reaction. The complete replacement of the one conditioned reflex by the other required about 30 reinforcements by the new unconditioned stimulus. After a considerable practice of the conditioned reflexes to acid the conditioned stimuli were once more transformed back again into alimentary ones ; the transformation occurred rapidly and only a few reinforcements were needed. This indicates that the original alimentary connection was still preserved in spite of the establishment of a new connection with the reflex to acid.

However, the main interest of the experiments of Dr. Friedman lay in the investigation whether a differentiation which had been established for the conditioned stimulus to one reflex would be preserved after its transformation. A detailed description of an experiment will be given in respect to one dog only, since the experiments with all three dogs gave identical results. The alimentary conditioned stimulus in this dog was given by the tone of 2600 d.v. ; a precise differentiation from this tone was established to the neighbouring tone of 2324 d.v. The positive conditioned alimentary reflex was now transformed into a conditioned reflex to acid, and when the differentiation was tested it was found from its very first application to be complete and to exert the same inhibitory after-effect as before. A new and more precise differentiation was now established on the basis of the " acid " reflex to a note a semitone higher than the original positive tone, i.e. 2760 d.v., and it was found that when the tone of 2600 d.v. was transformed back again into a conditioned alimentary stimulus this new and finer differentiation also retained its precision.

In the course of the preceding lectures we had occasion to refer to the fact that one and the same point of the cortex could, in accordance with the given experimental conditions, be a point of origin either of excitation or of inhibition. These transformations of the physiological significance of a definite cortical point are attained with comparative ease and are effected with considerable rapidity both in respect of positive and of negative stimuli (experiments with induction, p. 194), and in respect of their ultimate connection with one or another unconditioned reflex (experiments just described). However, amongst our material we have a number of cases in which the definite positive or negative quality of some region of the cortex, or even a temporary correlation between the two processes, assumed an exceedingly persistent character which could be changed only with great difficulty, or even failed to be changed. These cases were met with in the experiments of Dr. Frolov upon conditioned positive and negative trace reflexes. The results of these experiments were of such unique character that it is necessary to describe them in detail. In the case of one dog a trace conditioned reflex to acid was established to a tone of 1740 d.v. produced by an organ pipe : the tone was continued for 15 seconds and the acid was administered after a pause of 30 seconds. This trace reflex was repeated 994 times in the course of one year and nine months. Its latent period, counting from the beginning of the tone, was equal to very nearly 25 seconds (10 seconds reckoned from the cessation of the tone). After the termination of the investigation originally planned it was resolved to abolish the trace character of the reflex and to give it the character of a delayed reflex, evoking the positive secretory effect during the action of the tone, and not some time after its termination. For this purpose acid was administered at the 15th second after the beginning of the tone. After twenty reinforcements with this new interval it was still found that, not only did the reflex fail to appear during the 15 seconds of the isolated action of the tone, but even the administration of acid at the 15th second evoked a secretion only after the old latent period of 25 seconds from the beginning of the tone. The use of other auditory stimuli in place of the tone did not alter the result, and when the tone and the other auditory stimuli were protracted for 45 seconds without the administration of acid the secretion always started at about the 25th second from the beginning and then increased rapidly, giving about 10 drops during the remaining 20 seconds of isolated action of the conditioned stimulus. After this failure to diminish the latent period, the stimulus was reinforced practically simultaneously, i.e. two seconds after the beginning of the tone preceding the reinforcement. Nevertheless, even after several score of repetitions the conditioned secretion started only after a latent period of 20-25 seconds from the beginning of the tone ; this latent period could not be changed whether the acid was administered at the 2nd second or whether the tone was continued singly for a much greater length of time. The last experiment performed in this series is given in the following table:

Time	Length of time of isolated action of the conditioned stimulus before reinforcement with acid	Latent period of the Salivary Secretion in seconds
1.12 p.m.	30 seconds	26
1.24 ,,	2 ,,	29
1.31 ,,	45 ,,	23
1.40 ,,	2 ,,	32
1.54 ,,	15 seconds followed by a pause of 30 seconds	25

A conditioned alimentary reflex to a tone f sharp of a tone variator was now developed in this dog, but the latent period of this reflex also could not be reduced below 24 seconds, and it was only when a tactile stimulation was used as a conditioned stimulus and reinforced with acid after 2 seconds that a closer approximation to a simultaneous alimentary reflex was at last obtained. At the twenty-fourth test the reflex was measured by 12 drops during 30 seconds, with a latent period of 2 seconds.

A similar persistence of a thoroughly established cortical inhibition was observed in the case of another dog. The trace of a tone of 1740 double vibrations produced by an organ pipe was used as a conditioned inhibitor to the positive conditioned stimulus of a metronome beating at a rate of 104 per minute. The trace of the tone even after one minute still exerted a full inhibition upon the reflex to the metronome. Such an inhibition had to be developed of course gradually, starting with recent traces of only a few seconds. The experiments were conducted with this conditioned inhibition for well over two years, and the tone, besides serving as a conditioned trace inhibitor, was also differentiated from other tones, which, of course, led to an extreme intensification of its inhibitory properties. At the termination of these experiments the animal was used for another research in which it was desired to develop a positive conditioned reflex to a sound of a microphone which happened to be practically identical in pitch with the tone which had served as the conditioned inhibitor in the first series of experiments. The positive conditioned reflex refused for a long time to develop, and when the metronome was tested shortly after the sound of the microphone had been applied a most powerful conditioned inhibition was revealed. The experiments were now modified so that the inhibitory combination of the microphone with the metronome was directly reinforced by the unconditioned stimulus ; in other words, a procedure was adopted which exactly reversed that employed for the development of the conditioned inhibition to the original trace of the tone. The inhibitory combination now quickly acquired excitatory properties, and somewhat later the sound of the microphone applied singly acquired a positive significance of its own. However, the tone of the organ pipe which had been originally developed as the conditioned inhibitor did not acquire a positive character ; neither did it lose its inhibitory properties : these had to be destroyed by the same method as was used for the destruction of those of the microphone, but the process occupied a much longer time.

These cases of extreme stability of the inhibitory process must be regarded as exceptional. It is very probable that the intensity of inhibition in these cases was favoured by some special conditions of the experiments, and it is possible that this exceptional persistence of the inhibitory process can be correlated with the experiments upon hypnotism and sleep which will be described further on.

Along with these cases of an extremely stable " inhibitability " of definite points of the cerebral cortex must be placed a case of a similarly stable excitability. In an experiment by Dr. Bierman a well-established conditioned alimentary reflex, to the tone of 256 double vibrations produced by an organ pipe, was differentiated from twenty-two separate and distinct tones ranging in pitch from 768 d.v. to 85 d.v., the tone of 256 d.v. (c′) being always accompanied by food while all the others remained unreinforced. The positive tone was contrasted in each experiment several times with one or other of the negative tones. In this manner the positive cortical point became surrounded by a series of inhibitory points. However, this apparent encircling of the positive point by inhibitory ones did not lead to a diminution of the effect of the positive tone ; on the contrary it led to its extreme intensification. When in subsequent experiments the animal was experimentally subjected to a profound physiological sleep, so that, for example, shrill whistling and banging on the door of the experimental room containing the dog did not awaken it, the positive conditioned tone awakened the animal immediately and evoked a full conditioned secretion. Experimental proof will be given in further lectures that sleep itself is nothing but a form of internal inhibition, and from this point of view the experiment just described must be regarded as a case of extreme stability of the excitatory process in a definite point of the cerebral cortex which successfully resists the surrounding inhibition.

The foregoing discussion of the experimental evidence permits us to regard the activities of the cerebral hemispheres as a true mosaic of functions. All the numerous individual cortical points, each at any definite moment, have some very definite physiological significance, while the whole mosaic of functions is integrated into a complex dynamic system and perpetually achieves a unification of the individual activities. Every new localized influence playing upon it influences to a greater or less extent the entire system. Consider, for example, a dog which possesses at any given moment a definite number of conditioned reflexes. The addition of new positive, and especially of new negative, reflexes exercises, in the great majority of cases an immediate, though temporary, influence upon the older reflexes [experiments of Dr. Anrep]. Further, even when no new reflexes are added, and it is only a rigidly adopted sequence of their order which is changed, their magnitude undergoes distinct diminution, showing a considerable predominance of inhibition. In the following experiment by Dr. Soloveichik a dog was subjected at intervals of 10 minutes to the conditioned alimentary stimuli of a metronome, an electric lamp, a whistle and a tactile stimulus, always repeated in this order in every experiment. The following table gives the results of the final experiment with this order of the stimuli:

Time	Conditioned stimulus during 15 seconds	Salivary Secretion in drops during 15 seconds
3.9 p.m.	Metronome	4
3.19 ,,	Electric lamp	4
3.29 ,,	Whistle	4
3.39 ,,	Tactile	4
3.49 ,,	Metronome	5
3.59 ,,	Electric lamp	3
4.9 ,,	Whistle	$1\frac{1}{2}$
4.19 ,,	Tactile	2

In an experiment on the following day the order of the stimuli was changed.

Time	Conditioned stimulus during 15 seconds	Salivary Secretion in drops during 15 seconds
2.24 p.m.	Electric lamp	$2\frac{1}{2}$
2.34 ,,	Whistle	Trace
2.44 ,,	Tactile	2
2.54 ,,	Metronome	1
3.4 ,,	Electric lamp	2
3.14 ,,	Whistle	$\frac{1}{2}$
3.24 ,,	Tactile	0
3.34 ,,	Metronome	Trace

The diminution in the magnitude of the conditioned reflexes observed when the order of their administration is changed sometimes appears immediately, as in the foregoing experiment, and in other cases becomes more obvious in the succeeding experiment when the stimuli are again applied in their usual order. The diminution continues for several days, and then the reflexes quickly return to their normal magnitude. Such a diminution in the strength of the reflexes as occurred towards the end of the first experiment given above (3.59, 4.9, 4.19 p.m.) is of frequent occurrence and will be more fully discussed in the next lecture.

LECTURE XIV

The development of inhibition in the cortex under the influence of conditioned stimuli.

CONDITIONED stimuli, acting as they undoubtedly do through the intermediation of definite cortical cells, provide the obvious means whereby the physiological characteristics of these cortical cells can be studied. One of the most important of these properties is that under the influence of conditioned stimuli they pass, sooner or later, into inhibition. In the previous lectures upon internal inhibition it was shown that in all cases when a positive conditioned stimulus repeatedly remains unreinforced, it acquires inhibitory properties, *i.e.* the corresponding cortical cells enter under its influence into a state of inhibition. The present lecture will be devoted to the study of the intimate mechanism of this phenomenon, and of the part played therein by the unconditioned reflex and by other conditions which retard or accelerate the development of this inhibitory state.

The transition of the cortical cells into an inhibitory state is of much more general significance than could be inferred from the facts which have been discussed up to the present, concerning the development of internal inhibition. The development of inhibition in the case of conditioned reflexes which remain without reinforcement must be considered only as a special instance of a more general case, since a state of inhibition can develop also when the conditioned reflexes are reinforced. The cortical cells under the influence of the conditioned stimulus always tend to pass, though sometimes very slowly, into a state of inhibition. The function performed by the unconditioned reflex after the conditioned reflex has become established is merely to retard the development of inhibition.

The following is the most commonly occurring example of this phenomenon : We are dealing, we will suppose, with a conditioned reflex which is delayed by 30 seconds, *i.e.* a reflex in which the conditioned stimulus acts singly for exactly 30 seconds before the addition of the unconditioned stimulus. Let us suppose that when the reflex is well established its so-called latent period—the interval of time from the beginning of the conditioned stimulus to the onset of the secretion—is equal to five seconds. Now this latent period remains practically unaltered for a certain length of time, which varies greatly in different dogs. As time goes on the latent period lengthens out, and finally during the 30 seconds of the isolated action of the conditioned stimulus no trace of salivary secretion is produced. It is, however, only necessary to delay the administration of the unconditioned stimulus by a further 5-10 seconds for secretion again to be obtained during the prolongation of the isolated action of the conditioned stimulus. On continuing the experiment for some time as before, *i.e.* with a delay of 30 seconds, and then again introducing a delay increased by a further 5-10 seconds, no conditioned secretion is obtained any more. In order to obtain a conditioned secretion the administration of the unconditioned stimulus must be delayed for a still greater length of time. Finally a stage is reached when no conditioned secretion can be obtained during any length of isolated action of the conditioned stimulus. This gradual disappearance of the conditioned secretion in reflexes with a constant delay occupies very different periods of time in different dogs. In some it takes only days or weeks, and in others it takes several years. The conditioned secretion disappears later with tactile, than with thermal, later still with visual, stimuli and latest of all with auditory stimuli, especially if the latter are discontinuous.

The following is an example of the relative differences between the various conditioned stimuli with respect to the rapidity of transition of the cortical elements into an inhibitory state under the influence of a definite delay [experiments of Dr. Shishlo]. The first conditioned stimulus which was developed in a particular dog was one belonging to the tactile analyser : the administration of food was usually delayed 10 seconds from the beginning of the tactile stimulus, but on rare occasions a 30 seconds' delay was introduced. The reflex first appeared at the 27th stimulation, and within five weeks, after 179 stimulations, the reflex became stable at 8 drops during one minute. The development of a second alimentary conditioned reflex to a thermal cutaneous stimulus of 45° was now commenced, the normal period of delay being as before 10 seconds. This reflex developed quickly, and when at the twelfth stimulation a delay of 30 seconds was introduced a secretion of 4 drops was obtained. On continuation of the usual reinforcement applied 10 seconds after the beginning of the thermal stimulus the reflex rapidly diminished in strength and at the 33rd test, when the delay was specially prolonged to one minute, only one drop of secretion was obtained.

The following observation leaves no doubt that the disappearance of the conditioned reflex, notwithstanding its invariable reinforcement, is an expression of a progressive development of inhibition in the cortical elements. When an effective positive conditioned stimulus is applied shortly after the application of a conditioned stimulus which has, as described, just lost its positive properties, the resulting reflex suffers a diminution. Similarly, when one among a number of conditioned stimuli has lost its positive effect its disuse in the experiments leads to an increase in the effect of the remaining stimuli. To my mind such results can only be interpreted on the assumption that real inhibitory properties have been acquired by those stimuli which have lost their positive effect. This phenomenon should not be confused with what was previously described as the result of internal inhibition of delay. The inhibition of delay is revealed by the so-called latent period which is observed in every conditioned reflex and which remains unchanged for a considerable period of time. The phenomenon which is being described here, on the other hand, is characterized by its invariable progressiveness. The inhibitory state of the cortical elements under the influence of conditioned stimuli develops more quickly with longer delayed reflexes; the longer the isolated application of the conditioned stimulus the quicker the development of the inhibition. For example, it often happens that a reflex with a delay of 10 seconds remains unchanged in its strength for a very considerable time and thus permits of exact experimentation ; the same reflex when delayed to 30 seconds quickly becomes unsuitable for experiments through the progressive development of inhibition. Such a case is taken from experiments by Dr. Petrova :

A dog has a conditioned alimentary reflex established to the sound of a metronome, and throughout the whole period of work the reflex which has been delayed for 10 seconds remains constant in strength. The following experiment has been chosen at random :

Time	Conditioned stimulus applied during 10 seconds	Salivary Secretion in drops during 10 seconds
3.0 p.m.	Metronome	0
3.35 ,,	,,	1
3.47 ,,	,,	2
4.2 ,,	,,	2
4.9 ,,	,,	3
4.20 ,,	,,	2

As soon as the isolated application of the conditioned stimulus is prolonged to 30 seconds the reflex becomes inconstant in strength, and on repetition diminishes to zero during the time of one single experiment.

Time	Conditioned stimulus applied during 30 seconds	Salivary Secretion in drops during 30 seconds
2.55 p.m.	Metronome	6
3.5 ,,	,,	17
3.20 ,,	,,	4
3.30 ,,	,,	4
3.35 ,,	,,	2
3.45 ,,	,,	0

The above two experiments were conducted with an interval of one day.

In view of the great variations existing between individual dogs it has been found very useful, and sometimes essential, to employ in different dogs, reflexes which are delayed by different lengths of time. It now becomes obvious why the long-delayed reflexes develop only with difficulty and why during the beginning of our work they could be obtained only in some of the dogs. Moreover, it becomes easy to understand why in many of the experiments previously described the positive alimentary conditioned reflexes diminish during a single experiment and in some cases after only a single application—as in the experiment on page 232 of the previous lecture. This diminution is due to the repetition of the conditioned stimulus and not to any other factor, such, for example, as a gradual satiation of the animal during the experiment in the case of alimentary reflexes. The latter is obviously not the case, since on repeating any one of the established conditioned stimuli, only the effect produced by that one becomes diminished, while other conditioned stimuli may preserve their full effect up to the very end of the experiment. When a definite positive conditioned stimulus has already shown a tendency to assume inhibitory properties, then after a short interval in the experiments, or even at the beginning of a day's experiment, its first application produces a considerable secretion, but on repetition the stimulus quickly diminishes in its effect and becomes inhibitory in spite of its being reinforced at every application.

It is in the interest of the experimenter for most of the experiments to have at his disposal reflexes of a constant intensity. To obtain such reflexes it is necessary in many cases to fight against the progressive tendency of conditioned reflexes to undergo inhibition. At first on purely empirical grounds, and subsequently more rationally, a number of ways of combating this inconvenience were evolved. For obvious reasons the more effective of these methods were such as established conditions exactly the reverse of those which led to the progressive diminution of the conditioned reflexes. Foremost among such methods was the introduction of an occasional abrupt shortening of the length of isolated action of the conditioned stimulus. If, for example, the reflex originally has been delayed 30 seconds, the practice is now adopted of reinforcing at the 3rd to 5th second. Of course, during this short period of time the conditioned stimulus cannot evoke a measurable reflex, and very often no salivary secretion whatever can be observed during so short a period of delay. The short delay, however, is only introduced as a temporary expedient, being, so to speak, only a therapeutic measure applied for the purpose of regenerating the conditioned reflex. Afterwards, when the usual 30 seconds' delay is restored, it is found that the reflex is as strong and as constant as in the beginning. It is useful to make this return from the short-delayed reflex to the long-delayed one by stages, only gradually increasing the length of the isolated action of the conditioned stimulus. The efficacy of this method, measured by the permanence of the reconstituted reflex, depends upon the degree of weakening of the conditioned reflex, upon the time during which this weakness is allowed to persist, and upon the length of time during which the short delay is practised as a therapeutic measure. A short period of practice restores the reflexes only to a small degree and for a short time. Where a profound weakening of the reflex has been allowed to persist for a very long time, the method which has just been described, and which is, generally speaking, very effective, no longer suffices, as will be shown presently, to restore the reflex.

A conditioned reflex which has become weakened in the course of long practice can be helped towards recovery by avoiding any numerous repetitions of the conditioned stimulus within a single experiment, and, if possible, confining the use of the stimulus to single applications. A similar beneficial effect results from a simple interruption, even for a few days, in the work upon the weakened conditioned reflexes.

Besides these there are several subsidiary methods, as, for example, to increase the strength of some of the conditioned stimuli or to increase their number, by the summation of positive induction, or finally by increasing the strength of the unconditioned stimuli. At present, however, interest centres mainly in the direct methods referred to above.

There are cases where the extent of the diminution in the strength of conditioned reflexes is such that none of the above methods can be of any help—all positive conditioned reflexes simply disappear. The animal grows inert in the stand during the experiment, and even declines the food which is given after application of the conditioned stimulus. This can be observed even with dogs which have served, on account of the stability of the conditioned reflexes, for extremely exact experimentation during a period of many years.

What is to be done with an animal in such a condition ? In the earlier period of our work such a dog would undoubtedly have been discarded as one which could be of no further use for our purpose. Now, on the other hand, the condition of such a dog is regarded as calling for further investigation, which, as a matter of fact, can easily be carried out. It is sufficient to stop the use of all the old conditioned stimuli, and to develop instead conditioned reflexes to new stimuli, for the seemingly insurmountable difficulty to disappear. The new conditioned reflexes develop extremely quickly, and this is not surprising since all the extraneous reflexes which originally interfered with the development of conditioned reflexes have long since disappeared. The newly developed reflexes quickly attain a maximal and constant strength, and the animal entirely returns to its original condition and can be used for further experimentation. In view of the extreme importance of this fact I shall describe in greater detail the history of one of the dogs [experiments by Dr. Podkopaev].

Experiments with this dog were started in June, 1921. One after another different positive and negative conditioned reflexes were established. Among these were several reflexes to tactile stimulation of different places of the skin (designated by numbers in the succeeding tables). All the reflexes were extremely constant in their magnitude and in the length of their latent period, and the dog was used during several years for experiments on various problems. The following example illustrates the strength of the positive reflexes as tested in an experiment of 30th August, 1922 :

Time	Conditioned stimulus applied during 30 seconds	Salivary Secretion in drops during 30 seconds	Latent period in seconds
12.30 p.m.	Tactile No. 1	14	2
1.10 ,,	Tactile No. 2	$14\frac{1}{2}$	3
1.20 ,,	Tactile No. 3	14	3
1.25 ,,	Metronome	$14\frac{1}{2}$	3
1.33 ,,	Tactile No. 4	$13\frac{1}{2}$	6
1.39 ,,	Tactile No. 4	13	3

An experiment performed on the 6th August, 1923, involving various positive stimuli and a conditioned inhibitor gave the following results :

Time	Conditioned stimulus applied during 30 seconds	Salivary Secretion in drops during 30 seconds	Latent period in seconds
10.20 a.m.	Tactile No. 4	11	2
10.28 ,,	Tactile No. 8 + tone	0	–
10.33 ,,	Tactile No. 5	$11\frac{1}{2}$	5
10.40 ,,	Tactile No. 5	10	5

An experiment of 12th June, 1924, with the positive reflexes and a negative one (conditioned inhibition, but with a different inhibitor) resulted as follows :

Time	Conditioned stimulus applied during 30 seconds	Salivary Secretion in drops during 30 seconds	Latent period in seconds
10.33 a.m.	Tactile No. 1	$3\frac{1}{2}$	7
10.42 ,,	Tactile No. 8 + lamp	0	–
$10.43\frac{1}{2}$,,	Tactile No. 1	3	10
10.49 ,,	Metronome	$5\frac{1}{2}$	7
10.56 ,,	Tactile No. 8	2	12
11.8 ,,	Tactile No. 8	1	23

Towards the end of 1924 the stimuli very often had a zero effect and the dog no longer took immediately the food which was presented. Several expedients were tried in order to get rid of this increasing inhibition. Instead of tactile stimuli auditory ones were mainly used, and instead of long delays very short ones ; intervals of as much as a month and a half were made between experiments ; an increase in the strength of the unconditioned stimuli was tried ; and the animal was kept on the floor during the experiments, instead of in the stand. Any beneficial effect produced by these methods was only fleeting : the animal became more and more languid and often altogether declined food given after the application of conditioned stimuli. This state of the animal persisted throughout the whole of the year 1925. At the end of 1925 the use of all the old conditioned stimuli was abandoned and new ones were introduced. This procedure led to a quick and definite change in the condition of the animal. It again became alert, and immediately took food on presentation at the end of the application of the new conditioned stimuli. The conditioned reflexes were quickly established and reached a constant and considerable strength, while the latent periods returned to normal. These results remained steady in subsequent experimentation. The following is an early experiment during this phase, performed on the 21st January, 1926. The reflexes in this experiment are delayed by 15 seconds, and an attempt is made to reinstate among the new conditioned stimuli one of the old ones to the sound of a metronome.

Time	Conditioned stimulus applied during 15 seconds	Secretion in drops during 15 seconds	Latent period in seconds
9.43 a.m.	Intermittent flashes of lamp	3	3
9.55 ,,	Bubbling sound	6	2
10.4 ,,	Crackling sound	$2\frac{1}{2}$	6
10.10 ,,	Metronome	4	2
10.15 ,,	Bubbling sound	3	4
10.22 ,,	Intermittent flashes of lamp	3	3

The differences in the magnitude of the conditioned reflexes in the above experiment depend to a certain extent on the different stages of development which they have reached.

The general significance of these experiments is obvious. The isolated action of the conditioned stimulus, even though followed by the unconditioned, leads to the development of a state of inhibition in the cortical elements, and this development is the quicker the greater the length of isolated action of each single conditioned stimulus and the more often such a stimulus is used. It thus becomes apparent that the difference between the process of development of inhibition as studied in the early lectures with respect to different cases of internal inhibition and in those cases which have just been described is not of fundamental importance; although in most cases very substantial it is obviously only one of degree. In those cases in which the conditioned stimulus remains unreinforced the inhibitory process develops very quickly; in those cases with reinforcement which have just been described the development of the inhibitory process is usually delayed—sometimes so considerably that its development may even remain unsuspected. Only in very rare cases is the rate of development of inhibition in both groups of experiments nearly or completely identical.

We now come to the problem as to the mechanism by which unconditioned stimuli retard the development of the type of inhibition which we are now considering. In the second lecture we saw that conditioned reflexes do not develop when the unconditioned stimulus precedes the neutral agent which is required to be made into a conditioned stimulus. This is probably a result of external inhibition, the strong excitation produced by the unconditioned stimulus leading to inhibition of that cortical area which is but weakly excited as a result of the application of the neutral stimulus. If this be the case, the question arises whether the unconditioned stimulus similarly produces external inhibition of the cortical areas corresponding to an already established conditioned reflex. To test this point experiments were performed as follows :

A firmly established conditioned stimulus was superimposed on the background of the reinforcing unconditioned stimulus, i.e. the unconditioned stimulus was applied first and the previously established conditioned stimulus was applied only after the effect of the unconditioned stimulus had become apparent. This mode of experimentation was continued for several weeks or months on many dogs. The results were without exception uniform : the conditioned reflex never kept its original strength, but either weakened considerably or else disappeared altogether.

The stronger and the more practised the conditioned reflexes were, the more slowly they disappeared under this treatment, whereas weak and recently established reflexes lost their conditioned properties very quickly. The following experiment by Dr. Solovaichik gives an illustration of this case.

The dog employed had many strongly developed alimentary conditioned reflexes, each of which gave upwards of 20 drops of saliva during 30 seconds.

The establishment of a new reflex to a hissing sound was now begun. This reflex developed very quickly, and counting from the sixth application to the eleventh it gave secretions of 10, 8, 13, 9, 9 and $10\frac{1}{2}$ drops during 30 seconds. Altogether only eleven reinforcements were made, after which the conditioned stimulus of the hissing sound was superimposed upon the unconditioned. The application was repeated in this way fifty-four times in the course of thirty-two successive days. The following table shows the trial of the hissing sound after the fifty-fourth superimposition:

Time	Conditioned stimulus applied during 30 seconds	Salivary Secretion in drops during 30 seconds	Motor reaction
2.28 p.m.	Buzzer	20	Alimentary
2.35 ,,	Flashes of lamp	9	,,
2.44 ,,	Hissing sound after administration of food	—	—
2.53 ,,	Hissing sound before administration of food	0	Investigatory reflex only
3.2 ,,	Metronome	16	Alimentary
3.10 ,,	Whistle	11	,,

It is thus clear that the administration of the unconditioned stimulus results in an inhibitory state of those cortical elements on which the conditioned reflex depends—these cortical cells becoming temporarily unresponsive to their normal exciting stimulus. The above experiment does not, however, disclose the inner mechanism determining the difference in rate of development of inhibition of the cortical elements in the case of reinforcement and non-reinforcement.

The sum of all the periods of action of a positive stimulus required for the development of inhibition without reinforcement is usually incomparably less than that of the periods of isolated action of the same stimulus with reinforcement. It follows therefore that the transition of the excited cortical elements into an inhibitory state is not determined by the aggregate duration of the isolated stimulus. It is, however, probable that the excitation in the case of non-reinforcement persists for a long time after the cessation of the isolated action of the conditioned stimulus, while in the case of reinforcement the excitation is curtailed from the beginning of the unconditioned stimulus. The aggregate duration of the excitation produced by the stimulus may, therefore, be the determining factor, but other explanations are possible and the matter cannot be decided without further experimentation.

The fundamental fact in all these experiments, which repeats itself time after time, is the transition sooner or later into inhibition of the state of the cortical elements acted upon by the conditioned stimulus. So far as concerns all the experimental evidence at our disposal up to the present, this transition must be regarded as depending on a functional exhaustion of the cortical elements as a result of their activity in response to a stimulus. Such an exhaustion would obviously be dependent upon the duration and intensity of this activity. On the other hand it is also obvious that the process of inhibition cannot be regarded as identical with such functional auto-destruction of the cortical elements, since a state of inhibition which is initiated in an active cell spreads to other cortical elements which were not active and which were not therefore functionally exhausted.

The rate at which cortical elements become subjected to inhibition in the case without reinforcement fits in with the extreme sensitivity which they exemplify in their extreme need for constant nutrition, being, as is well known, finally and irreparably destroyed by an arrest of the blood supply far sooner than any other tissue of the body. It is in complete harmony also with the conception of the cerebral cortex as a signalling apparatus. The fact that the unconditioned stimulus which is signalled induces during its action an inhibition in the cortex is only an artistic finishing touch to the efficiency of the machine. I may permit myself to use the analogy of an efficient and watchful signalman who after having performed his responsible duties has to be provided with an immediate rest during which he is refreshed, so that he may afterwards perform his task again with the same efficiency as before.

Another question arises whether there exists such a minimal period of isolated action of a conditioned stimulus as does not lead in time to a progressive development of inhibition in the cortical elements. The details of this problem are receiving a full experimental investigation in our laboratories at present, but there are some experiments already performed which have a probable bearing upon it. In dogs which had had for a very considerable time conditioned reflexes delayed by 30 seconds, and in which the conditioned stimuli still retained their full effect, all the reflexes were transformed into almost simultaneous ones by reinforcement 1 to 2 seconds after the beginning of the conditioned stimulus. This modification in the procedure immediately began to reflect itself on the secretory and motor components of these reflexes, bringing about also a disturbance of the previous balance in strength between positive and negative conditioned reflexes. The magnitude of the positive reflexes increased considerably, while the negative reflexes were to a large extent dis-inhibited ; in other words excitation began to predominate over inhibition [experiments of Dr. Petrova and Dr. Kreps]. The following is the method used by Dr. Kreps :

The dog, in view of an especially exaggerated tendency to inhibition, was not kept in its stand during the experiments, but was kept on the floor. Among other conditioned reflexes this dog possessed a positive alimentary reflex to 132 beats per minute of a metronome, while a rate of 144 beats per minute served as the stimulus to a precise and stable differentiation. A considerable time before the experiment a conditioned inhibition had been established in which flashes of a lamp acted as the conditioned inhibitor to a rate of 120 beats per minute of the metronome. The conditioned inhibition was absolute, but had not been used for a considerable time. All the reflexes were delayed 30 seconds. These delayed conditioned alimentary reflexes were now transformed into simultaneous ones, the food being presented one second only after the administration of the conditioned stimulus. The modification in the mode of reinforcement led to a disappearance of the conditioned inhibition, which could not be re-established in spite of 100 applications of the inhibitory combination during 36 days. The differentiation of the metronome, which was absolute before the transformation of the reflexes into simultaneous ones, was also dis-inhibited, and in the succeeding 33 repetitions which were performed within 13 days the differentiation continued to be unsatisfactory (3 drops as against 6 to 7 of the positive reflex). On returning to the delay of 30 seconds with all the reflexes, the differentiation again became absolute during the very first day, and the conditioned inhibition was completely re-established after 3 days, as shown by the following table :

Time	Conditioned stimulus during 30 seconds	Secretion in drops during 30 seconds
1.6 p.m.	Metronome, 120 beats	7
1.10 ,,	,, ,,	5
1.20 ,,	,, ,,	6
1.26 ,,	,, ,, + flashes of lamp	0
1.33 ,,	Metronome, 120 beats	6
1.38 ,,	,, ,,	6
1.45 ,,	,, ,, + flashes of lamp	0

On transforming the reflexes again into simultaneous ones the conditioned inhibition was almost completely dis-inhibited after only three repetitions of the simultaneous reinforcement.

It remains still to be determined whether in the experiments just described, in which the conditioned stimulus is almost immediately followed by the unconditioned, there will be no tendency towards a progressive development of inhibition with prolonged practice, or whether the apparent vigour of the reflexes will be only temporary and will, though much later, nevertheless be superseded by inhibition.

Hand in hand with the exhaustion of the cortical elements there goes of course their recovery. We should expect, therefore, that the inhibition which appears to stand in some kind of relation to functional exhaustion of the cortical elements should disappear with their functional recovery. This expectation fits the case of spontaneous recovery of extinguished conditioned reflexes which after some interval of time return to their normal strength. Regarded from this point of view it becomes more easy to understand how the slowly developing inhibition on repetition of the reinforced conditioned reflexes is replaced by a temporary return of the delayed reflexes to their original strength when a period of very short delays is introduced or when a considerable interval is made between experiments. By shortening the period of isolated action of the conditioned stimulus in the one case, or by completely avoiding for a time any repetition of the excitation in the other case, the functional exhaustion of the cortical elements is diminished and a better opportunity is afforded for complete recovery.

Experiments are now being performed with the object of specially studying the restoration of conditioned reflexes in the case of experimental extinction, and in the case of the gradual spontaneous development of inhibition occurring in spite of reinforcement. An example of such an experiment may be taken from a research by Dr. Speransky.

Amongst others the following serve as positive conditioned alimentary stimuli : beats of a metronome, intensification of the general illumination of the room, the sound of a whistle, and the appearance of a circle. The acoustic reflexes were somewhat stronger than the visual ones, giving 10 to 12 drops during 30 seconds preceding reinforcement while the visual ones gave only 6 to 8 drops. The stimuli were all applied at intervals of 10 minutes and always in the above order. In every experiment all the stimuli were repeated once or twice. Following a series of experiments of this type the next experiment would consist in stimulation by the metronome alone. Twelve successive applications were made at intervals of 10 minutes, each being reinforced. The first two applications gave 12 and 11 drops of salivary secretion respectively during their isolated action, while the last two gave 9 drops each. It is thus seen that simple repetition of the stimulus led to a diminution in its effect by 25%. On the following day a similar experiment was conducted, but the interval between the stimuli was made very much shorter, being only $1\frac{1}{2}$ minutes. The use of such short intervals was possible only because in this particular dog the secretion caused by the reinforcement with food finished extremely quickly and, as had been found by previous determinations, well within the $1\frac{1}{2}$ minutes. In this variation of the experiment the reflex which measured 11 drops on the first stimulation became diminished to $4\frac{1}{2}$ drops on the third stimulation (diminution by 60%), to 2 drops on the 8th stimulation (diminution by 82%) ; passing with more or less regular undulations of 2, 5, and 7 drops, it gave on the 22nd stimulation only one drop and then no secretion at all, the dog even refusing food after the last three stimuli. When the visual stimulus of increased illumination of the room was applied $1\frac{1}{2}$ minutes after the last stimulation by the metronome a reflex of $2\frac{1}{2}$ drops of secretion was produced, and the animal took the food. Moreover, when food was given without a previous conditioned stimulus the animal devoured it with avidity. On the next day a return was made to the original method of application of all the conditioned stimuli at intervals of 10 minutes. The metronome was the first stimulus to be applied and gave $6\frac{1}{2}$ drops.

On introducing a second stimulation by the metronome as the 5th stimulus the secretion obtained was only $1\frac{1}{2}$ drops. Finally, introduced a third time as the 9th stimulus, the metronome did not produce any secretion at all. In this experiment the secretion given by the other stimuli, although slightly below normal on their first application, did not greatly diminish on repetition. The reflex to the metronome was found to be restored to its usual intensity on the following day, and now it showed no further tendency to diminish on repetition. The foregoing experiment presents many points of interest. It is seen that one and the same stimulus which is constantly reinforced and repeated many times at long intervals of time loses only little of its effect : the same stimulus when applied at short intervals of time quickly diminishes in its effect at first, then after a wave-like variation it ends by giving a complete zero of secretory and motor reactions, the animal declining food after the conditioned stimuli. In spite of this, another and usually much weaker stimulus immediately evokes both secretory and motor effects. The fact that the animal in the stand consumed with avidity a large amount of food when not preceded by the conditioned stimulus shows that satiety of the animal played no part. Relating the effect of the beats of the metronome to different states of the cortical elements it must be concluded that in the case of frequent stimulation these elements get functionally exhausted and have insufficient time for recovery, so that after a preliminary oscillation which may be regarded as a struggle between excitation and inhibition the cortical elements pass completely into inhibition. The weaker visual stimulus diminishes considerably in its effect after the disappearance of the conditioned reflex to the stronger stimulus of the metronome. On the following day the cortical elements which are stimulated by the metronome are still not fully recovered and pass again into inhibition when the stimulus is repeated. This inhibition is of the same character as the internal inhibition which has been described in previous lectures, and it exhibits the same properties of irradiating to other cortical elements which were not primarily involved. The experiment shows that the inhibition irradiating to neighbouring cortical elements standing in connection with other conditioned stimuli leads to a diminution of their positive effect, exactly as was described for internal inhibition. That the inhibition in the neighbouring cortical elements is really due to an irradiation of the primary inhibition is evidenced by the fact that on repetition of the stimuli they do not show such a rapid diminution in their effect as is observed in the case of the metronome. On the third day the cortical elements related to the metronome became almost entirely functionally restored.

The observations described in this lecture open up many important problems, and in the first instance the question of rapidity of recovery from the inhibitory effect of different stimuli during complete rest and during activity, the effect upon this recovery of reinforcement, and so on. Besides these comparatively straightforward problems there are more complex and more difficult ones. It is obvious that only certain cases of the development or disappearance of inhibition can be brought into relation with a supposed functional exhaustion and recovery of the cortical elements, and we cannot interpret in this fashion the cases of permanent and unvarying inhibitions in which the activity of the cortex is so rich—for example, all cases where an established inhibitory conditioned stimulus evokes an inhibition of the cortical elements directly and without a preceding phase of excitation—as, for instance, in the case of differentiation and conditioned inhibition. The problem presented by inhibitions of the latter type becomes still more complicated when we remember that those points of the cortex which become the centres of such direct inhibitions are never transformed into centres for excitation, even though the experiments are interrupted for weeks and months.

LECTURE XV

Internal inhibition and sleep as one and the same process with regard to their intimate mechanism.

In the last lecture we arrived at the very important conclusion that under the influence of our conditioned stimuli the cortical elements invariably enter sooner or later into an inhibitory state. With frequent repetitions of the stimuli this happens extremely quickly, and it may legitimately be regarded as an expression of the fact that the cortical elements, which represent the highest point of development of the nervous system, are extremely sensitive and therefore are functionally exhausted with comparative ease. The progressively developing inhibition, which itself cannot be regarded as a functional exhaustion, but which is a result of exhaustion, assumes the rôle of a protector of the cortical elements, preventing any excessive fatigue or dangerous functional destruction of this highly sensitive structure. During the period when the cells are in a state of inhibition, being free from activity the cortical elements recover their normal state. This applies to all the cellular structures of the cortex equally, and therefore under conditions in which a great number of cortical points are repeatedly entering into a state of excitation the whole of the cortex may be expected sooner or later to become subjected to inhibition. Such a state of widely spread inhibition actually does occur, exactly in the same manner as in the case of individual cortical elements, and is familiar to all of us as the common and everyday occurrence of sleep. The complete and continuous proof of this contention is spread over the whole of our twenty-five years' work upon the hemispheres, and at the present time no part of the physiology of the hemispheres studied by the method of conditioned reflexes is better substantiated. Drowsiness and sleep were met with in our experimental animals from the very beginning of our work, and we have been obliged to direct our attention towards them continually. This, of course, has led to the collection of an immense number of facts, which were bound in different phases of our experimentation to receive many different interpretations. However, already for many years all these varied interpretations have been fused into a final one harmonizing with all the facts at our disposal. This conclusion is, in essence, that sleep and what we call internal inhibition are one and the same process.

The fundamental condition of the appearance and development of internal inhibition and sleep is exactly the same. It consists in the more or less prolonged or many times repeated isolated action of a conditioned stimulus producing stimulation of the cellular structures in the cortex. In all cases of internal inhibition which were discussed in the fourth to the seventh lectures drowsiness and sleep were met with continually. In the case of extinction of a conditioned reflex some animals even at the first extinction showed not only a disappearance of the conditioned secretory and corresponding motor reaction but also a great dullness as compared with the normal state of the animal before the extinction. Repetition of extinctions, in the course of a number of days, even if all the conditioned stimuli were reinforced in between, led in every case to an obvious drowsiness and even sleep of the animal in its stand, though no such symptoms had ever previously been observed. The same happens, but to a much greater extent, in the development of differentiation. To take an example. An animal has conditioned reflexes established to different stimuli, including one to a definite musical tone. During the whole period of work the animal remains alert. The development of a differentiation of a tone close to the positive one is now started, and it is noticed that during the process the animal gets drowsy. The drowsiness gradually increases, and often culminates in a deep sleep with a complete relaxation of the skeletal muscles, and snoring, so that when now other positive conditioned stimuli are administered and reinforced by food it is necessary to stir up the animal and even to introduce the food forcibly into its mouth to initiate the act of eating. Exactly the same thing happens in the case of development of long-delayed reflexes (for example, with a delay of three minutes), and in the early period of our work this interfered with our researches, for, being not yet thoroughly familiar with the technique, it was impossible to obtain in some animals the reflex we required, on account of the development of sleep. The same happens also in the development of conditioned inhibition, but to a smaller extent.

In all the foregoing cases of internal inhibition sleep develops fairly rapidly, which depends on non-reinforcement of the conditioned stimulus. In the case of the slowly developing internal inhibitions produced by the repeated use of reinforced conditioned stimuli over a period of months or years, the development of sleep is proportionately slower and generally speaking stops short at one or other of the intermediate stages between the alert state and sleep itself, depending on the dog employed. In this respect the animals differ exactly as they differ in respect of rapidity of development of the common forms of internal inhibition.

It is not necessary to give any examples of individual experiments upon this transition of internal inhibition into sleep, since all our experiments abound with observations showing that internal inhibition invariably passes into sleep unless special precautions are taken. As there is practically no stimulus of whatever strength that cannot, under certain conditions, become subjected to internal inhibition, so also there is none which cannot produce sleep. Very powerful electric shocks applied to the skin, when used as conditioned alimentary stimuli, led, after many months of use in the experiments of Dr. Eroféeva, to a progressively increasing internal inhibition in spite of continuous reinforcement, and in the experiments of Dr. Petrova they became most effectual agents in inducing sleep. Similarly, different external agencies in their rôle of conditioned stimuli fall into an identical order of classification as regards the rapidity with which they lead to internal inhibition and to sleep. It was mentioned in the preceding lecture that internal inhibition develops most readily with thermal and least readily with auditory stimuli ; in exactly the same manner sleep develops quickly with thermal conditioned reflexes and more slowly and less frequently with auditory conditioned reflexes. The interference by sleep in the case of thermal conditioned stimuli was indeed so persistent and upset the work to so great an extent that in the early period of our research I had real difficulty in finding collaborators who would agree to work with these stimuli.

Finally, the length of isolated action of the conditioned stimulus was mentioned as a factor determining the development of internal inhibition ; so also it is a factor in determining the development of sleep. In some dogs, while the conditioned reflex was delayed only 10 or 15 seconds, the animal remained fully alert during experiments spread over years, but so soon as the reflex was delayed for 30 seconds drowsiness and sleep appeared. The results of this type of experiment are often truly striking, for the quick transition from full alertness into true physiological sleep, due to this seemingly insignificant change in the experimental conditions, is amazing. Examples with variable length of delay and with variable precision of results are strewn over our work in abundance.

All those methods described in the preceding lecture as retarding or abolishing that progressive growth of internal inhibition, which develops in the case of frequently repeated conditioned reflexes notwithstanding their constant reinforcement, can be used with equal efficiency for the purpose of resisting sleep.

At this point the following question naturally arises : If sleep so closely coincides in its appearance and disappearance with internal inhibition, how is it that the latter plays such an extremely important part during the alert state of the animal, serving for the most delicate physiological mechanism of equilibration of the higher organism with its environment ? To my mind all the facts which have been given in the preceding lectures dispose at once of the apparent contradiction. Internal inhibition during the alert state is nothing but a scattered sleep, sleep of separate groups of cellular structures ; and sleep itself is nothing but internal inhibition which is widely irradiated, extending over the whole mass of the hemispheres and involving the lower centres of the brain as well. Thus internal inhibition in the alert state of the animal represents a regional distribution of sleep which is kept within bounds by the antagonistic nervous process of excitation. Such a restricting antagonism has been illustrated already in the lectures upon the functional mosaic of the cortex and upon its analysing activity.

In the case of extinction the development of sleep is prevented only if after extinction the conditioned stimuli are systematically reinforced and extinction is not repeated too often. In differentiation of stimuli the developing internal inhibition—which tends at first to be accompanied by sleep—can only be definitely restricted within its own analyser by inserting the inhibitory conditioned stimuli between repeated applications of the positive conditioned stimulus. In this manner the process of excitation which is repeatedly being evoked antagonizes a universal spreading of internal inhibition. Exactly the same is observed in the case of conditioned inhibition and inhibition of delay. In all these cases if the experiment is conducted with forethought drowsiness and sleep appear only as phasic events during the time when the physiological demarcation between the areas of excitation and inhibition is not yet fully established. However, as soon as the conditions of the experiments lead to a prevalence of inhibition sleep again reappears. The following is a striking example : In the lecture upon the functional mosaic a dog was mentioned in which a tone served as the stimulus to a positive conditioned reflex, while twenty neighbouring tones up and down the scale were differentiated as stimuli for negative conditioned reflexes. This animal was never inclined to drowsiness or sleep when a balance was maintained between the number of repetitions of the positive and negative conditioned stimuli, and under these conditions the dog always gave full reflexes to the applications of the positive stimulus. As soon, however, as the inhibitory tones were used several times in succession, the dog quickly fell into such profound sleep that even most powerful extraneous stimuli failed to awaken it. When a return was made to the interposition of the negative conditioned stimuli between applications of the positive one, sleep was never observed to develop. In this respect, such experiments as have already been mentioned in connection with the mosaic character of cortical functions—especially those with the use of tactile stimuli—are very instructive. In spite of a tendency of tactile conditioned stimuli to favour the development of drowsiness and sleep, the dog used by Dr. Koupalov never exhibited any signs of drowsiness, although a conditioned tactile mosaic was practised in this dog for over two years (p. 223). This was obviously due to the inhibition being constantly limited and checked in its irradiation by the antagonistic excitatory process. Another method of combating any wide irradiation of inhibition is to increase the number of positive conditioned stimuli, and so check the spread of inhibition from its initial points of development.

The following observation of Dr. Petrova, which to some extent also bears on this subject, is more complicated. A long-delayed alimentary reflex to a metronome was being developed without the previous establishment of a simultaneous reflex : the length of the delay was 3 minutes. During several days the dog became more and more drowsy, and finally fell into a state of profound sleep. Obviously the inhibition which developed during the first period of action of the metronome was so powerful that it prevented the development of the phase of excitation which normally precedes reinforcement. Five new agencies were now used to develop further alimentary conditioned reflexes—these agencies together with the original stimulus were allowed to act for only 5 seconds before reinforcement. Drowsiness quickly disappeared and all the reflexes developed with ease. The delay before reinforcement was now gradually extended in all six reflexes by 5 seconds each day. Corresponding with the increase in delay before reinforcement the latent period of the reflexes became longer, and finally without any interference of sleep six long-delayed reflexes became firmly established, all with a preliminary period of inhibition of 1-1½ minutes. The process of excitation, originating in six different points of the cortex, allowed the inhibition to develop only gradually, limiting it both in time and space and preventing the development of sleep.

To the same group as the last belong some further observations which were made in only a few dogs, all of them very easily subjected to inhibition. These dogs developed drowsiness and sleep simply on account of limitation of movements when placed in the stand. Sleep could be avoided, at least for some length of time, by conducting the experiments with the animals free upon the floor. It is probable that under the latter condition stimuli originating within the motor apparatus and the skin provided fairly regular foci of excitation within the cortex which counteracted to some extent any wide irradiation of conditioned inhibition. However, another factor of probably greater importance also undoubtedly played a part, and to this we shall return later.

What has been shown to take place in the cortical elements with respect to the development of internal inhibition under the influence of conditioned stimuli, can be observed to the same extent in the case of stimulation of the cortical elements by agents which have no special conditioned physiological significance. As has previously been mentioned, among the different reflexes the investigatory reflex has a special importance. This reflex has a *point d'appui* in the cells of the cortex as well as in the lower parts of the brain. In the normal animal the reflex is undoubtedly produced with the active co-operation of the cortex. This view is supported by the exquisite sensitivity of the reflex, for it is evoked by any minutest change in the environment. This is made possible only through the presence of the higher analysing activity of the cerebral cortex and is wholly unattainable by the lower parts of the brain alone. The investigatory reflex, as we know, invariably weakens on repetition, and finally disappears altogether. Special experiments conducted in my laboratory by Professor Popov showed that the disappearance of the investigatory reflex is based on the development of inhibition, and is in all details analogous to extinction of conditioned reflexes.

If the agent which is responsible for the investigatory reflex ceases, on repetition at frequent intervals of time during one single experiment, to call forth the corresponding motor reaction, a prolongation of the interval in the same experiment restores the reaction exactly as in the case of extinguished conditioned reflexes. Similarly, a definite investigatory reflex which has only just disappeared on account of repetition of the stimulus becomes temporarily re-established by an application of some new extra stimulus calling forth another investigatory reflex. It follows, therefore, that the extinguished investigatory reflex undergoes dis-inhibition exactly as do the underlying positive reflexes in cases of internal inhibition. If the investigatory reflex to a definite agent is repeatedly evoked in the course of a number of days it permanently disappears, just as does a systematically non-reinforced conditioned reflex. Finally, such an extinguished investigatory reflex can be temporarily re-established by administration of stimulants (caffeine) exactly, for example, as in the case of conditioned differentiated reflexes (p. 127). The inhibition of the investigatory reflex invariably leads to drowsiness and sleep (even more easily than the inhibition of conditioned reflexes). In the following experiments by Dr. Chechoulin the development of inhibition and sleep in the case of the investigatory reflex was studied by means of conditioned stimuli.

The dog used for these experiments had a conditioned alimentary reflex established to a whistle. Hissing, bubbling, tactile stimulation of the skin and other stimuli were all applied for the first time to bring about the investigatory reflex.

Time	Conditioned stimulus applied during 30 seconds	Salivary Secretion in drops during 30 seconds	Latent period in seconds	Remarks
4.7 p.m.	Whistle	3	3	Reinforced
4.15 ,,	Whistle	4	3	Reinforced

Now, beginning from 4.21 p.m., the bubbling sound was repeatedly applied during periods of 30 seconds and at intervals of 2 minutes. During the first three applications there were movements of orientation of the animal in the direction of the sound, and these movements gradually became weaker. With the fourth application the first signs of drowsiness made their appearance. Up to the eighth repetition the sleep was interrupted at different moments of the stimulation. During the eighth and ninth stimulations all movements of the animal disappeared. At 4.43 p.m. the sound of bubbling was applied for 10 seconds, and then the whistle was added and kept on for 30 seconds. This brought about neither motor nor secretory reaction and the sleep continued. Administration of food awakened the animal; it took the food but even after that it still remained drowsy. The experiment with the conditioned stimulus continued as follows :

Time	Conditioned stimulus applied during 30 seconds	Salivary Secretion in drops during 30 seconds	Latent period in seconds	Remarks
4.53 p.m.	Whistle	$2\frac{1}{2}$	8	Reinforced
5.2 ,,	Whistle	3	7	Reinforced

It should be remembered that this dog was never observed to fall asleep in its stand during the usual experiments with conditioned reflexes. In the succeeding experiments new agents bringing about an investigatory reflex were repeated up to the point of sleep, or sometimes only until the stage of disappearance of the motor reaction. Twenty-one days after the experiment recorded above tactile stimulation of the skin was used as the extra stimulus for the investigatory reflex, the experiment proceeding as follows :

Time	Conditioned stimuli of different duration	Secretion in drops	Latent period in seconds	Remarks
2.5 p.m.	Whistle, 5 secs.	–	–	Reinforced
2.12 ,,	Whistle, 30 secs.	6	5	Reinforced
2.21 ,,	Whistle, 5 secs.	–	–	Reinforced

The conditioned reflex in the above experiment was twice reinforced after only five seconds of the action of the stimulus in order to maintain the normal strength of the reflex to the end of the experiment.

Starting from 4.25 p.m. an application of the tactile cutaneous stimulus was made during 30 seconds and similar applications were repeated at intervals of one minute. During the first three applications the animal turned its head towards the place on the skin where the tactile stimulus was applied. During the fourth and fifth repetitions there were no movements at all, but there was no drowsiness of the animal. Now, at 4.32½ p.m., the tactile stimulus was applied singly during 10 seconds, after which the whistle was added to it and both stimuli were continued together during 30 seconds. Fifteen seconds after the beginning of the action of the whistle there was a commencement of salivary secretion, but during the whole remaining period of stimulation only 2 drops were recorded. The experiment continued as follows :

Time	Conditioned stimulus applied during 30 seconds	Secretion in drops	Latent period in seconds	Remarks
2.45 p.m.	Whistle	5	7	Reinforced

The experiments show that on repetition the motor component of the investigatory reflex gradually diminished, and that, on continuing the repetitions further, drowsiness developed and became more and more profound, although in some experiments before drowsiness appeared the stimulus remained, during a certain interval of time, apparently without effect. Nevertheless, superimposition of a conditioned stimulus upon the extraneous stimulus showed that during the whole period of this apparent ineffectiveness the investigatory agent was exerting an inhibitory influence (the experiment with the tactile stimulus as extra stimulus). This inhibition of the conditioned stimulus was not due to external inhibition, for, so far from producing inhibition of the conditioned reflexes, a weakened investigatory reflex actually dis-inhibits them (compare the sixth lecture for the action of the investigatory reflex upon the two phases of delayed conditioned reflexes). It is obvious therefore that inhibition and sleep develop as a result of the repetition of the investigatory reflex, in the former case leading to a diminution and in the latter to a disappearance of the conditioned reflex (the experiment with the bubbling sound).

The same is very well shown also when the experiments are conducted on puppies [experiments of Dr. Rosenthal]. On monotonous repetition of a stimulus under constant environmental conditions the puppies fall asleep very quickly and often with surprising simultaneity. It is, I think, a common experience that man, when unused to an intensive mental life, usually falls into drowsiness and sleep when subjected to the accompanying monotonous stimuli, however unfortunate such drowsiness or sleep may be as to place and as to time. This means, of course, that the definite cortical elements which react to such protracted external stimuli become functionally fatigued and pass into a state of inhibition, which in the absence of a counteraction by an excitation of other places, spreads over the hemispheres and leads to sleep. The extreme rapidity with which the cellular structures of the cortex undergo functional fatigue and become subjected to inhibition can be contrasted with the persistence of function of the cellular structures of the spinal cord and medulla under identical conditions. Experiments by Dr. Zeliony in our laboratory showed that while in a normal dog an investigatory reflex to a definite sound quickly vanished, the same sound in a dog with extirpated cortex, under identical conditions, called forth an investigatory reflex in a stereotyped manner and for an unlimited number of times.

To return again to conditioned reflexes. The development of inhibition with its ultimate expression in the form of sleep is due to functional fatigue of the cellular structures of the cortex. This is borne out by the following observations which were made repeatedly in our laboratory. In dogs in which any analyser had been surgically damaged, positive conditioned stimuli related to this analyser could scarcely be continued even for a very short time singly, since they tended quickly to assume inhibitory properties ; quite often they never excited any preliminary positive action at all, but behaved as inhibitory stimuli from the start. This phenomenon is especially constant and easy of demonstration in the case of the damaged cutaneous analyser. After extirpation of the *gyri coronarius* and *ecto-sylvius anterior* (see Fig. 8), positive reflexes to tactile stimulation of the extremities, pelvis and shoulder became replaced for several months by inhibitory reflexes. That the reflexes were now truly inhibitory was proved by the fact that positive conditioned reflexes related to other analysers showed their full normal effect before the application of a tactile stimulus, but diminished in their positive effect or lost it altogether after the application of the tactile conditioned stimulus. At the same time tactile stimuli quickly and easily produced sleep even in dogs which never before the operation fell asleep in response to tactile stimuli. These facts often assumed the following extremely impressive form. A tactile conditioned stimulus which was applied to the part of the cutaneous surface related to the damaged portion of the analyser would lead to inhibition and sleep, but the same stimulus applied to the skin corresponding to the non-damaged portion of the analyser would give a full positive effect, leaving the animal fully alert [experiments of Dr. Krasnogorsky, Dr. Rosenkov and Dr. Archangelsky]. To the same group of observations belong those made in our laboratory during the period of shortage in Russia a few years ago. The semi-starved animals could not be used for experiments with conditioned reflexes, since all positive conditioned stimuli assumed inhibitory properties, and the dogs invariably developed sleep exactly in conjunction with the application of the conditioned stimuli. Obviously the general malnutrition of the dog had powerfully affected the functional resistance of the cortical elements [experiments of Dr. Frolov, Dr. Rosenthal and others].

In the examples enumerated up to the present we have had only cases of transition of inhibition into sleep, but the reverse can also take place, sleep passing into inhibition. To take an example. A conditioned reflex delayed by 3 minutes has been established. The animal is placed in the stand and is fully alert, but so soon as the conditioned stimulus is applied the animal becomes drowsy and no salivary secretion is evoked during the whole 3 minutes. When food is given at the end of the third minute the animal takes it but slowly and reluctantly. The stimulus is repeated several times in the same experiment with the usual variations of the interval between the applications; at each stimulation the dog becomes more alert and the secretion appears at first towards the end of the 3rd minute. On further repetition of the stimulation the secretion augments and finally the three-minute period of stimulation divides itself approximately into two equal parts. In the first part there is no secretion, although the animal remains entirely alert; in the second part there is a copious secretion, and at the end of the stimulation the animal takes the food promptly and eats it with avidity. In this case the widely irradiated inhibition (sleep), which appeared in the beginning on account of the preponderance of the inhibition initiated during the first part of the action of the conditioned stimulus, gets gradually concentrated into a restricted inhibition. This concentrating of the inhibition is brought about through the influence of the progressively increasing excitation determined by the second part of the action of the conditioned stimulus and by the dis-inhibitory effect of reinforcement.

It sometimes happens that the reverse, namely a pure replacement of inhibition by sleep, is obtained with the long delay of 3 minutes, or even with delays so short as 30 seconds. The animal, which has previously kept fully alert in its stand during the experiment, now falls asleep, each time exactly at the beginning of the action of the conditioned stimulus. The eyes close, the head droops, the whole body relaxes and hangs on the loops of the stand, and the animal emits an occasional snore. After the lapse of a definite period of time—in the short delay 25 seconds or in the case of the long delay $1\frac{1}{2}$-2 minutes—the animal quickly and spontaneously awakens and exhibits a sharp alimentary motor and salivary reaction. It is clear that in this case an inhibition which is generally concentrated becomes replaced by diffused inhibition, *i.e.* sleep.

Finally, it can also be shown [experiments of Dr. Foursikov] that a summation of two distinct and different inhibitions leads to sleep. For example, the dog has a well-established long-delayed conditioned reflex to a metronome : the length of the delay is 3 minutes. No salivary secretion occurs during the first two minutes of the stimulation, but at the end of the second minute the secretion appears, and reaches a maximum towards the end of the third minute. An extraneous stimulus of a weak hissing sound is now made to accompany the conditioned stimulus. The hissing sound dis-inhibits the inhibitory phase of the reflex, while a small motor reaction in the form of an investigatory reflex towards the hissing is observed. The conditioned reflex is reinforced. On a repetition of this com-bination not only does the investigatory reflex to the hissing disappear, but the alimentary reflex also, and the animal becomes obviously drowsy. This experiment can only be interpreted in the following way : The investigatory reflex to hissing undergoes extinction on its first application, and now, therefore, the hissing sound initiates an inhibitory process. This inhibitory process summates with the inhibitory phase of the delayed reflex and streng-thens it to such an extent that the excitatory phase of the reflex is never allowed to develop, being replaced by general drowsiness of the animal. That this is the true interpretation of the experiment appears abundantly in the sequel. On the next repetition of the conditioned stimulus, and without the addition of the weak hissing sound, a regular delayed reflex, with its two phases well pronounced, is obtained, and on repeating after this the combination of the metronome with the hissing sound the conditioned reflex again disappears and obvious drowsiness takes its place. The following are the actual figures of the experiment :

Time	Stimulus during 3 minutes	Secretion in drops during successive 30 seconds	Remarks
4.52 p.m.	Metronome + hissing	0, 3, $3\frac{1}{2}$, 1, 0, $3\frac{1}{2}$	Weak investigatory reflex
5.3 ,,	,, ,,	0, 0, 0, 0, 0, 0	No movements of animal; pronounced drowsiness
5.15 ,,	Metronome	0, 0, 0, 0, 1, 9	Normal alimentary reaction; the reflex is reinforced
5.28 ,,	Metronome + hissing	0, 0, 0, 0, 0, 0	Drowsiness

In this connection I conceive it useful to draw attention to the following interesting point. It is evident that the above experiment, together with that of Dr. Chechoulin mentioned previously (p. 256), reveals still another phase in the action of extra stimuli upon conditioned reflexes. A powerful extra stimulus, as will be remembered from the sixth lecture, at first brings about through the investigatory reflex a complete inhibition of the delayed reflex. On repetition, when the investigatory reflex considerably weakens, it brings about only dis-inhibition of the first phase of the delayed reflex. Finally, as we have just learned, the extra stimulus yet again inhibits the reflex, but now by another mechanism : it becomes itself a stimulus for a direct initiation of an inhibition in the cortex. A weak extra stimulus, as was just shown by the experiment of Dr. Foursikov, brings about at first a weak and transitory investigatory reflex and so leads on its very first application to dis-inhibition of the delayed reflex (4.52 p.m.). Afterwards, the weak extra stimulus itself initiates a second, and now direct, inhibition.

The following general properties of inhibition and sleep also uphold our view as to their identity. In the preceding lectures abundant evidence was given to establish the fact of irradiation and concentration of the inhibitory process within the mass of the cerebral cortex, and it was shown that the development of the inhibition was extremely slow, being measured by minutes. Moreover, it varied in respect to rate in different animals and under different conditions. There is no question but that sleep also does not develop instantly. We know from our own experience how drowsiness and sleep overtake us only gradually, and how sometimes they spread only slowly and with difficulty ; and some investigators, indeed, have endeavoured to study experimentally the problem of the gradual involving of the activity of the different sense organs, and its more complex mental concomitants. We know also how variable is the rate of transition in human beings between sleep and waking, and the same variability has been observed in our experimental animals. Moreover, during our lectures it has constantly been mentioned how inhibition, which at first develops with difficulty, gets reproduced with greater and greater ease upon practice and repetition and by using different forms of inhibition. Exactly in the same manner, extra stimuli, and conditioned stimuli which upon repetition bring about a state of sleep, with practice bring about this state more and more easily.

The following is of special interest. As was discussed previously, inhibition induces excitation. Corresponding with this, in some animals in which the inhibitory phase of a delayed reflex is replaced by sleep, this appearance of sleep is on some occasions preceded by a short period of a slight but definite general excitation of the animal. The phenomenon is still more obvious and constant when sleep is induced under the action of a repeated and prolonged neutral extra stimulus. It was often observed in the experiments by Dr. Rosenthal, that, when the neutral stimulus evoked definite drowsiness in a puppy, and before the animal completely fell asleep, it passed through a fleeting phase of excitation, moved about uneasily, scratched itself, and barked without any obvious reason, holding its nose up into the air. A similar state of general excitation preceding sleep, as is well known, often occurs in children. It is legitimate to regard such phenomena as an effect of induction. The excitation in initial stages of anaesthesia could also perhaps be interpreted from this point of view.

I believe the aggregate of facts given in the present lecture can be taken as sufficient proof of the view that sleep and internal inhibition are fundamentally one and the same process. I personally do not know, up to the present, of a single fact in all our researches which contradicts this conception. It is to be deplored, however, that we have as yet no reliable graphic method of registration of sleep. On some occasions we tried to apply for this purpose a graphic registration of the position of the head of the animal. A perfection of some such method for the graphic registration of sleep is greatly to be desired, so that the whole evidence regarding sleep can be expressed in an exact quantitative manner.

The details of our normal everyday existence are in full agreement with the foregoing interpretation of sleep. Our daily work, for some of us a round of exceeding monotony and for others extremely rich and varied, in either case must in the end determine an appearance of sleep. A prolonged stimulation of one and the same point in the cortex leads to a great and profound inhibition, and this irradiates widely so as to involve the whole of the cortex and the lower parts of the brain. In the case of a varied activity, although no given point of the cortex attains such a profound depth of inhibition, yet the great number of inhibitory points leads to a widely distributed inhibitory state even without wide irradiation, and this also descends to affect some of the lower centres of the brain. Of course a great number of quickly changing stimuli following in succession may often exert a very prolonged and powerful resistance to the general dissemination of inhibition over the hemispheres, thus delaying the onset of sleep. A well-established rhythm in the changes from wakefulness to sleep and from sleep to wakefulness may determine a beginning of sleep even without a sufficient functional fatigue of the cellular structures of the cortex. Both cases have had sufficient illustration in our experiments, in the analogous relations between the excitatory and inhibitory processes.

LECTURE XVI

Transition stages between the alert state and complete sleep : hypnotic stages.

In the last lecture an abundant array of facts was brought forward showing that sleep is nothing but internal inhibition which has become diffused continuously (*i.e.* without intervening fields of excitation) over the entire cortex and has descended also to some of the lower parts of the brain.

Since, as we know, the spread of inhibition is a gradual process involving first a smaller and then a greater area we should expect to find different extensities as well as different intensities of sleep or, in other words, transition stages between the fully alert state and complete sleep. Such transition stages actually exist ; we had many opportunities to observe them and to produce them experimentally.

In our experiments we came across not only the usual form of sleep, which is evidenced by an absence of the normal function of the cortex and a relaxation of the skeletal muscles (closure of the eyes, drooping of the head, sagging limbs, and body limply hanging in the loops of the stand), but also a quite different form, so far, at any rate, as could be judged by the condition of the skeletal muscles. In this form the activity of the hemispheres is also absent : all conditioned stimuli remain without effect, and different extraneous stimuli, unless exceptionally powerful, fail to evoke any reaction. Nevertheless the animal preserves an entirely alert posture ; it stands with wide open immovable eyes, head up, extremities extended, not seeking support in the loops, remaining motionless sometimes for minutes and sometimes for hours. On changing the position of an extremity such extremity retains the new position. The flexor reflex evoked by touching the planta assumes the character of a contracture. The presentation of food brings no reaction and the animal continues to remain quite still. This form of inhibition was noticed only in a small number of dogs, and up to the present we are not in a position to define the special conditions of experimentation or the special peculiarities of the nervous system which are necessary for its production. My collaborator, Dr. Rojansky, has made most careful observations upon the transition of dogs from the alert state to sleep, and he finds that the condition just described is present in all dogs, though usually only in a fleeting form.

It seems that the physiological interpretation of this state should not present any great difficulty : we are dealing with a complete inhibition confined exclusively to the cortex, without a concurrent descent of the inhibition into the centres regulating equilibrium and maintenance of posture (centres of Magnus and de Kleijn) ; in other words the animal is in a state of catalepsy. Thus in this form of sleep the plane of demarcation between the inhibited regions of the brain and the regions which are free from inhibition seems to pass just beneath the cerebral cortex. A similar demarcation of excitable areas from areas which have undergone complete inhibition may exist also between different large areas of the cortex itself, producing what may be called a localized sleep. This form of sleep was met with frequently, and we are now able to produce it experimentally as well. On the first occasion it was observed as follows [experiments of Dr. Voskressensky] : A dog in which work had hitherto proceeded without any interference by sleep began to show signs of drowsiness—due to its being frequently left in the stand in the experimental room for hours at a stretch without any application of conditioned or any other stimuli. Obviously the monotony of the stimulation by the constant surroundings led finally to a development of an intense inhibition involving finally the whole of the brain. The inhibitory effect of the environment became so strong that the mere introduction of the dog into the experimental room had an immediate and obvious inhibitory effect which became still more pronounced after the animal was placed in the stand. It had to be roused up in all manner of ways to keep it from falling fast asleep before the preparations for the experiment had been completed (a matter of only a few minutes). When the experimenter left the room and closed the door in order to start the experiment from outside, and then without losing a minute began to apply one or another conditioned stimulus, the normal conditioned reflex was fully present ; a normal secretion of saliva was obtained and the animal immediately took the food. When, however, after leaving the room an interval was made of 4-5 minutes before the application of the first stimulus, this stimulus now produced the following re-markable result. The conditioned secretory effect was present and the salivary secretion was sharply augmented on food being presented; the animal however did not take the food, which in order to effect adequate reinforcement had to be placed in its mouth. During this time no relaxation of the skeletal muscles could be observed. When an interval of ten minutes was made after leaving the room no conditioned alimentary reflex could be obtained, and the animal was found fast asleep with a relaxed musculature and occasional snoring. Only one possible explanation of these observations suggests itself. The inhibition must have spread in the first place only over the motor area of the cortex, so that excitation could be initiated by a conditioned stimulus belonging to any other analyser and could spread to the salivary gland but not to the muscles—with a resulting one-sided alimentary reflex lacking its motor component. Later the inhibition spread over the whole mass of the cortex and over the lower parts of the brain, bringing about complete sleep with a relaxation of the skeletal muscles. In this experiment the stages of a gradually developing sleep were brought about under the influence of the protracted action of neutral stimuli upon the hemispheres, but more usually this effect appeared as the result of numerous applications within a single experiment of negative or positive conditioned stimuli, especially if, in the latter case, either the intensity of the stimulus was weak or the period of application prolonged. The following two examples may serve in illustration :

In the first example the subject of the experiment was a dog which has already been mentioned in previous lectures (p. 231). A tone of 256 d.v. was used as a positive conditioned alimentary stimulus, while ten neighbouring tones up and ten down the scale were differentiated [experiments of Dr. Bierman].

Time	Conditioned stimulus during 30 seconds	Secretion in drops during 30 seconds	Remarks
3.50 p.m.	Tone, 256 d.v.	13	Takes the food
4.0 ,,	,, 426 d.v.	0	⎫ The animal gradually becomes drowsy
4.5 ,,	,, 160 d.v.	0	⎬ dually be-
4.10 ,,	,, 640 d.v.	0	⎭ comes drowsy
4.13 ,,	,, 256 d.v.	9	Does not take the food

The second example is taken from experiments upon a dog which had many exceptionally constant alimentary conditioned reflexes.

In this case the dissociation between the motor and the secretory response was more permanent and occurred even in experiments in which the causative inhibitory stimulus was not used.

A fresh reflex, to the appearance of a grey screen, was established and a series of experiments were performed, in each of which the new stimulus was repeated many times in succession at short intervals. It was now observed that on application of any of the old stimuli, though the conditioned secretion was often still considerable, the animal did not touch the food presented to it in reinforcement [experiments by Dr. Rosenthal].

Time	Conditioned stimulus during 30 seconds	Salivary Secretion in drops during 30 seconds	Remarks
3.15 p.m.	Metronome	5	
3.18 ,,	Flashes of lamp	7	The animal does not
3.21 ,,	Sound of bubbling	7	touch the food
3.24 ,,	Buzzer	7	

This condition was independent of any application of the grey screen in the particular experiment and lasted for a considerable time. During the experiment the dog remained almost motionless, but there were no obvious signs of sleep. Food presented to the animal in the same stand and under precisely the same environmental conditions, but without a previous application of a conditioned stimulus, was taken with avidity.

The following chance observation belongs to the same group of phenomena. A dog which served for experiments with conditioned alimentary reflexes, and which never showed any dissociation of the secretory and motor components of the reflex, nor any signs of sleep while in the stand, was placed for the very first time in front of a large audience for the purpose of a demonstration. The unfamiliarity of the surroundings had a big effect upon the animal; it shivered slightly, and became as though spellbound. On administration of the conditioned stimulus the normal secretory effect was obtained, but the dog did not take the food, and in a relatively short time fell into profound sleep in its stand, right in front of the audience, with complete relaxation of the skeletal muscles. Evidently in this case the powerful, unusual and protracted extraneous stimulus produced at first a partial inhibition affecting only the motor area of the cortex ; then the inhibition spread over the whole cortex and descended also to the lower parts of the brain. The experiment on the whole is similar to those by which so-called animal hypnotism is usually demonstrated. For example, a rapid immobilization of an animal held on its back also leads to an inhibition which spreads to a varying degree in different animals. In some cases a complete or partial catalepsy is produced (immobility of the body, but with movements of the eyes, head and neck) ; in others it leads to the development of profound sleep. In our laboratory this was observed on several occasions. An extremely unruly animal, for example, vigorously resisting the preparations for the experiment, would be rapidly immobilized by a powerful grasp, associated of course with considerable mechanical stimulation, and would fall asleep in its stand almost immediately.

We see in this manner that a partial as well as a complete sleep can be produced by weak and protracted neutral stimuli, by short but vigorous stimuli, and by negative as well as positive conditioned stimuli. I shall have an opportunity of discussing certain further details in the next lecture.

The above experiments demonstrate that the extent of the spread in the brain of the diffused inhibition can be small or great, and that there may exist different transition stages in the depth of the inhibition, or, in other words, different intensities of the diffuse inhibition (sleep).

In the eighth lecture I discussed the mechanism by which, in the case of simultaneous conditioned stimuli, a stimulus from one analyser is overshadowed by a stimulus from another, and the suggestion was put forward that this overshadowing might be dependent upon the different strengths of the stimuli belonging to the different analysers (p. 141). Experiments which have since been performed entirely uphold this suggestion. When we intentionally produced a considerable change in the strength of our usual conditioned stimuli, the auditory being made weaker and the others either remaining unchanged or being made stronger, there was a definite reversal of the relations previously obtained, the auditory stimuli now participating in the stimulatory compound to a smaller extent than the other stimuli, *i.e.* on isolated application of an auditory stimulus a much smaller effect was obtained than on application of any other stimulus belonging to the compound. The following are some of the experiments :

In one dog a compound simultaneous conditioned stimulus consisted of a tactile and an auditory component, the auditory being considerably weakened. The compound stimulus, when well established, gave 4-4½ drops of saliva during 20 seconds' isolated action. When used separately the auditory component gave a secretion of 1-1½ drops and the tactile 2½-5 drops [experiments of Dr. Rickman].

In another dog the compound simultaneous conditioned stimulus was made up of a 100 candle-power lamp together with the sound of a musical tone which was considerably damped. The compound stimulus when fully established gave 7-8 drops of saliva during 30 seconds ; the visual stimulus applied singly gave 5 drops, and the auditory gave 2½ drops. In an exactly similar manner a thermal cutaneous stimulus of 0° C., which was employed with a very weak tone to form a compound simultaneous conditioned stimulus, gave when applied singly a much greater effect than the tone [experiments of Dr. Gantt and Dr. Koupalov].

Thus we see that the difference in the intensity of the reflexes evoked by the various conditioned stimuli belonging to the different analysers is determined by the strength of the stimulus and not by any functional difference in the nervous elements of the analysers. These experiments give us a method of comparing the intensity of stimuli which belong to different analysers.

Bearing these facts in mind we can begin to study the different stages through which the diffused inhibition passes in its development. The starting-point for these investigations was provided by a case of a pathological state of the nervous system which had been brought about experimentally by means of a purely " functional (non-surgical) interference." Experimentally produced pathological states of the nervous system will be dealt with fully in succeeding lectures ; in the present lecture I shall describe only the experiment which induced us to pursue the further investigation of normal animals.

Positive conditioned alimentary reflexes [experiments by Dr. Rosenkov] were established to the sound of a whistle, beats of a metronome, rhythmic tactile stimulation of the skin at a rate of 24 per minute, and flashes of an electric lamp ; several negative reflexes were also established by differentiation, including one to tactile stimulation of the same skin area at the rate of 12 per minute. The following table gives the figures for the normal effect of the positive stimuli :

Time	Conditioned stimulus during 30 seconds	Salivary Secretion in drops during 30 seconds
2.3 p.m.	Tactile (24 per minute)	3
2.10 ,,	Whistle	5
2.21 ,,	Lamp	2
2.32 ,,	Metronome	$3\frac{1}{2}$

On the basis of the previous discussion we may take the strength of the stimuli in order from strong to weak as whistle, metronome, tactile stimulation and lamp.

The experiment now proceeded as follows : In between the different positive stimuli the differentiated tactile stimulus of 12 per minute was introduced, being applied during 30 seconds and followed without any interval by the positive tactile stimulus of 24 per minute which was also continued for 30 seconds and then reinforced as usual. This seemingly small factor produced an extraordinary effect. On the day following this experiment and on the succeeding nine days all conditioned reflexes had disappeared excepting only for a very occasional small secretion. This period was followed by a series of definite successive changes in the conditioned activity of the brain. The first of these extremely peculiar changes is illustrated by the next experiment.

Time	Conditioned stimulus during 30 seconds	Salivary Secretion in drops during 30 seconds
11.10 a.m.	Whistle	0
11.19 ,,	,,	$\frac{1}{3}$
11.32 ,,	Lamp	3
11.48 ,,	Metronome	1
12.6 p.m.	Tactile (24 per minute)	$5\frac{1}{2}$

The experiment shows exactly the reverse of what was observed during the normal state of the animal. The strong stimuli have either no effect or only a very small one ; the weak stimuli have a greater effect than normal. All positive stimuli were, of course, reinforced. This state of the cortex we called the *paradoxical phase.* The paradoxical phase in this dog continued for fourteen days and was then succeeded by the following change :

Time	Conditioned stimulus during 30 seconds	Salivary Secretion in drops during 30 seconds
10.40 a.m.	Tactile (24 per minute)	4
10.48 ,,	Metronome	$4\frac{1}{2}$
10.58 ,,	Whistle	4
11.10 ,,	Lamp	4

This was called the *phase of equalization,* since all the stimuli became equal in their effect. The phase of equalization lasted for seven days and was then succeeded by still another phase during which the effect of stimuli of medium strength was greatly increased ; the effect of the strong stimulus was slightly diminished, while the weak stimulus had no effect. After seven days more, all the reflexes had returned to their normal value. In the succeeding experiments on the same problem, in order to be quite certain, we used different intensities of one of the positive stimuli. The results obtained were exactly comparable with the results of the previous experiments. It thus became obvious that the difference in the reaction to stimuli in all these different phases is determined by the relative strength of the stimuli.

In the manner just described was secured the first direct evidence that the cellular structures of the cortex undergo a series of definite stages of transition between complete inhibition and normal excitability, stages which are divulged by the peculiar reactions of the cortical elements to the stimuli of different strengths. After the study of these transition stages in this obviously pathological state, the question arose whether the same stages would be found normally during the transition from the alert state to sleep and the reverse. It was thought probable that the pathological case just described consisted only in an exaggeration and prolongation of events which in the normal animal were transient and not so evident, just as was the case with catalepsy. Special experiments conducted in this direction led to a definitely positive result. The following are some illustrations :

Twenty neighbouring tones had been differentiated from the tone acting as a positive stimulus. This dog had also, among many others, two positive conditioned reflexes, differing greatly in intensity, to a weak and to a loud crackling sound. The following table gives the normal intensity of these two reflexes :

Time	Conditioned stimulus during 30 seconds	Salivary Secretion in drops during 30 seconds
2.10 p.m.	Loud crackling sound	$12\frac{1}{2}$
2.20 ,,	Weak crackling sound	$4\frac{1}{2}$
2.30 ,,	Loud crackling sound	11

The actual experiments proceed as follows. By repeated application of the differentiated tones the animal is rendered definitely drowsy ; the weak crackling sound is now applied. The secretory effect is absent. The dog awakens during the reinforcement with food, which it begins to eat. The next application of the weak crackling sound evokes a secretion which is yet small. The reflex is again reinforced. A third application of the weak crackling sound produces a normal, or in some cases even a supernormal, secretory effect, and the reflex is again reinforced. The strong crackling sound is applied next ; its effect is either less than or equal to the last effect of the weak sound. It is only somewhat later, when the alert state has been fully recovered, that the strong crackling sound evokes its full normal effect, and that the normal quantitative relations between the two reflexes become restored. The following gives one of the actual experiments :

Time	Conditioned stimulus applied during 30 seconds	Salivary Secretion in drops during 30 seconds
2.48 p.m.	Strong crackling sound	13

Sleep is now induced in the dog by repeated application of the differentiated inhibitory tones.

Time	Conditioned stimulus	Salivary Secretion
3.17 p.m.	Weak crackling sound	$\frac{1}{2}$
3.22 ,,	,, ,,	$3\frac{1}{2}$
3.26 ,,	,, ,,	7
3.32 ,,	Loud crackling sound	6
3.40 ,,	Weak crackling sound	5
3.50 ,,	Loud crackling sound	10

In some experiments repetition of these stimuli instead of leading to a temporary predominance of the effect of the weaker stimulus resulted only in an equalization of the effects of the strong and weak crackling sounds. Evidently during the gradual dispersion of sleep under the action of repeated brief feedings the cortical elements pass through the paradoxical phase and the phase of equalization. It follows that these experiments are exactly comparable to the pathological case which was previously described, excepting that the change which took under normal conditions a few minutes required in the pathological case many days.

In another dog a slight drowsiness developed on account of too prolonged experimentation. This was accompanied by a complete obliteration of the differences in the intensities of the reflexes to the different stimuli, so that all the positive conditioned reflexes now became equal. With the help of injections of a suitable dose of caffeine the dog was brought back to its usual condition of wakefulness, and with this all the normal relations between the intensities of the different conditioned reflexes returned. Both experiments [by Dr. Zimkin] are given below :

Time	Conditioned stimulus applied during 30 seconds	Salivary Secretion in drops during 30 seconds
12.50 p.m.	Loud beats of metronome	8
12.57 ,,	Lamp	$7\frac{1}{2}$
1.4 ,,	Loud buzzing sound	8
1.11 ,,	Weak buzzing sound	8

On the following day the animal received subcutaneously 8 cc. of a 2% solution of caffeine eighteen minutes before the experiment. At the time of the experiment the animal was fully alert.

Time	Conditioned stimulus applied during 30 seconds	Salivary Secretion in drops during 30 seconds
12.18 p.m.	Lamp	7
12.25 ,,	Loud beats of metronome	10
12.32 ,,	Weak buzzing sound	6
12.39 ,,	Weak beats of metronome	$7\frac{1}{2}$
12.46 ,,	Loud buzzing sound	$8\frac{1}{2}$

In the animal which was previously mentioned in this lecture as showing dissociation of the secretory and motor reactions, it was often observed that during the period of this dissociation the weakest conditioned stimulus (the lamp) was the only one which evoked on some occasions a strong salivary reflex, sometimes even bringing about both reactions—a normal secretion and motor response, and acceptance of the food on reinforcement. It is thus seen that a paradoxical phase could be observed also in these cases of a limited extent of diffusion of the inhibition [experiments by Dr. Rosenthal].

A further and quite peculiar condition was observed in some cases of intense drowsiness which fell just short of changing into complete sleep. When positive conditioned stimuli had nearly lost their effect, well-developed negative stimuli, on the other hand, acquired definite excitatory properties. The following is an example of such an experiment by Dr. Shishlo :

Positive conditioned alimentary reflexes were established to tactile stimulation of the shoulder and of the thigh, and to a thermal cutaneous stimulus of 45° C. ; a very constant negative conditioned stimulus was also established to a tactile stimulation of a definite skin area on the back. The effect of the positive tactile stimuli ranged normally from 15-18 drops during one minute. The thermal conditioned stimulus began relatively soon to induce drowsiness and sleep. The experiment to be described commenced with an application of the thermal cutaneous stimulus which led to drowsiness. The experiment then proceeded as follows :

Time	Conditioned stimulus during one minute	Salivary Secretion in drops during one minute	Remarks
12.29 p.m.	Tactile stimulation of shoulder	1	The dog remains drowsy in spite of reinforcement of the reflexes
12.39 ,,	Tactile stimulation of thigh	2	
12.50 ,,	Tactile stimulation of back (inhibitory)	12	

A similar conversion of negative stimuli into positive ones was also on several occasions observed in pathological conditions. This effect is given the name of the *ultra-paradoxical phase*.

It thus becomes evident that during the transition from the alert state to complete sleep the hemispheres pass through several different stages. Since sleep is nothing but a widely distributed internal inhibition, we should expect at least some of these stages to appear during the ordinary inhibitory after-effect, which was discussed at length in the earlier lectures upon internal inhibition. So far only one case has been investigated, namely, conditioned inhibition, and this would appear to realize our expectation [experiments by Dr. Bikov] :

Five positive conditioned reflexes were established—to a metronome, a loud tone, the same tone damped down, the appearance of a disc of cardboard, and tactile stimulation of the skin. A conditioned inhibition was developed to a combination of a sound of bubbling with the action of the tactile stimulus. The mean figures of the secretory effect of the five positive stimuli, averaged from a great number of experiments, were in the above-mentioned order of the stimuli—metronome 22, loud tone $18\frac{1}{2}$, soft tone $16\frac{1}{2}$, disc $13\frac{1}{2}$, and tactile stimulus 10 drops during 30 seconds. The conditioned inhibition having been firmly established, all the conditioned stimuli in turn were tested 10 minutes after the application of the inhibitory combination. The metronome gave $16\frac{1}{4}$, the loud tone 16, the damped tone 20, and the disc 18 drops. Taking into consideration the possible interferences of irradiation of inhibition and of induction, the only point of importance in the present connection is that the effect of the weaker tone was considerably above normal, while that of the stronger tone was below normal. This reversal in the effect of the strong and weak tones can be regarded as evidence of a paradoxical phase, since the tone was the same, differing only in strength, and both stimuli therefore were obviously related to the same point of the cortex. This investigation is at present being continued with other types of internal inhibition.

In the lecture upon mutual induction a suggestion was made that external inhibition might be due to negative induction, *i.e.* to an inhibition which is induced in cortical areas neighbouring on the area of excitation. Expressed in another fashion, it was suggested that the intimate mechanism underlying external inhibition is identical with that underlying internal inhibition. It was hoped to test this theory by determining whether external inhibition causes similar changes in the reactions of the cortex to those which have just been described in the case of internal inhibition. For the purpose of this investigation a stimulus was needed which would produce a protracted effect of external inhibition, and use was made of the introduction into the animal's mouth of rejectable substances which, as was mentioned previously, produces a prolonged after-effect. The experiments were performed upon two dogs, both of which had well-established alimentary conditioned reflexes.

In the first dog [experiments by Dr. Prorokov], after introduction of a solution of sodium carbonate, strong and weak conditioned stimuli were tested immediately on termination of the secretion due to the alkali itself. It was found that at first all the conditioned reflexes were inhibited to the same extent, but that within the next 15-20 minutes the reflexes to the weak stimuli returned to normal or even exceeded the normal value, while the strong stimuli were either equal in effect to the weaker ones or even gave a considerably smaller effect. In the experiment given below a solution of sodium carbonate was introduced into the dog's mouth at 9.41 a.m.

Time	Conditioned stimulus during 30 seconds	Salivary Secretion in drops during 30 seconds
9.46 a.m.	Lamp	0·4
9.51 ,,	Tactile	6·2
9.56 ,,	Loud buzzer	3·0

Under the usual conditions without administration of the alkali the effect of the buzzer was about 8 drops during 30 seconds, while the effect of the tactile stimulus was 4 drops during 30 seconds.

In a second dog [experiments by Dr. Anokhin] there were, however, somewhat different results. After the introduction of the rejectable substance into the dog's mouth and the termination of the resulting secretion, all the conditioned stimuli, when tested at frequent intervals up to the end of the experiment, showed an equalization in their effect. Concurrently with this there was observed as the experiment continued a step-like diminution in the strength of the reflexes. In control experiments performed previously the reflexes were proportional to the strength of the stimuli, the stronger buzzer giving the largest effect and the lamp the smallest. In the following example a solution of sodium carbonate was introduced into the dog's mouth at 11 a.m., and the resulting secretion of saliva continued for ten minutes.

Time	Conditioned stimulus during 30 seconds	Salivary Secretion in drops during 30 seconds
11.10 a.m.	Lamp	12·5
11.15 ,,	,,	10·5
11.20 ,,	Loud buzzer	10·5
11.25 ,,	Metronome	6·3
11.30 ,,	Weak buzzer	6·8

Although the results obtained in the two dogs would appear to corroborate the suggestion that internal and external inhibition are fundamentally one and the same process, yet the complexity of the problem necessitates a repetition and greater variation of the experiments with more critical attention to other possible interpretations of the results.

In the course of our investigation we became greatly interested in the effect upon conditioned reflexes of different narcotics in the first stages of their action, in complete narcosis, and again during the period of recovery. Urethane and chloral hydrate were used for this purpose. In the case of the action of narcotics as compared with the effect of inhibition a different sequence of events was observed : there was a gradual weakening of all conditioned reflexes, the weak conditioned stimuli naturally becoming ineffective before the strong ones. This state was given the name of the *narcotic phase*. The following experiment is taken from a research by Dr. Lebedinsky :

Positive conditioned reflexes were established to loud buzzing, metronome, weak buzzing, tactile stimulus, and intermittent flashes of an electric lamp. With regard to the intensities of their effect the stimuli followed in the order given. The animal, after being placed in the stand, received at 10.9 a.m. two grammes of chloral hydrate dissolved in 150 cc. of water in the form of an enema. The experiment proceeds as shown in the table on the opposite page.

We thus see that with the development of narcosis the effect of all the stimuli progressively diminished, and on return to the alert state the stimuli progressively recovered their normal conditioned effect. The only exception, out of the twenty stimuli, was presented by the weak buzzing sound which at 11.53 a.m. produced an abnormally large effect.

Thus in different healthy animals under different conditions there were found many different phases of transition in the reactions of the cortex to conditioned stimuli. An obvious question arises as to how far all these different phases, including also the narcotic phase,

Time	Conditioned stimulus during 30 seconds	Salivary Secretion in drops during 30 seconds	
10.14 a.m.	Metronome	11	Dog takes the food, yawns and stands shakily
10.21 ,,	Lamp	3½	Takes the food ; hangs down in the loops of the stand
10.29 ,,	Strong buzzing	7	Takes the food
10.38 ,,	Tactile	0	Takes the food
10.45 ,,	Weak buzzing	2	Slowly raises itself from the loops and takes food
10.53 ,,	Strong buzzing	0	Sleeps ; does not take food
11.6 ,,	Metronome	0	Sleeps ; does not take food
11.13 ,,	Weak buzzing	0	Sleeps ; does not take food
11.19 ,,	Strong buzzing	5½	Wakes up, takes the food
11.26 ,,	Tactile	0	
11.35 ,,	Lamp	0	
11.45 ,,	Metronome	5	
11.53 ,,	Weak buzzing	9½	
12 noon	Tactile	4	
12.7 p.m.	Strong buzzing	8½	Takes the food
12.15 ,,	Lamp	6	
12.24 ,,	Metronome	9½	
12.34 ,,	Strong buzzing	13	
12.42 ,,	Weak buzzing	10	
1.3 ,,	Tactile	5½	

appertain to every single animal under the usual conditions of life. In investigating this problem we were fortunate to have at our disposal an unusually reactive type of animal, the special features of which will be discussed in the succeeding lectures. (This dog was used for the experiments described towards the end of the fourteenth lecture, p. 247). Given constant conditions, the dog was remarkable for the constancy of its highest nervous activity as expressed in the form of conditioned reflexes, and fully merited its nickname of " an animated instrument." The dog had ten different conditioned reflexes. There were six positive ones—to a buzzer, metronome, whistle, increase in illumination of the room, appearance of a small toy horse ; and four negative ones—to a different rate of metronome, a diminution in the illumination of the room, the appearance of a square, and the appearance of a toy rabbit approximately of the same size and colour as the toy horse. For some time prior to the following experiments the buzzer had not been used, while out of the differentiated stimuli the metronome had been employed practically exclusively. The auditory stimuli usually, and in the early experiments always, gave a secretion 30 to 50% greater than that given by the visual stimuli. After two years' work in the laboratory with this dog the positive conditioned reflexes showed some tendency to diminish and began to vary in their relative intensity, as frequently happens in the case of continuous and prolonged use of the same conditioned stimuli. During this state of the animal we could find all the definite transition stages of the cortical activity which were described earlier in this lecture as different phases of the progressive diffusion of the inhibitory process over the hemispheres. Each of these phases either lasted during the whole course of a single experiment or else, under the action of different influences produced experimentally, changed into some other phase [experiments by Dr. Speransky]. The only phase which could not be observed in this dog was the ultra-paradoxical, but the conditions were not such as to favour the appearance of this phase as the animal never became very drowsy. The experiments taken from different periods of the work are shown on the opposite page.

When the reflexes deviated very much from normal they were strengthened and corrected by the method discussed in the fourteenth lecture, namely, by abbreviating the interval between the beginning of the conditioned stimulus and its reinforcement. The spontaneous transition from one phase to another in the two last experiments was most probably due to repeated reinforcement. We had, however, two special methods at our disposal by the use of which we could produce an immediate interchange of phases. One of these methods consisted in the application of the completely differentiated inhibitory rate of the metronome. Most probably the effect of this inhibitory stimulus was due to concentration of the diffuse inhibition, or to an induction of the antagonistic process of excitation.

Time	Conditioned stimulus during 30 seconds	Salivary Secretion in drops during 30 seconds
	Normal Experiment.	
10.30 a.m.	Metronome	8
10.40 ,,	Increased illumination	5
10.50 ,,	Whistle	8
11.0 ,,	Disc	5
11.10 ,,	Metronome	9
11.20 ,,	Increased illumination	5
11.30 ,,	Whistle	8
11.40 ,,	Disc	6

Experiment showing phase of equalization.

Time	Conditioned stimulus during 30 seconds	Salivary Secretion in drops during 30 seconds
9.0 a.m.	Metronome	7
9.10 ,,	Increased illumination	5
9.20 ,,	Whistle	5
9.30 ,,	Disc	$4\frac{1}{2}$
9.40 ,,	Metronome	5
9.50 ,,	Increased illumination	5
10.0 ,,	Whistle	5
10.10 ,,	Disc	4

Experiment showing paradoxical phase and its transition into the normal phase.

Time	Conditioned stimulus during 30 seconds	Salivary Secretion in drops during 30 seconds
10.0 a.m.	Metronome	4
10.11 ,,	Increased illumination	6
10.22 ,,	Whistle	4
10.33 ,,	Disc	7
10.43 ,,	Metronome	4
10.54 ,,	Increased illumination	$2\frac{1}{2}$
11.3 ,,	Whistle	7
11.12 ,,	Disc	$4\frac{1}{2}$
11.22 ,,	Metronome	$8\frac{1}{2}$
11.33 ,,	Increased illumination	5

Experiment showing complete inhibition and transition into the narcotic phase.

Time	Conditioned stimulus during 30 seconds	Salivary Secretion in drops during 30 seconds
10.0 a.m.	Metronome	0
10.9 ,,	Increased illumination	0
10.19 ,,	Whistle	3
10.31 ,,	Disc	0
10.42 ,,	Metronome	3
10.52 ,,	Increased illumination	0
11.3 ,,	Whistle	$3\frac{1}{2}$
11.12 ,,	Disc	0

The second method consisted in the application of an extra stimulus, viz. the entry of the experimenter into the animal's room. The following experiments serve as examples of the effect of each method :

Time	Conditioned stimulus during 30 seconds	Salivary Secretion in drops during 30 seconds	Remarks
9.30 a.m.	Metronome (positive)	0	Does not take the food
9.37 ,,	Toy horse	0	Does not take the food
9.45 ,,	Metronome (inhibitory)	0	(Not reinforced)
9.52 ,,	Metronome (positive)	4	⎫
9.59 ,,	Increased illumination	9	⎪
10.10 ,,	Whistle	$6\frac{1}{2}$	⎪
10.18 ,,	Toy horse	11	Takes the food
10.30 ,,	Metronome	$12\frac{1}{2}$	⎪
10.38 ,,	Disc	$8\frac{1}{2}$	⎭

The phase of complete inhibition with absence of the secretory and motor reactions is transformed in the above experiment first into the paradoxical, and then into the normal, phase by the application of the inhibitory rate of the metronome.

Time	Conditioned stimulus during 30 seconds	Salivary Secretion in drops during 30 seconds	Remarks
10.0 a.m.	Metronome (positive)	0	Does not take the food

The experimenter enters and remains in the room with the dog.

10.9 a.m.	Metronome (positive)	9	Takes the food
10.18 ,,	Increased illumination	$3\frac{1}{2}$	Takes the food

The presence of the experimenter in the room with the dog immediately changed the phase of complete inhibition to normal.

The question whether all these different stages in the activity of the hemispheres can be arranged in a definite order, and if so in what kind of order, must remain for the present entirely open. A consideration of all the experiments at our disposal shows that the sequence of the different phases was fairly variable, and it is not clear, therefore, whether the different states of the hemispheres in different animals are strictly successive or whether they may occur as parallel events. Only further experimentation can explain why a given phase undergoes transition directly into one or another of the remaining phases.

It is hardly possible to doubt that all these different states of the hemispheres bear a strong resemblance to the different stages of what is generally known as hypnotism. The relation between the experimental results described here and hypnotism as observed in man will form the subject of the last lecture.

LECTURE XVII

The different types of nervous system.—Pathological disturbances of the cortex, result of functional interference.

WE have been dealing up to the present with the normal activity of the cerebral cortex. It was noticed in passing, however, that the experiments to which our animals were subjected led in some instances to chronic disturbances of this normal activity. This was especially liable to occur in the early stages of our work, since in planning the experiments we had at first not even the slightest idea as to the limitations and the natural resistance of the cortex. The present lecture will be devoted to a description of those disturbances in the higher nervous activity which are of a purely functional origin, and not due to surgical interference or trauma. From some of these disturbances the animal recovers gradually and spontaneously under the influence of rest alone, on discontinuance of the disturbing experiments; in other cases the disturbances are so persistent as to require special therapeutic measures. In many instances we were able to make observations during the actual period of transition from the normal physiological state of the cortex to a pathological state, and then to study its therapy. The pathological state of the hemispheres in different individual animals from the action of injurious influences varies greatly. One and the same injurious influence causes severe and prolonged disorders in some dogs; in others the disorders are only slight and fleeting; while yet other dogs remain practically unaffected. In many cases the deviation from normal produced by the same causative agent assumes in different dogs quite different aspects. The type and the degree of pathological disturbance that develops from some definite cause was found in all cases to be determined primarily by the character of the individual nervous system of the animals. Therefore, before describing the different pathological states it is important to say a few words about the different individual types of nervous system found in our dogs. The systematic investigation of the higher nervous activity has enabled us to outline even at present certain definite criteria which when expanded in the future will lead up to an exact definition of the different types of nervous system of individual animals. Such criteria when perfected should greatly assist the development of a strictly scientific experimental investigation of the hereditary transmission of different aspects of nervous activities in animals.[1] At present, however, I shall not go beyond a general classification of our dogs. Two definite types, which may be regarded as extremes, stand out with special prominence.

The first type was met with practically from the beginning of our investigation, and the researches on animals belonging to this type led in our early experiments to much confusion. At a time when we were still quite unfamiliar with the subject of conditioned reflexes, we met in some of the experiments with considerable difficulties on account of a drowsiness, which developed from the use of certain conditioned stimuli and under certain conditions of experimentation, and which we were not able to overcome. We thought to get rid of this drowsiness by choosing for our experiments dogs which outside the experimental conditions were very lively. Animals were selected which were extremely vivacious, always sniffing at everything, gazing at everything intently, and reacting quickly to the minutest sounds. Such animals when they get acquainted with men, which they do very quickly and easily, often become annoying by their continuous demonstrativeness. They can never be made to keep quiet either by orders or by a mild physical punishment. It was, however, soon found that these very animals when placed in the stand and limited in their movements, and especially when left alone in the experimental room, were the quickest to become drowsy, so that their conditioned reflexes quickly diminished or even disappeared altogether, in spite of frequent reinforcement by food or acid. Indeed, our repeated stimuli when they had not yet acquired stable positive conditioned properties immediately, and in a most unequivocal fashion, produced drowsiness and even sleep in dogs which at the commencement of the experiment were wide awake.

[1] Experiments which have been communicated briefly at the Edinburgh International Congress of Physiology (1923) upon hereditary facilitation of the development of some conditioned reflexes in mice have been found to be very complicated, uncertain and moreover extremely difficult to control. They are at present being subjected to further investigation under more stringent conditions. At present the question of hereditary transmission of conditioned reflexes and of the hereditary facilitation of their acquirement must be left entirely open.

In some animals this happened even when they were not placed in the stand during the experiments, but were left free on the floor, the experimenter remaining quietly in the room ; nevertheless the dogs on administration of a conditioned stimulus soon got sleepy, closed their eyes and finally lay down on the floor. This often happened immediately after the reinforcement of a conditioned stimulus. At first we despaired of achieving anything with these animals ; later we learned how to get over the difficulties. In dogs of this type many conditioned reflexes must be developed concurrently, and with a great variety of stimuli ; no stimulus must be repeated more than once in a single experiment, and long pauses between the applications of the various stimuli must be avoided ; not only excitatory but also inhibitory reflexes must be developed. In short, when we make rapid and considerable variations in the experimental environment such dogs become quite satisfactory subjects for the experiments. It is an interesting point, but one which cannot be pursued here, whether this type represents a higher or lower stage of nervous development.

Until a rigid scientific classification is fully established for all the various types of central nervous system I think we may be permitted to make use of the ancient classification of the so-called temperaments. The animals just described must be regarded in the light of the ancient classification as belonging to the pure " sanguine " type. Under quick changes of stimuli they are energetic and highly reactive, but with the slightest monotony of the environment they become dull, drowsy and inactive.

Our second type of dog is also very definite, and must be placed at the other end of the classical series of temperaments. In every new and slightly unfamiliar set of surroundings such animals are extremely restrained in their movements. They slink along close to the wall in a cringing fashion, and often at the smallest movement or sound from outside—a shout or a threatening movement—they immediately cower to the floor. Everybody who sees such an animal would immediately judge it a great coward. These animals get used to their experimental surroundings and the associated manipulation very slowly, but when they become thoroughly familiar with the new conditions they make invaluable subjects for experimentation. The animal described at the end of the last lecture as " a living instrument " belonged to this type. Such animals do not sleep in their stands when the experimental conditions remain more or less constant ; on the contrary their conditioned reflexes, especially the inhibitory ones, remain extremely stable and regular. We are engaged at present in our laboratory with a most exaggerated representative of this type. This dog—a bitch—was born at the institute and was always treated with the utmost gentleness. When she was about twelve months old she was occasionally brought into the laboratory, and during every experiment in the stand only very few stimuli were given. When brought to the laboratory five years after its first introduction this dog still behaved in exactly the same manner as on the first occasion, and until quite recently never got used to the laboratory conditions in the slightest degree. She slinks along behind the experimenter on the way to the experimental rooms, always with her tail between her legs. On meeting members of the staff (some of whom constantly try to make friends with her and pet her) she invariably and quickly dodges them, draws back and squats down on the floor. She reacts in the same manner to every slightly quicker movement or slightly louder word of her master, and behaves towards all of us as if we were her most dangerous enemies from whom she constantly and most severely suffers. In spite of all this, when she at last got used to her own experimental room many extremely regular and constant positive and negative conditioned reflexes were developed. This was so unexpected by us that the animal was flatteringly given the name of " Brains." It would not be an exaggeration to bring this animal under the type of " melancholic." I shall return to this animal later. Both the above types are obviously extremes. In the first the excitatory process predominates in the extreme, and in the second the inhibitory. Both, therefore, are limited types, with, so to speak, a narrow scope of vital expression. The first needs a continuous and novel succession of stimuli, which may indeed often be absent in the natural surroundings ; the other, on the contrary, needs extremely uniform conditions of life and therefore suffers from being unable to react to a sufficient number of stimuli to ensure a full use and development of its nervous organization.

It has, no doubt, occurred to some that these two types present a contradiction to the theory of the identity of sleep and internal inhibition, in that the type with a predisposition to excitation tends to fall asleep under the conditions of our experiments, while the type with a predisposition to inhibition remains fully awake. If, however, as can reasonably be supposed, functional exhaustion of the cortical elements serves as an impetus to a development of an inhibitory process, it is easy to understand that in the first type the excess of excitability of the cortical elements leads to their precipitate functional exhaustion, and so, when the cortical elements are exposed to prolonged monotonous stimuli, especially favours a development of inhibition which irradiates widely over the whole cortex. Only a quick succession of new stimuli acting upon different groups of nerve cells can neutralize the tendency of this type of animal towards inhibition. In the second type, on the other hand, though the inhibition of the motor area of the cortex is so easily initiated (passive defence reflex) the inhibition does not irradiate over a wide area, some considerable parts of the cortex remaining unaffected; the parts which remain in an active state resist the diffuse spread of inhibition, *i.e.* sleep, and thereby make possible the restitution of the active state of the whole cortex as soon as the cause which initiated the initial inhibition has disappeared. In the first case the biologically unprofitable tendency is checked by the excitatory effect of a quickly changing environment, in the second by the restriction of the actual spread of inhibition in the cortex. In fact the limitation of the irradiation of the inhibition in the latter case seems to be a special protective mechanism of an otherwise defective nervous system. There is a parallel to such limitation in the case of a man who has trained himself to sleep even while walking, *i.e.* to limit the inhibition to the cortex, so that it does not descend to the subcortical areas.

In between the extremes just described can be found numerous intermediate types which present a greater balance between excitation and inhibition, types on the whole better adapted to the natural conditions of life and therefore biologically more resistant. Those that approximate to the first type are lively and active, and in most cases aggressive ; those that approximate to the second type are quiet and restrained. I remember in particular one dog of the latter type whose behaviour was in many respects extraordinary. I have never noticed it to lie down on the floor while it waited for the experiment after being fetched from the kennel to the laboratory. It reacted as if most disinterested in what happened around, and did not enter into either friendly or antagonistic relations with anybody, even its master. In its stand it never showed any signs of drowsiness, and its positive or negative conditioned reflexes were always extremely precise. The dog undoubtedly had a definite tendency towards inhibition ; it was, however, also capable of considerable excitation. I succeeded in disturbing the placid calm of this animal by making most extraordinary sounds with a toy trumpet and having a frightful animal mask over my face. The dog lost all its usual restraint, began to bark determinedly and tried to get at me—a most " phlegmatic " but powerful type.

Another group of dogs belongs to a more excitable type, and may be regarded as corresponding to the " choleric " type of the ancient classification. Inhibitory conditioned reflexes in these animals are less stable.

It is obvious that a large number of animals cannot be placed definitely in any one of these four types, but broadly speaking all the dogs which we used could be divided into two groups—those with an excessive or moderate tendency to excitation, and those with an excessive or moderate tendency to inhibition.

After this digression I can now proceed to the description of the functional disturbances in the cortical activities which were either observed accidentally or produced experimentally. The first observation was made under the following conditions. As was mentioned in the third lecture, a conditioned alimentary reflex can be developed to a most severe electrical stimulus applied to the skin— a stimulus which would normally evoke the inborn defence reaction but to which the animal now responds by an alimentary reaction, turning its head towards the place where the food appears, licking its lips and producing a secretion of typical " alimentary " saliva [experiments of Dr. Eroféeva, p. 29]. In the case which is being described the development of this reflex had been started with the use of a very weak current, which was gradually increased in strength until finally it was extremely powerful. The conditioned alimentary reflex developed in this way remained stable for many months. The electric current was occasionally replaced by cauterization or mechanical injury of the skin, both evoking the same reflex. The animal remained perfectly normal throughout a long period of the experiments, but after a certain time this peculiar conditioned stimulus, similarly to any other, began to acquire inhibitory properties, the onset of the secretory effect becoming more and more removed from the beginning of the conditioned stimulus. On rare occasions the electrical stimulus had been applied to places other than the one for which the reflex had been originally developed. Now, however, we resolved to generalize the reflex by a systematic application of the stimulus to new places. For some time the electrical stimulus continued, when applied to the different places of the skin, to produce the same conditioned alimentary reflex without any interference of a defence reaction. A limit, however, was suddenly reached. When a still further place was added to those already successfully generalized everything underwent an abrupt and complete change. No trace of the alimentary reaction was left : instead only a most violent defence reaction was present. Even an extremely weak current, which before the development of the alimentary conditioned reflex remained entirely without effect, now when applied to the original place of stimulation or to any other brought about the most violent defence reaction. The experiment was repeated on two other dogs. In one of them the outburst of excitation occurred on the application of the stimulus of the electric current to a ninth new place. In the other the application to a thirteenth new place did not yet bring about any explosion of excitation. When, however, the electric stimulus was applied in the same experiment to several of these places on the same day, and not, as before, to a single place only, the same explosive change occurred.

In all three dogs nothing could be done to restore at once the alimentary reflex to the electrical stimulus. The animals became restless and excited in an extreme degree, which they had never been before. In one dog it was only after an interval of three months that it was possible to start a fresh development of the original alimentary conditioned reflex to the stimulus of the electric current. This was a much more difficult operation than before, but the reflex was finally restored. In the other two dogs an even longer interval did not help. Obviously the nervous system had been brought into a chronic pathological state. At the time of these experiments, unfortunately, we had not begun to take account of the type of nervous system of our dogs.

Possibly on account of the special nature of the stimulus used in these experiments all these facts did not attract sufficient attention on our part ; but some time afterwards the same phenomenon was observed under more usual conditions of experimentation. The experiments in question were made to determine the limits of the analysis of shapes of different objects [experiments of Dr. Shenger-Krestovnikova]. A projection of a luminous circle on to a screen in front of the animal was repeatedly accompanied by feeding. After the reflex had become well established a differentiation between the circle and an ellipse with a ratio of the semi-axes 2 : 1, of the same luminosity and the same surface area, was obtained by the usual method of contrast. A complete and constant differentiation was obtained comparatively quickly. The shape of the ellipse was now approximated by stages to that of the circle (ratios of the semi-axes of 3 : 2, 4 : 3 and so on) and the development of differentiation continued through the successive ellipses. The differentiation proceeded with some fluctuations, progressing at first more and more quickly, and then again slower, until an ellipse with ratio of semi-axes 9 : 8 was reached. In this case, although a considerable degree of discrimination did develop, it was far from being complete. After three weeks of work upon this differentiation not only did the discrimination fail to improve, but it became considerably worse, and finally disappeared altogether. At the same time the whole behaviour of the animal underwent an abrupt change. The hitherto quiet dog began to squeal in its stand, kept wriggling about, tore off with its teeth the apparatus for mechanical stimulation of the skin, and bit through the tubes connecting the animal's room with the observer, a behaviour which never happened before. On being taken into the experimental room the dog now barked violently, which was also contrary to its usual custom ; in short it presented all the symptoms of a condition of acute neurosis. On testing the cruder differentiations they also were found to be destroyed, even the one with the ratio of the semi-axes 2 : 1. A fresh development of the latter differentiation up to its previous exactness progressed twice as slowly as at first, but during the re-establishment of this crude differentiation the animal gradually became quieter, returning finally to its normal state. The development of the finer differentiations now occurred even more quickly than before. The 9 : 8 ellipse at its first application was completely discriminated from the circle, but from the second application onwards no trace of a discrimination was obtained, and the animal again entered a state of extreme general excitation with the same results as before. No further experiments were performed with the animal. Some of the different stages of these experiments are given on page 292.

In the first experiment given below the ellipse with ratio of the semi-axes 4 : 3 was fully discriminated. In the second experiment the ellipse with the ratio 9 : 8, in its first stage of development, gave only 1 drop of salivary secretion. After repeating it in the course of the succeeding two weeks its effect, as shown in the third of the experiments given below, became equal to that of the circle. After this even the ellipse with a ratio of 2 : 1 failed to become fully discriminated, as shown in the fourth experiment; and only in the fifth of the given experiments, performed $1\frac{1}{2}$ months after the beginning of the work, did it again produce a zero secretion.

Time	Conditioned stimulus applied during 30 seconds	Salivary Secretion in drops during 30 seconds
Experiment of 4th August, 1914.		
4.10 p.m.	Circle	4
4.22 ,,	,,	6
4.37 ,,	4 : 3 ellipse	**0**
4.55 ,,	Circle	4
Experiment of 2nd September, 1914.		
1.10 p.m.	Circle	2
1.27 ,,	,,	8
2.6 ,,	,,	10
2.16 ,,	9 : 8 ellipse	**1**
2.30 ,,	Circle	6
2.48 ,,	,,	8
Experiment of 17th September, 1914.		
3.20 p.m.	Circle	4
3.31 ,,	,,	7
3.54 ,,	9 : 8 ellipse	**8**
4.9 ,,	Circle	9
Experiment of 25th September, 1914.		
2.17 p.m.	Circle	9
2.47 ,,	2 : 1 ellipse	**3**
3.8 ,,	Circle	8
3.22 ,,	,,	8
3.46 ,,	2 : 1 ellipse	**3**
Experiment of 13th November, 1914.		
10.55 a.m.	Circle	10
11.5 ,,	,,	7
11.30 ,,	2 : 1 ellipse	**0**
11.44 ,,	Circle	5

After these experiments we paid considerable attention to pathological disturbances in the cortical activity and began to study them in detail. It became obvious that under certain conditions the clashing of excitation with inhibition led to a profound disturbance of the usual balance between these two processes, and led in a greater or less degree and for a longer or shorter time to pathological disturbances of the nervous system. In the first example, with the development of an alimentary reflex to the strong electric stimulus, it was the inborn defence reflex which had to be inhibited ; in the second example, with the visual stimuli, as we know already from the seventh lecture, the differentiation which had to be established also depended on a development of inhibition. In both cases a balance of the two antagonistic processes was satisfactorily maintained until a certain critical stage was reached, when, under the stress of the delicate antagonistic relations of the stimuli, the further adjustment of the balance became impossible and finally gave way to an undisputed predominance of one of them (as will be shown later), producing a pathological state.

In further experiments dogs were intentionally selected which possessed different types of nervous system, in order to find out the different pathological disturbances which would be produced by functional (*i.e.* non-surgical) interferences with the cortical activity. The first of these experiments [Dr. Petrova] were performed on two dogs, representatives, as judged by their general behaviour, of the two extreme types of nervous system. These dogs were those already described in the lecture upon sleep, the drowsiness, which they exhibited at first, being successfully removed by the administration in rapid succession of six different conditioned reflexes with an interval of 5 seconds between the beginning of the conditioned and the unconditioned stimuli (p. 254). Besides abolishing sleep the experiments provided very clear and definite illustration of the essential differences between the types of nervous system of the two dogs, successfully corroborating the diagnosis of their respective types which was previously made by general observation. In the course of the experiments the conditioned reflexes, which to begin with were practically simultaneous, were transformed into long-delayed reflexes with an interval of 3 minutes between the conditioned and the unconditioned stimuli. The transformation of the reflexes was performed gradually by prolonging the length of isolated action of the conditioned stimulus by 5 seconds daily ; correspondingly the so-called latent period of the reflexes—*i.e.* the interval of time between the beginning of the conditioned stimulus and the onset of the salivary response—became gradually more and more prolonged. All six reflexes were being treated in this manner at the same time.

The dog with a predominant tendency to inhibition mastered the problem of developing the longer delay straight ahead, and without any nervous disturbances ; the dog with a predominant tendency to excitation reacted to the problem in a quite different manner. When the delay of the reflexes reached two minutes the animal began to enter into a state of general excitation, and with a further prolongation of the delay to 3 minutes the animal became quite crazy, unceasingly and violently moving all parts of its body, howling, barking and squealing intolerably. All this was accompanied by an unceasing flow of saliva, so that although the secretion increased during the action of the conditioned stimuli all traces of the delay completely disappeared. Obviously the development of the inhibitory phase of delay required by many conditioned reflexes at one time was too difficult a problem for the excitable nervous system of this dog. It should be added that certain difficulties in the way of a successful development of a balance between the two antagonistic processes, difficulties in the form of hyper-excitation, were met with in many dogs, but in no other dog did this general excitation reach so great an intensity. However, the problem set to this animal was much more than usually complicated, since it was required to set up a balance of the two antagonistic processes in many points of the hemispheres at one and the same time. Eventually there was nothing to be done, other than to relinquish the experiments in this form. It is interesting that the problem which so far seemed impossible of resolution by the nervous system of this dog was nevertheless quite satisfactorily achieved when another method of experimentation was employed. We restricted our work to one of the conditioned stimuli only. The animal became quiet again, and even began to get sleepy during the experiment not only when kept in the stand but also when kept free on the floor. All the conditioned stimuli were now applied again, but with only 5 seconds' delay. Once more the isolated action of each conditioned stimulus was gradually prolonged from day to day until the delay of 3 minutes was reached. On this occasion definite long-delayed reflexes were developed without any disturbances. During the $1\frac{1}{2}$-2 minutes after the beginning of the conditioned stimulus the animal was asleep, but towards the end of the second minute or at the very beginning of the third it quickly roused up from its relaxed posture and a very sharp alimentary motor as well as secretory reaction appeared. The final stage of these experiments was described in the fifteenth lecture (p. 261).

In this manner, with the help of suitable periods of rest and by patient practising of the reflexes, that satisfactory balance of the two processes, which failed to appear at the first attempt was achieved. The differences in the nervous systems of the two dogs was thus made clear and we could now proceed with the main object of our experiments. This time, however, the investigation was carried out in a manner slightly different from that of those accidentally observed cases which were described previously. The effect of different forms of inhibition (differentiation, conditioned inhibition and extinction) was tested upon long-delayed reflexes. We hoped that as a result of such a complex presentation of different inhibiting influences a disturbance of the normal relations between the two antagonistic nervous processes would occur, as had already happened in the first establishment of the long-delay. Such a disturbance of the balance between the two processes did not, however, occur. What did happen was that these experiments, with the various forms of internal inhibition, always brought out more and more forcibly the essential differences between the two dogs. The development of every new inhibition was accompanied in the excitable dog by a temporary period of excessive general excitation, while the other dog evinced practically no difficulties. Since we failed to produce a disturbance of the equilibrium in the manner described we had recourse to the procedure which had proved successful with the dog previously described. We therefore commenced a development of a conditioned alimentary reflex to an electric stimulus applied to the skin. This reflex was fully established and practised with some intervals for a considerable length of time. A chronic functional disturbance of the nervous system occurred in both dogs even without the application of the electric stimulus to new places. It is probable that this disturbance of the normal balance between excitation and inhibition was favoured by the complexity of the inhibitory activity already established. The new and important point is that the disturbance of the normal activity of the nervous system found an opposite expression in the two animals : in the excitable dog it was the inhibitory reflexes which suffered, in the other it was the excitatory reflexes, and only much later the inhibitory ones. The following is a detailed description of these experiments.

Positive alimentary conditioned reflexes were established in the excitable dog to metronome, buzzer, bubbling sound, and tactile stimulation of the thigh ; and negative reflexes to a combination of a hissing sound with the metronome (the hissing sound preceded the metronome by 5 seconds), and to a tactile stimulation of the shoulder (differentiation). All the positive conditioned reflexes were delayed for three minutes.

Experiment of 15th March, 1923
(before the development of the conditioned reflex to the electric stimulus).

Time	Conditioned stimulus applied during 3 minutes	Salivary Secretion in drops during successive minutes from the beginning of the conditioned stimulus
3.0 p.m.	Metronome	0, 5, 16
3.25 ,,	Hissing + metronone (inhibitory)	0, 0, 0
3.45 ,,	Bubbling	0, ·1, 14
3.54 ,,	Buzzer	3, 0, 17
4.0 ,,	Tactile stimulation of thigh	0, 2, 12
4.13 ,,	Tactile stimulation of shoulder (inhibitory)	0, 0, 0

In reference to this experiment it should be mentioned that in excitable dogs the commencement of conditioned stimuli, especially strong ones, always elicits a brief investigatory reflex. On this account, in the case of delayed reflexes, there is often observed an initial short dis-inhibition of the inhibitory phase (3.54 p.m.).

The development of the conditioned reflex to the electric stimulus was begun towards the end of March. In April it was already fully established. During the whole time before the electric stimulus had been given any considerable strength all the forms of inhibition remained practically unaffected. In August the electric current was considerably increased in strength, and now the delayed reflexes became disturbed and the conditioned inhibition became incomplete. In order to diminish the inhibitory stress all conditioned stimuli excepting the buzzer were now allowed to act for 30 seconds only, instead of three minutes, before reinforcement. In spite of this, and in spite of the disuse of the " alimentary " electric stimulus, the gradual weakening of all inhibitory processes continued. The delay disappeared altogether ; the hissing, which, when preceding by 5 seconds the action of the metronome had established an inhibitory combination, now itself acquired excitatory properties, *i.e.* became a conditioned stimulus of the second order. Even the differentiation of the tactile stimuli was now considerably disinhibited.

Experiment of 29th September, 1923 (final period of work).

Time	Conditioned stimulus	Salivary Secretion in drops
3.15 p.m.	Bubbling, 30 seconds	5
3.26 ,,	Tactile stimulation of thigh, 30 seconds	8
3.40 ,,	Tactile stimulation of shoulder (inhibitory), 30 seconds	3
4.0 ,,	Metronome, 30 seconds	6
4.12 ,,	Hissing + metronome (inhibitory), 30 seconds	10
4.35 ,,	Buzzer, 3 minutes	16, 12, 13
4.46 ,,	Tactile stimulation of thigh, 30 seconds	8
5.0 ,,	Tactile stimulatiou of shoulder (inhibitory), 30 seconds	3

In the case of the inhibitable dog the conditioned stimuli were the same. The following experiment illustrates the conditioned reflexes as they were before the development of the reflex to the electric stimulus :

Experiment of 21st March, 1923.

Time	Conditioned stimulus applied during 3 minutes	Salivary Secretion in drops during successive minutes
3.18 p.m.	Bubbling	0, 2, 6
3.54 ,,	Buzzer	0, 0, 12
4.13 ,,	Metronome	1, 5, 15
4.35 ,,	Hissing + metronome (inhibitory)	1, 0, 0
4.42 ,,	Buzzer	0, 6, 14
4.55 ,,	Hissing + metronome (inhibitory)	0, 0, 0
5.3 ,,	Tactile stimulation of thigh	0, 3, 9
5.15 ,,	Tactile stimulation of shoulder (inhibitory)	0, 0, 0

The development of the conditioned reflex to the electric stimulus was begun in this dog also towards the end of March. The reflex developed easily and soon reached a magnitude of 7 drops during 30 seconds. The defence reaction occasionally returned when the

current was increased in strength, but finally it disappeared altogether and was entirely replaced by a typical alimentary reaction.
It was soon noticed on repeating the already established reflex to the
electric current that its secretory effect began to diminish, while the
secretory effect of other stimuli had practically disappeared, being present only at the beginning of the experiment and in a very weak form.

The following serves as an illustration of this period of the
experiments :

Experiment of 30th April, 1923.

Time	Conditioned stimulus during 3 minutes	Salivary Secretion in drops during successive minutes
3.25 p.m.	Buzzer	0, 0, 2
3.35 ,,	Metronome	0, 0, 5
3.47 ,,	Buzzer	0, 0, 0
4.3 ,,	Tactile stimulation of thigh	0, 0, 0
4.20 ,,	Tactile stimulation of shoulder (inhibitory)	0, 0, 0
4.25 ,,	Bubbling	0, 0, 0
4.37 ,,	Metronome	0, 0, 0
4.48 ,,	Buzzer	0, 0, 0

The animal started at this time to lose weight and became very
dull. All experiments were therefore interrupted for a considerable
time, and the dog was given plenty of food and cod-liver oil. It
soon picked up weight, and its general alertness also increased.
After this period of interruption all the long-delayed conditioned
reflexes excepting the one to the buzzer were shortened to delays
of 30 seconds. The ultimate result remained, however, unchanged.
No more than indications of the positive reflexes were obtained.
The electrical stimulus still evoked a considerable secretion, but on
increasing its strength the reflex again diminished and finally
disappeared altogether. The other positive conditioned reflexes
had long since disappeared, and now all the forms of internal inhibition began gradually to disappear also, a salivary secretion being
evoked on some occasions by the inhibitory stimuli.

The following experiment illustrates this condition and shows
that the stimulus for the long-delayed reflex (buzzer) produced a
positive effect during the formerly inhibitory phase and had no
effect during the formerly positive phase.

Experiment of 6th December, 1923.

Time	Conditioned stimulus	Salivary Secretion in drops
12.48 p.m.	Tactile stimulation of thigh (positive), 30 seconds	0
1.0 ,,	Tactile stimulation of shoulder (inhibitory), 30 seconds	0
1.7 ,,	Bubbling (positive), 30 seconds	1
1.20 ,,	Metronome (positive), 30 seconds	0
1.40 ,,	Buzzer (positive long delayed), 3 minutes	3, 2, 0
1.51 ,,	Tactile stimulation of thigh (positive), 30 seconds	0
2.0 ,,	Tactile stimulation of shoulder (inhibitory), 30 seconds	0
2.11 ,,	Metronome (positive), 30 seconds	0
2.42 ,,	Hissing + metronome (inhibitory), 30 seconds	0
2.53 ,,	Metronome (positive), 30 seconds	0

The positive effect of the formerly inhibitory stimuli did not depend upon a weakening of the inhibitory process but was determined by disturbances in the excitatory process, appearing in the form of the ultra-paradoxical phase of the cortical elements (see p. 275).

The general condition of the dog during this period of the experiments was quite satisfactory. It was found in other experiments that the differentiation and the conditioned inhibition were also weakened, giving place to a salivary secretion.

The experiments just described show that in these two dogs, with different types of nervous system, prolonged disturbances of the higher nervous activity which developed under precisely identical injurious influences took quite different directions. In the excitable dog the inhibitory function of the cortical elements became extremely weakened. In the quiet dog it was the excitation of the corresponding cells (since the stimuli were identical) which became extremely weak. In other words, two quite different types of neurosis were produced.

The experimentally developed neuroses were in both cases extremely persistent and prolonged, and even after a break in the experiments they showed no tendency to improve. It was now resolved in the case of the excitable dog to employ a valuable therapeutic agent, namely, bromides, since in our early experiments [Drs. Nikiforovsky and Deriabin] a strengthening of inhibition was sometimes observed under the action of bromides in cases where the internal inhibition was weak. Therefore, after the state of neurosis had continued for several months the animal was given 100 cc. of 2% solution of potassium bromide daily in the form of an enema. It was soon observed that all the forms of internal inhibition began quickly to re-establish themselves and in a definite sequence. The first to recover completely was the tactile differentiation ; this was followed by the conditioned inhibition, and finally by the delay. All the reflexes had returned to normal by the tenth day of the treatment.

Experiment of 5th March, 1924.

Time	Conditioned stimulus	Salivary Secretion in drops
3.0 p.m.	Metronome (excitatory rate), 30 seconds	5
3.12 ,,	Hissing + metronome (inhibitory), 30 seconds	0
3.28 ,,	Bubbling, 30 seconds	8
3.37 ,,	Buzzer, 3 minutes	2, 12, 16
3.44 ,,	Metronome, 30 seconds	8
3.55 ,,	Metronome (inhibitory rate), 30 seconds	0
4.10 ,,	Bubbling, 30 seconds	7
4.16 ,,	Buzzer, 3 minutes	2, 1, 9
4.25 ,,	Buzzer, 3 minutes	0, 8, 21

It must be noted that as a result of administration of bromides there was no diminution in the magnitude of the positive reflexes. On the contrary they were extremely constant. According to these and all our previous experiments bromides should not be regarded as sedatives diminishing the excitability of the central nervous system : they simply regulate the activity of the nervous system by strengthening the intensity of internal inhibition.

Bromides were administered for eleven days only, but the cure of the neurosis was permanent and all reflexes remained normal for the remaining $2\frac{1}{2}$ months of our experimentation. The state of neurosis of the " phlegmatic " dog was not improved by the administration of bromides, nor by other therapeutic measures which were tried. The animal was therefore left alone for a very long time, and little attention was paid to it. At the end of this period we were surprised to find that the animal had spontaneously and completely recovered. We shall come across further experiments with this dog in the next lecture.

LECTURE XVIII

Pathological disturbances of the cortex, result of functional interference
(continued).

In the present lecture we shall discuss further experiments and observations upon the pathological states of the cerebral cortex. The inquiry is one of particular interest, not only on account of the special attention devoted to this subject at the present time, but also on account of several fortuitous occurrences. It has become possible to trace how, as a result of different injurious influences, the activity of the cortex gradually and by scarcely noticeable stages deviates from normal and becomes pathological ; often also the pathological states can be made use of for inquiry into nervous processes taking place under purely physiological conditions, since under pathological conditions different aspects of the nervous processes which are screened off from us by the unified and balanced complexity of the normal physiological state become dissociated or accentuated. In the lecture upon the hypnotic states occurring under normal conditions it was mentioned that the most interesting of these were subjected to experimental investigation only after they had previously been observed in exaggerated form in a pathological case.

In one of our dogs which, it will be remembered (p. 270), had several positive and negative conditioned reflexes, a tactile stimulation at the rate of 24 per minute had been established as a positive stimulus and a stimulation at the rate of 12 per minute as a negative one : moreover, as usually under normal conditions, the relative intensity of the positive reflexes was directly determined by the relative strength of their conditioned stimuli. In one of the experiments the positive rate of the tactile stimulation was made to follow the inhibitory rate without any interval of time. This apparently small modification of the experiment was sufficient to create a pathological disturbance of the cortical activities in this dog. At first, for a few days, all positive conditioned reflexes disappeared completely ; this was followed by a series of different modifications in the strength of the reflexes, a state of affairs which lasted for many days, the relation between the magnitudes of the reflexes and the intensities of the stimuli gradually changing from one phase to another. The entire disturbance lasted for $5\frac{1}{2}$ weeks, after which the reflexes returned to normal. Obviously this dog falls into one group with the inhibitable dog (described at the end of the preceding lecture), in which functional interferences with the cortical activities produced a profound nervous disturbance which was accompanied by a disappearance of all positive conditioned reflexes for many months. In the dog just described the same type of disturbance was produced, but lasted for only thirty-six days, within which period the activity of the cortex passing through different stages finally returned to normal.

It becomes clear on considering all the pathological cases so far described, that the underlying cause of their development is in every instance the same. Broadly we can regard these disturbances as due to a conflict between the processes of excitation and inhibition which the cortex finds difficult to resolve.

Besides these pathological cases we have at our disposal others which present features of perhaps even greater interest, firstly on account of certain intrinsic peculiarities, secondly on account of peculiar features in the mode of their origination. The case which is to be described first was studied from day to day during many months, and in view of the considerable interest it presents the description will be given in detail [experiments of Dr. Rickman]. The experiments were carried out on a dog which was exceedingly inhibitable. The animal had served in the laboratory for different experiments for a very long time, and it had among others an inhibitory alimentary conditioned reflex to a metronome rate of 60 beats per minute, while a rate of 120 beats per minute served as a positive stimulus. The strength of the various positive reflexes was definitely related to the strength of their respective conditioned stimuli. The inhibitory conditioned reflex, which at the time of the experiments had been repeated 266 times, was constant and precise, being so concentrated that its inhibitory after-effect upon the positive reflexes was very short. The strength of the reflexes during this normal period is represented in the table shown on the opposite page.

The dog belonged to a group which can be called " expert at inhibition," in view of the fact that in this group all the types of internal inhibition develop with great ease and precision. We now determined to investigate in further experiments the degree of stability of the inhibitory process in this dog. For this purpose it was decided to transform the negative conditioned stimulus into a positive one by the method which is usually the most effective, namely, repeated reinforcement of the inhibitory stimulus without any intermediate introduction of the positive stimuli (see p. 198). However, the destruction of the inhibition in this dog proceeded extremely slowly. The hitherto inhibitory stimulus was followed by reinforcement 4-7 times in succession on each of three successive

Experiment of 1st December, 1925.

Time	Conditioned stimulus applied during 20 seconds	Salivary Secretion in drops during 20 seconds	Motor reaction and general behaviour
10.37 a.m.	Metronome, 120 per minute	8	⎫ Lively ali-
10.45 ,,	Electric light	4	⎬ mentary
10.49 ,,	Strong tone	6	⎭ reaction
10.56 ,,	Metronome, 60 per minute	0	The dog re-mains mo-tionless
11.0 ,,	Buzzer	9	⎫ Lively ali-
11.5 ,,	Weak tone	$3\frac{1}{2}$	⎬ mentary ⎭ reaction

days. The first sign of any destruction of the inhibition was observed at the seventeenth application with reinforcement, in the form of a very small secretion without any accompanying alimentary motor reaction. At the twenty-seventh reinforcement the salivary secretion was already considerable. No definite disturbances in the other positive stimuli could be observed at this period, excepting a certain tendency to equalization of the secretory effect of strong and weak positive conditioned stimuli. The experiment of the 14th December on page 304 shows the strength of the reflexes at this time.

The secretory reaction thus established to the rate of 60 beats of the metronome did not, however, remain constant, but in spite of continued reinforcement quickly declined and at its thirtieth repetition fell to zero. Moreover, it was now noticed that immediately after an application of the metronome at the rate of 60 practically none of the positive reflexes could be elicited (18th December).

Experiment of 14*th December*, 1925.

Time	Conditioned stimulus applied during 20 seconds	Salivary Secretion in drops during 20 seconds	Motor reaction and general behaviour
10.56 a.m.	Metronome, 60 per minute (formerly the inhibitory rate)	$5\frac{1}{2}$	Investigatory in character rather than alimentary
11.3 ,,	Electric lamp	5	
11.10 ,,	Metronome, 120 per minute	5	
11.17 ,,	Buzzer	8	Alimentary reaction
11.24 ,,	Weak tone	5	
11.31 ,,	Metronome, 120 per minute	$5\frac{1}{2}$	
11.38 ,,	Buzzer	7	

Experiment of 18*th December*, 1925,
showing the general disturbance of the conditioned reflexes.

Time	Conditioned stimulus applied during 20 seconds	Salivary Secretion in drops during 20 seconds	Motor reaction and general behaviour
12.4 p.m.	Electric lamp	$4\frac{1}{2}$	Alimentary reaction ; takes the food with avidity
12.9 ,,	Metronome, 60 per minute (formerly the inhibitory rate)	1	Investigatory reflex
12.14 ,,	Strong tone	0	At first turns the head away but subsequently takes food
12.23 ,,	Buzzer	0	Turns itself right away and declines food
12.30 ,,	Electric lamp	0	Takes the food after some delay
12.38 ,,	Weak tone	0	Alimentary reaction ; takes the food at once

In its general behaviour the animal appeared to be perfectly healthy and when free on the floor it consumed the same food as that offered during the experiment with great avidity, just as it did in the above experiment after the conditioned stimulus applied before the metronome (12.4 p.m.).

In succeeding experiments, though some of the positive effect of the metronome rate of 60 per minute returned, its strong inhibitory effect upon other conditioned reflexes nevertheless continued as before.

In all those experiments, however, in which the metronome was not used all the reflexes were perfectly normal, excepting that the weaker stimuli gave a somewhat smaller secretion towards the end of an experiment than usual.

Experiment of 24th December, 1925
(without application of the metronome).

Time	Conditioned stimulus applied during 20 seconds	Salivary Secretion in drops during 20 seconds	Motor reaction and general behaviour
11.2 a.m.	Buzzer	9	
11.10 ,,	Electric lamp	$5\frac{1}{2}$	
11.15 ,,	Strong tone	7	
11.20 ,,	Weak tone	5	Lively
11.28 ,,	Buzzer	$6\frac{1}{2}$	alimentary
11.32 ,,	Electric light	3	reaction
11.39 ,,	Strong tone	6	
11.44 ,,	Weak tone	$3\frac{1}{2}$	

I have intentionally given several experiments with the initially positive reflexes in order to show how long and how persistently the normal relations were retained in spite of the disturbing influence of the metronome during the intervals between these particular experiments. On continuing the experiments further the general relation between the strength of the reflexes and the strength of the stimuli continued to be maintained in all experiments in which the metronome was not used. In those experiments, however, in which either of the rates of the metronome—which themselves gave a secretion varying from $\frac{1}{2}$ to $7\frac{1}{2}$ drops—was used there was invariably a disturbance of all conditioned reflexes following within the given experiment—a disturbance in the form of complete inhibition or of one of its intermediate stages. It is of interest that the metronome rate of 120 per minute often produced a greater disturbance than the formerly inhibitory rate of 60. The experiments given below are taken from this period of experimentation.

Time	Conditioned stimulus applied during 20 seconds	Salivary Secretion in drops during 20 seconds	Motor reaction and general behaviour

Experiment of 28th December, 1925 (Phase of Equalization).

Time	Conditioned stimulus	Salivary	Motor reaction
10.56 a.m.	Buzzer	10	Alimentary reaction
11.7 ,,	Electric lamp	6	,, ,,
11.13 ,,	Metronome, 60 per minute	2	,, ,,
11.20 ,,	Weaker tone	5	,, ,,
11.28 ,,	Metronome, 120 per minute	4½	Weak alimentary reaction
11.33 ,,	Strong tone	5	Alimentary reaction
11.40 ,,	Buzzer	4½	,, ,,
11.47 ,,	Electric lamp	5½	,, ,,

Experiment of 5th January, 1926 (Narcotic Phase).

Time	Conditioned stimulus	Salivary	Motor reaction
12.53 p.m.	Metronome, 60 per minute	6	Delayed alimentary reaction
1.0 ,,	Electric lamp	3½	Alimentary reaction
1.5 ,,	Strong tone	6	,, ,,
1.10 ,,	Metronome, 120 per minute	3	,, ,,
1.18 ,,	Weak tone	0	Weak alimentary reaction
1.25 ,,	Buzzer	4½	Alimentary reaction
1.30 ,,	Electric lamp	0	Turns head away, declines food
1.35 ,,	Buzzer	6	Definite alimentary reaction : takes food immediately

Experiment of 20th January, 1926 (Paradoxical Phase).

Time	Conditioned stimulus	Salivary	Motor reaction
10.44 a.m.	Strong tone	8	Alimentary
10.49 ,,	Electric lamp	3	,,
10.57 ,,	Metronome, 60 per minute	½	Investigatory
11.2 ,,	Weak tone	5	Lively alimentary
11.7 ,,	Buzzer	4½	Weak alimentary
11.14 ,,	Weak tone	5	Lively alimentary
11.21 ,,	Buzzer	2½	Weak alimentary
11.26 ,,	Electric lamp	3½	Lively alimentary
11.31 ,,	Strong tone	1	Alimentary

Time	Conditioned stimulus applied during 20 seconds	Salivary Secretion in drops during 20 seconds	Motor reaction and general behaviour	

Experiment of 21st January, 1926
(Complete Inhibition).

11.9 a.m.	Strong tone	6	Alimentary	⎫
11.14 ,,	Electric lamp	4½	,,	During the
11.22 ,,	Metronome, 120 per minute	3½	,,	intervals between
11.27 ,,	Weak tone	0	,,	the stimuli
11.32 ,,	Buzzer	3	,,	the animal
11.39 ,,	Weak tone	0	,,	remains
11.47 ,,	Buzzer	0	,,	perfectly
11.52 ,,	Electric lamp	0	Weak alimentary	still
11.57 ,,	Strong tone	0	,, ,,	⎭

Experiment of 26th January, 1926
(without the use of the metronome).

11.18 a.m.	Electric lamp	6	Lively alimentary
11.28 ,,	Strong tone	6½	,, ,,
11.33 ,,	Buzzer	7½	,, ,,
11.40 ,,	Weak tone	4½	,, ,,
11.48 ,,	Buzzer	6	,, ,,
11.53 ,,	Electric lamp	2	Weak alimentary
12.2 p.m.	Strong tone	3½	,, ,,

In the last experiment, though the relative strength of the reflexes remained unchanged, a general diminution in the strength of all the reflexes became apparent towards the end of the experiment. In view of this tendency all the stimuli were for several days reinforced after a very much shorter delay and the use of the metronome was discontinued. Subsequently to this, the delay was extended again, but only to 15 seconds instead of to 20 seconds as previously. Moreover, a new conditioned reflex to a bubbling sound was established ; the stimulus belonged in this dog to the group of strong stimuli. As a result of this treatment the reflexes increased in strength and now showed no diminution towards the end of an experiment. After eleven days of such experimentation the rate of 120 beats per minute of the metronome was again tried :

Experiment of 2nd March, 1926.

Time	Conditioned stimulus during 15 seconds	Salivary Secretion in drops during 15 seconds	Motor reaction and general behaviour
10.44 a.m.	Bubbling	$6\frac{1}{2}$	Alimentary
10.54 ,,	Weak tone	$5\frac{1}{2}$	,,
11.2 ,,	Metronome, 120 per minute	6	Investigatory reflex followed by alimentary reflex
11.7 ,,	Electric lamp	$4\frac{1}{2}$	Alimentary
11.15 ,,	Buzzer	$4\frac{1}{2}$	,,
11.23 ,,	Bubbling	$3\frac{1}{2}$	,,
11.31 ,,	Weak tone	$5\frac{1}{2}$	Lively alimentary
11.38 ,,	Buzzer	$4\frac{1}{2}$	Alimentary

It was seen that the administration of the metronome led to an immediate disturbance of all the succeeding conditioned reflexes, which entered into a phase of equalization passing into the paradoxical phase. The disturbance, however, went much deeper than this. On the following day and for a long time afterwards the cortex was unable to withstand any kind of strong stimulus without undergoing complete inhibition. The fact that the maximum disturbance in the central nervous activity does not appear immediately on administration of the causative stimulus, but after one or more days has been observed in many animals. The following is an experiment which was performed on the day following the last administration of the metronome :

Experiment of 3rd March, 1926.

Time	Conditioned stimulus applied during 15 seconds	Salivary Secretion in drops during 15 seconds	Motor reaction and general behaviour
3.41 p.m.	Buzzer	5	Weak alimentary
3.46 ,,	Electric lamp	$\frac{1}{2}$	Delayed alimentary
3.55 ,,	Strong tone	0	Declines food
4.2 ,,	Weak tone	$\frac{1}{2}$	Alimentary ; takes the food
4.7 ,,	Buzzer	0	Declines food
4.10 ,,	Administration of food without any conditioned stimuli	—	Takes the food immediately

To all appearance the dog was at this time perfectly healthy.

The cortical disturbance continued for 11 days without showing signs of any improvement, and we therefore determined to avoid any further use of the strong tone and to damp down the sounds of buzzer and bubbling. The following is the first experiment :

Experiment of 15th March, 1926.

Time	Conditioned stimulus applied during 15 seconds	Salivary Secretion in drops during 15 seconds	Motor reaction and general behaviour
10.20 a.m.	Electric lamp	$6\frac{1}{2}$	
10.27 ,,	Weak tone	5	
10.32 ,,	Weak sound of bubbling	$3\frac{1}{2}$	
10.40 ,,	Weak buzzer	$6\frac{1}{2}$	Alimentary reaction
10.48 ,,	Weak tone	$4\frac{1}{3}$	in every case
10.56 ,,	Weak sound of bubbling	$4\frac{1}{2}$	
11.4 ,,	Weak buzzer	5	
11.12 ,,	Electric lamp	4	

The experiments gave similar results on nine successive days. After this the strong stimuli were again applied, with the following result :

Experiment of 27th March, 1926.

Time	Conditioned stimulus applied during 15 seconds	Salivary Secretion in drops during 15 seconds	Motor reaction and general behaviour
4.2 p.m.	Strong buzzer	4	Alimentary
4.9 ,,	Electric lamp	$\frac{1}{2}$	,,
4.16 ,,	Strong sound of bubbling	0	Turns head away, and declines the food
4.23 ,,	Weak tone	0	Takes the food reluctantly
4.30 ,,	Strong buzzer	0	Signs of general excitation ; takes the food reluctantly
4.37 ,,	Electric lamp	$1\frac{1}{2}$	Takes the food reluctantly

When free upon the floor the animal behaved quite normally and took the food with avidity. After an interval of one day an experiment was performed again with the use of only weak stimuli, and all the reflexes were found to be present.

Experiment of 29th March, 1926.

Time	Conditioned stimulus applied during 15 seconds	Salivary Secretion in drops during 15 seconds	Motor reaction and general behaviour
3.57 p.m.	Weak tone	$6\frac{1}{2}$	
4.5 ,,	Weak bubbling	6	
4.10 ,,	Electric lamp	$4\frac{1}{2}$	
4.19 ,,	Weak buzzer	6	Alimentary reaction in every case
4.26 ,,	Weak bubbling	$6\frac{1}{2}$	
4.31 ,,	Electric lamp	3	
4.40 ,,	Weak buzzer	5	

To sum up, these experiments show that the transformation of an inhibitory point of the acoustic analyser into an excitatory one occurred only gradually and imperfectly. Moreover, and this is more important, it rendered this point abnormal so that its stimulation by the conditioned stimulus of the metronome immediately led to a profound disturbance in the activity of the entire cortex, leading finally to an inability to withstand any strong conditioned stimuli without passing into different phases of inhibition, including the phase of complete inhibition. At first the normal activity of the cortex was comparatively quickly restored on discontinuing all stimulation of the abnormal point. At a later period, with further stimulation of this point, the disturbance took on a more permanent character. Since other auditory stimuli continued at this time to act quite normally the disturbance must be regarded as a result of a strictly localized functional interference in the acoustic analyser, a chronic functional lesion of some circumscribed part, the stimulation of which produces an immediate effect upon the function of the whole cortex, and finally leads to a protracted pathological state.

These observations to my mind reveal once more in an almost tangible form the mosaic character of the cortical activities which has been discussed already.

The disturbance in the activity of the entire cortex which has just been described can be regarded as being produced in either of two ways. First, it is possible that the excitation evoked by stimuli acting upon the area of cortical disturbance now rapidly passes over into inhibition. Such a transition into inhibition is at first restricted to the immediate area around the original point of cortical disturbance but ultimately irradiates to involve the whole of the cortex. Second, it is possible that the stimuli act upon the area of cortical disturbance as injurious agents, so that, exactly as in the case of any injurious agents acting on any other part of the body, the entire cortical activity becomes inhibited on account of external inhibition.

In either case it is obvious that the localized disturbance of the acoustic analyser is again the result of a clash between excitation and inhibition.

Besides those cases which have been related in the present and in the preceding lectures many others have been observed in which a similar clashing of the two antagonistic nervous processes led sometimes to a temporary, sometimes to a more prolonged disturbance of the normal activity of the cortex, in the form of a lasting predominance of one or the other process. In many cases these pathological disturbances could not be remedied by any of the measures which were applied. These abnormal conditions developed either during the establishment of very difficult differentiations— especially in the case of successive compound stimuli [experiments of Dr. Ivanov-Smolensky, Dr. Eurman and Dr. Zimkina]—or on immediate transition from inhibitory cutaneous stimuli to excitatory ones—especially when the differentiation depended upon a definite rate of stimulation of one and the same place on the skin. When in the latter case the experiments were performed on an excitable and aggressive type of animal [experiments of Dr. Federov] the general excitation reached such an intensity that it became impossible to continue the experiments. The animal was, however, cured by prolonged administration of bromides and by disuse of both positive and negative tactile stimuli. In a dog of more inhibitable type [experiments of Dr. Petrova] there developed under similar conditions an abnormal focus, to all appearance strictly localized, in the cutaneous analyser, just as in the experiments of Dr. Rickman with the acoustic analyser. The positive stimulation of this point invariably led to a diffuse spreading of inhibition which persisted throughout the given experiment or even during a few subsequent days. Further experiments with this dog were prevented on account of its falling ill of nephritis.

With regard to the pathology of the cortex, there remain to be mentioned another set of cases in which the disturbances verge almost impreceptibly into the normal. These cases are the result of a permanent congenital weakness of the nervous system of the animal, which under definite conditions is rendered abnormal, while a more resistant nervous system remains normal. However, before describing these it is necessary, for the sake of clearness, to discuss briefly those external stimuli which directly lead to inhibition of the cortical elements. These are of three kinds—monotonously recurring weak stimuli, very strong stimuli and unusual stimuli. All these can result either from the appearance of some new stimulus or from a new grouping of old stimuli. The conditions of our lives as well as of the lives of animals provide many occasions for the action of such stimuli, and it is not necessary to give any special examples. The biological significance of the development of cortical inhibition in response to such stimuli can easily be perceived. If stimuli of considerable strength, and especially continually changing stimuli, determine—as they must do in order to maintain the delicate equilibration of the organism in its surroundings—an alert state of the cortex, then it is quite reasonable to suppose that weak and monotonous stimuli which do not call forth any activity should tend towards inhibition so as to rest the cortical elements and give them time for recovery after a preceding activity. The inhibitory influence of very strong stimuli can be regarded as a reflex of " passive self-defence," as, for instance, in the case of hypnosis. The immobility of the animal makes it less noticeable to the enemy, and thus abolishes or diminishes the aggressive reaction of the enemy. It has been seen that the presence of something unusual also leads to a limitation of movement, which again may possess " survival value " for the animal, since in the new conditions its usual reactions might not be appropriate and might lead to some injury. Of course in the case of a new, even small, change in the environment, two reflexes appear —a positive one, the investigatory reflex, and a negative one, which might be described as a reflex of caution and restraint. Whether these two reflexes are independent or whether the second is a sequence to the first and results from external inhibition or negative induction cannot be settled at present. The second supposition seems to me the more probable. The mechanism by which these three different types of stimuli bring about inhibition will be discussed in a further lecture.

A big flood which occurred in Petrograd on the 23rd September, 1924, afforded us an opportunity to observe in our dogs prolonged neuro-pathological disturbances which developed as a result of the extremely strong and unusual external stimuli consequent on the flood. The kennels of the animals which stood on the ground at about a quarter of a mile's distance from the main building of the laboratory were flooded with water. During the terrific storm, amid the breaking of the waves of the increasing water against the walls of the building and the noise of breaking and falling trees, the animals had to be quickly transferred by making them swim in little groups from the kennels into the laboratory, where they were kept on the first floor, all huddled up together indiscriminately. All this produced a very strong and obvious inhibition in all the animals, since there was no fighting or quarrelling among them whatever, otherwise a usual occurrence when the dogs are kept together. After this experience some of the dogs on their return to the kennels showed no disturbance in their conditioned reflexes. Other dogs—those of the inhibitable type—suffered a functional disturbance of the cortical activities for a very considerable period of time, as could be disclosed by experiments upon their conditioned reflexes.

One of the dogs has already been mentioned in these lectures [experiments by Dr. Speransky]—a strong healthy animal, but very easily subjected to inhibition, with all conditioned reflexes normally of considerable magnitude, very constant and very precise so long as the environing conditions were kept rigidly constant. This dog had ten alimentary conditioned reflexes, six positive and four negative (differentiations). Out of the positive reflexes three were auditory and three visual. The buzzer, which was the strongest of the auditory stimuli, evoked the largest secretion. The three visual reflexes were equal in their secretory effects and smaller by about one-third than the auditory. A week after the flood the dog was brought in to the experimental room and placed in its stand. The animal was abnormally restless and all conditioned reflexes were practically absent, and, though usually very ready for food, the animal now would not touch the food and even turned its head away. During three days while the animal was purposely left without food its general behaviour during the experiments remained unaltered. On considering various possible interpretations we reached the conclusion that this extraordinary behaviour of the animal must still be an after-effect of the flood, and the following method of combating the disturbance was adopted : Instead of leaving the animal alone during the experiment the experimenter now remained in the same room with it, while I myself conducted the experiment from the outside. All the reflexes showed an immediate restoration in the first experiment and the animal took the food with avidity, but it was sufficient for the experimenter to leave the animal alone for all the abnormal symptoms to recur. In order to re-establish the reflexes permanently it was necessary to adopt the above course, of alternately leaving and entering the room, for a considerable period of time. On the eleventh day of this treatment a conditioned stimulus which had not been employed since before the flood was now for the first time again employed, namely, the buzzer, which was the strongest stimulus, and which before the flood constantly evoked the largest secretion. After the application of the buzzer all the remaining conditioned reflexes almost completely disappeared, the animal again declined the food, became very restless and continuously stared at the floor. Under the influence of the same special stimulus, namely, the presence of the experimenter in the room with the animal, the reflexes were again gradually restored, but repetition of the buzzer after an interval of five days produced the disturbance afresh. The buzzer was then applied only when the experimenter was in the room with the animal, but even so, normal relations only returned gradually and very slowly. On many occasions a phase of equalization of the reflexes was observed after administration of the buzzer, the reflexes often diminishing and the animal declining the food. Perfectly normal reflexes were at last obtained after forty-seven days of experimentation, i.e. two months after the flood. We now made the following experiment. A small stream of water was allowed to trickle silently beneath the door into the animal's room. The water formed a small pool on the floor next to the table on which the dog stood in its stand. This experiment, which is represented in full on page 315, was conducted in the absence of the experimenter from the animal's room.

Several months after, when the reflexes were perfectly normal and the buzzer had intentionally not been used for a considerable length of time, a first fresh application of the buzzer gave a reflex which was of greater intensity than the reflexes to the other stimuli, but on repeating the stimulus of the buzzer once every day for several days the secretory effect gradually diminished, and finally the buzzer became not only entirely ineffective of itself, but its applications now led also to a diminution of all the other reflexes. It is of interest that at this stage of the experiment the presence not

Experiment of 17th November, 1924.

Time	Conditioned stimulus applied during 30 seconds	Salivary Secretion in drops during 30 seconds	Remarks
10.15 a.m.	Metronome, 120 per minute	15½	⎫
10.24 ,,	Strong illumination of room	9	⎬ Takes the food with avidity
10.36 ,,	Buzzer	17	
10.46 ,,	Appearance of a circle	9	
10.59 ,,	Whistle	15	⎭
11.11 ,,	Metronome, 80 per minute (inhibitory)	0	—
11.20 ,,	Metronome, 120 per minute	12½	Takes the food with avidity
11.30 ,,	Appearance of a square (inhibitory)	0	—
11.41 ,,	Appearance of a circle	9	⎫ Takes the food with avidity
11.50 ,,	Buzzer	17	⎭
11.59 ,,	—	—	A small stream of water is allowed to trickle noiselessly into the animal's room and form a pool on the floor
12.2 p.m.	Strong illumination of the room	0	The animal jumps up quickly, gazes restlessly at the floor, tries to get off the stand and breathes heavily
12.7 ,,	Metronome, 120 per minute	0	
12.15 ,,	Whistle	0	The conditioned stimuli serve only to increase the general excitation; the animal declines the food
12.25 ,,	Buzzer	0	
12.32 ,,	Appearance of a circle	0	

only of the experimenter in the animal's room but even of his clothes placed somewhere out of sight (*i.e.* olfactory stimulus) was sufficient to restore the reflexes.

Evidently under the effect of an extremely powerful and unusual stimulus the cortical cells, which in this dog already had a tendency to inhibition, now permanently became still more susceptible to inhibition. Stimuli to which the dog had already for a considerable time been indifferent (the general environment of the experiment), and also strong agencies which had acted before as powerful conditioned stimuli (buzzer), produced a strong inhibitory effect upon the cortical elements, the resistance of which was now diminished. Minutest components of the extraordinary stimulus of the flood were sufficient to evoke the same abnormal reaction.

The dog upon which the experiments described in detail at the beginning of the present lecture were performed had also passed through the experience of the flood, with resulting disturbances, which, though based on a similar predisposition to inhibition, assumed a somewhat different character from those observed in the first dog. Two experiments are given below, the one performed the day before the flood (22nd September, 1924), the other on the third day after the flood (26th September, 1924).

(The experiments by Dr. Rickman upon the same dog, given in the first part of this lecture, were performed, it will be remembered, much later than this, December 1925—March 1926.)

Time	Conditioned stimulus applied during 30 seconds	Salivary Secretion in drops during 30 seconds

Experiment of 22nd September, 1924.

12.53 p.m.	Metronome, 120 per minute	6
12.58 ,,	Tactile	$3\frac{1}{2}$
1.3 ,,	Metronome, 60 per minute (inhibitory)	0
1.13 ,,	Electric lamp	4
1.23 ,,	Strong tone	$7\frac{1}{2}$

Experiment of 26th September, 1924.

2.42 p.m.	Metronome, 120 per minute	$2\frac{1}{2}$
2.50 ,,	Tactile	2
2.55 ,,	Metronome, 60 per minute (inhibitory)	$3\frac{1}{2}$
3.2 ,,	Metronome, 120 per minute	$1\frac{1}{2}$
3.6 ,,	Tactile	0
3.16 ,,	Metronome, 120 per minute	$2\frac{1}{2}$

In the experiment of the 26th September the animal accepted the food, but the positive conditioned reflexes were diminished and the maximum secretory effect was obtained by the negative stimulus (2.55 p.m.—ultra-paradoxical phase). Experiments were now performed in which for a very long time the inhibitory rate of the metronome was not used. The positive reflexes were satisfactory and approached the normal, but even now on a single fresh application of the inhibitory stimulus, in any experiment, all conditioned reflexes were greatly diminished or even abolished, not only in the given experiment but during several succeeding days. The following are two examples :

Time	Conditioned stimulus applied during 30 seconds	Salivary Secretion in drops during 30 seconds
Experiment of 6th October, 1924.		
12.3 p.m.	Metronome, 120 per minute	5
12.10 ,,	Strong tone	5
12.20 ,,	Tactile	2
12.25 ,,	Strong tone	4
12.33 ,,	Metronome, 60 per minute (inhibitory)	0
12.36 ,,	Metronome, 120 per minute	0
12.43 ,,	Tactile	0
Experiment of 20th October, 1924.		
11.41 a.m.	Weak tone	6
11.46 ,,	Metronome, 120 per minute	$7\frac{1}{2}$
11.51 ,,	Metronome, 60 per minute (inhibitory)	0
11.56 ,,	Strong tone	0
12.1 p.m.	Buzzer	3
12.6 ,,	Electric lamp	0
12.11 ,,	Metronome, 120 per minute	$1\frac{1}{2}$

During the period of recovery of the conditioned reflexes when the inhibitory stimulus was not used all the different phases of transition between complete inhibition and the normal positive effect were observed. In the beginning the recovery was favoured by the usual method of interrupting the experiments for a few days and shortening the isolated action of all the conditioned stimuli. Soon, however, these methods became of no further use. The first one or two reflexes in the beginning of an experiment were generally very weak, and all the rest failed altogether. The animal grew lethargic and persistently declined the food. As a final measure the experiments were conducted with the animal kept free on the floor instead of in its stand. The beneficial effect of this method lies partly in the removal of the inhibitory influence of the stand, and partly in the introduction of additional excitatory impulses from the muscles and joints. The measure proved efficacious. The reflexes began gradually to return and progressively gained in strength. The animal accepted the food and normal relations became finally re-established. The administration of the negative stimulus led during the first seven days to a disappearance of the reflexes for the rest of that particular experiment. This inhibitory effect was not so apparent at the beginning of the experiment on the following day. In the course of the succeeding two weeks the prolonged inhibitory after-effect gradually disappeared and the inhibitory stimulus could now be practised during a single experiment more often. The differentiated inhibitory stimulus was repeated several times in every experiment, and concentration of the inhibition was accelerated by the immediate application of the corresponding positive stimulus. But it was only after two months of experimentation with the animal on the floor, and eight months after the flood, that it was found possible to return to the usual experiments with the animal in the stand.

It is thus seen that the powerful and unusual stimuli arising from the flood increased the susceptibility of the cortical elements to inhibition to so great an extent that even a comparatively minute intensification of inhibition from the outside, in the form of a conditioned inhibitory stimulus, rendered impossible for a long time any existence of positive conditioned reflexes under ordinary experimental conditions.

All these experiments clearly bring out the fact that a development of a chronic pathological state of the hemispheres can occur from one or other of two causes : first a conflict between excitation and inhibition which the cortex finds itself unable to resolve ; second the action of extremely powerful and unusual stimuli.

I have still to describe the pathological state of another animal [experiments of Dr. Vishnevsky], but unfortunately I cannot state definitely whether its present state depends only upon a congenital defect which has been accentuated by its general conditions of life

—age, pregnancy and so on—or whether it was produced as a result of the flood, as in the case of the two preceding animals. This animal was described in the preceding lecture (p. 287) as belonging to an extremely inhibitable type. Previously to the flood it had been left for a long time without observation, and it was not until four months after the flood that experiments with the dog were resumed. It has already been mentioned that a long time before the flood this dog served for a considerable number of valuable experiments. Now, in spite of all the therapeutic measures which have been applied, the animal still cannot be employed for experiments upon our usual problems. All that I can do, therefore, in the present lecture is to describe its condition. The scope of the normal life of the animal, at any rate under laboratory conditions, has narrowed down considerably. In the laboratory it reacts to the minutest stimuli either by a passive defence reaction (an investigatory reflex which is immediately followed by inhibition of all movements and even refusal of food) or, as an exception to its type, it sleeps. Only in two ways can any return to normal conditions of life be brought about in this dog : either there must be adopted a quick transition from the conditioned stimulus to its reinforcement with food (within 1-2 seconds from its beginning), or else the experiments must be conducted with the animal on the floor and with the experimenter constantly moving about in the same room. In the latter case the animal trots after the experimenter during the whole of the experiment, but even so the reinforcement of the conditioned stimulus must not be too much delayed. Both methods effect improvement in the same manner, the animal now ceasing to react to small changes in the environment in the same way that it did before, so that it is now able to take the food unless disturbed by stimuli of unusual strength. Conditioned reflexes begin, under these conditions, to return. It is, however, only necessary to delay reinforcement until 5-10 seconds from the beginning of the conditioned stimulus for the animal quickly to grow drowsy and even fall asleep over its plate while taking the food. This truly extraordinary state of the nervous system may be pictured as a state of extreme exhaustion— a perfect example of the so-called *faiblesse irritable*. The disturbance obviously has its seat in the cortical elements, since the delicate reactions of the nervous analysers are essentially an intrinsic function of the cerebral cortex. A more detailed investigation of this dog is being conducted at the present time.

LECTURE XIX

Pathological disturbances of the cortex, result of surgical interference : (a) General disturbances of the cortical activity. (b) Disturbances of the acoustic analyser.

HAVING attained, on entirely objective lines, to a measure of understanding concerning at least the main aspects of the physiological activity of the cortex, we naturally became interested to apply the method of conditioned reflexes to the study of cortical localization of functions in an endeavour to determine the importance of different parts of the brain for the normal functioning of the cortex as a whole. Experiments were made in this direction even in the early stages of our research (see my communication at the International Medical Congress at Madrid, 1903). The only method so far available for such a study consists in observing the effects of partial destruction or complete extirpation of different parts of the cortex. This method naturally suffers from fundamental disadvantages, since it involves the roughest forms of mechanical interference and the crude dismembering of an organ of a most exquisite structure and function. Imagine that we have to penetrate into the activity of an incomparably simpler machine fashioned by human hands, and that for this purpose, not knowing its different parts, instead of carefully dismantling the machine we take a saw and cut away one or another fraction of it, hoping to obtain an exact knowledge of its mechanical working ! The method usually applied to the study of the hemispheres or other parts of the central nervous system is essentially as primitive as this. Hammer and chisel, the saw and the drill ; these are the instruments which must be used to open up the strong protective skull. Then we tear through the several layers of enveloping protective membranes, rupturing many blood-vessels, and finally, we injure or destroy whole lumps of the delicate nervous tissue in different mechanical ways—concussion, pressure and incision. But such is the marvellous functional resistance and the peculiar vitality of the living substance, that, in spite of all these gross manipulations, within the lapse of only a single day it is sometimes impossible without special and exact investigations to observe anything abnormal in animals submitted to cerebral operations. Accordingly, even by these primitive methods, some insight into the functions of the cortex can be gained. But the obvious usefulness of these crude methods should on no account satisfy the physiologist. He should strive to apply new advances of technical science and to seek ever new and more appropriate methods for the study of the exquisite mechanism of the hemispheres. Naturally the methods available for the investigation of the cortex at present, by means of extirpation of different parts, can but lead to entangled pathological states, and even the most guarded deductions with regard to the constitution of the cortex cannot therefore be ensured against a high probability of error. Indeed, since the special function of the cortex is to establish new nervous connections and so to ensure a perfect functional correlation between the organism and its environment, every disturbance of any part of it will be reflected upon the whole mechanism. Besides this direct influence of the operative procedure, which may reasonably be expected with time to diminish spontaneously, there is another very serious complication of the operation which appears later on—namely, the development of a scar at the place of cerebral lesion which now becomes a source of irritation and leads to further destruction of the surrounding parts. On the one hand the scar, owing to its mechanical irritation of the surrounding normal parts of the brain, sets up recurrent outbursts of nervous excitation ; on the other hand, owing to pressure, distortion and rupture, it progressively disintegrates the hemispheres. I have been unfortunate in attempting to improve the operative technique, having made, as I now think, a big mistake. In order to obviate haemorrhage during the operation I used to remove in the dogs, long before the operation on the brain, the temporal muscles which cover the skull ; this resulted in a partial atrophy of the bones of the skull, so that these could now be opened, often without the loss of a single drop of blood. But the dura mater in these cases also undergoes considerable atrophy, becomes dry and brittle, so that in most cases it is impossible to make use of it to close up the cerebral wound completely. As a result the wound was left after the operation in direct communication with the more external tissues, which led to the formation of a very hard scar ultimately penetrating and growing into the cerebral tissue. Almost every animal that was operated upon suffered from attacks of convulsions which on some occasions occurred so soon as five to six weeks after the operation. A few animals died during the first attack, but more usually the convulsions were not severe in the early stages and occurred at infrequent intervals. In the course of several months they recurred more frequently and increased in force, finally either proving fatal or else leading to a new and very profound disturbance of the cortical activity. Therapeutic measures in the form of repeated anaesthesia or extirpation of the scar were found to be unreliable, though sometimes they were unquestionably effective.

Besides the difficulties arising on account of the purely surgical interference itself, the experimenter has to take into serious account a further difficulty which is especially pronounced in the case of the cerebral hemispheres. In the living organism we constantly discover different mechanisms by means of which functional compensation of damaged and destroyed parts is effected. In the nervous system such vicariation and compensation of function occur in the most extreme degree. It is well known in the spinal cord—where it is facilitated by the complicated and varied course of the nerve fibres—and also in the peripheral nervous system. The effect of mechanical destruction of localized parts is thus neutralized to a considerable extent by compensation. In the highest parts of the central nervous system, which regulate the major part of the internal and external activity of the organism, the principle of compensation and vicariation must be still more pronounced.

Having at our disposal the method of conditioned reflexes, related to different individual analysers, we attempted to determine and study the pathological disturbances affecting the entire cortex following the extirpation of one or another part, and also to use this study so far as possible in investigating the problem of the general construction of the hemispheres and the significance of its separate parts.

The first change which follows the extirpation of some part of the cortex is the almost invariable disappearance of conditioned reflexes ; but in the majority of cases it is only the " artificial " conditioned reflexes which disappear, i.e. those which were established in the laboratory, being therefore relatively recent and little practised. If the " natural " conditioned reflexes have also disappeared they are always the first to reappear ; but usually no disappearance of the natural conditioned reflexes could be observed even though tested immediately after the recovery from the anaesthetic administered during the operation. Examples of the greater resistance of conditioned reflexes to " natural " stimuli as compared with those established to " artificial " stimuli occur in every research upon partial extirpation of the cortex and there is therefore no need to give any special examples. As a rule the conditioned reflexes disappear after the operation, whether it is performed on one or both of the hemispheres and on whatever portion of them it is carried out. The absence of " artificial " reflexes persists for different lengths of time, varying from a single day to several months.

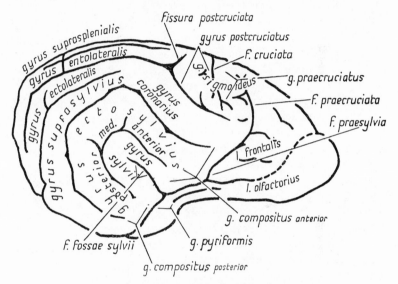

Fig. 8.—Dog's brain showing the outer surface.
The nomenclature used is that of Ellenberger and Baum.

Usually the greater the lesion the more prolonged is the absence of the reflexes ; but considering the whole number of our experimental animals we find in this respect not a few exceptions. Even in animals in which the operations were apparently identical as to the place and extent of the lesion, there are great variations as to the length of time during which conditioned reflexes are absent. It is highly probable that, apart from the skill and neatness with which the operation was performed, the ultimate extent of the irritation and the destruction of the tissue depend upon the anatomical and functional peculiarities of the operated animal. After the operation the conditioned reflexes never return all at once, but in sequence, depending not only, as already mentioned, upon the stability of the reflex, but also upon the locality of the lesion. Generally speaking, reflexes belonging to those analysers which are most distant from the place of the lesion recover quickest. For example, after the removal of the *gyrus pyriformis* [experiments of Dr. Zavadsky] the conditioned reflex from the surface of the mouth (the "water reflex" which will be discussed later) reappeared on the eleventh day, the reflex to the smell of camphor on the eighteenth day, the reflex to an increase in the general illumination of the room on the twenty-fifth day, while the reflexes to conditioned tactile stimuli failed to recover even by the thirty-fifth day. The experiments demonstrate a certain disturbing influence which has spread from the point of lesion over the mass of the hemispheres and has then receded to the point of origin. This disturbing influence is, of course, generally speaking, due to the irritation caused by the lesion. It has already been shown that the influence of very strong stimuli, and even a conflict between nervous processes of opposite sign, lead to a prolonged inhibitory after-effect. It is, therefore, only natural to expect the same to result from a surgical destruction of a portion of the cerebral cortex itself.

When the conditioned reflexes finally get re-established they are found not only to regain their normal strength but often to exceed it, often also becoming considerably more stable than before. The inhibitory process, on the other hand, grows weaker. Many examples of this can be quoted from the experiments at our disposal. Thus, after extirpation of a part of the acoustic area of H. Munk in two dogs (see Fig. 13), the conditioned alimentary reflexes not only made a complete recovery but considerably increased in strength, and kept constant throughout every single experiment, whereas before the operation they used to decrease considerably towards the end of an experiment [experiments of Dr. Eliason]. The increase in the strength of the conditioned reflexes was still more conspicuous in another dog, after removal of the occipital lobes. The alimentary reflexes in this dog measured before the operation 1-2 drops during the isolated action of the conditioned stimuli ; after the operation 13 drops [experiments of Dr. Koudrin]. In many dogs there is observed after an operation a very definite prolongation of the salivary secretion which follows the administration of an unconditioned stimulus : the length of time required for complete extinction of the reflex also becomes in many dogs very prolonged : the development of differentiations and conditioned inhibitions becomes more difficult and very often salivary secretion is observed in between the application of the stimuli—this never happening before. This last is most probably to be accounted for by dis-inhibition of the reflex to environment (see the seventh lecture). It is an open question whether this weakening of the inhibitory effect is the result of an increase in the intensity of the excitatory process or whether the excitatory process is revealed on account of weakening of inhibition itself.

Another peculiarity with respect to inhibition is observed after surgical interferences. The inhibitory process becomes inert ; and so to speak inflexible. As we saw before, in normal animals the inhibitory after-effect becomes with practice concentrated with regard to its duration as well as its extent. In the post-operative period this concentration proceeds extremely slowly and is imperfect. This inertia of the inhibitory process is observed not only in the reflexes belonging to the analyser which has been surgically damaged, but also in reflexes belonging to other analysers [experiments of Dr. Krasnogorsky].

In this manner the endeavour to demonstrate by means of experiments with extirpation the disappearance out of the normal cortical activity of the functions related to the extirpated part is complicated in the first period after operation by the general effect which the operation has upon the hemispheres as a whole. Although this unfortunate complication slowly and gradually disappears, it is followed, as already mentioned, by a second complication which also affects the hemispheres as a whole, and which depends on the development of scar tissue. The effect of the scar varies widely in different cases. After one and the same operation the injurious effect of the scar develops in some cases quickly and is severe ; in other cases it is slow and feeble. Unfortunately the former was much the more common case in our experiments. The most usual effect of the scar consists in recurrent attacks of convulsions, sometimes affecting the whole body, and sometimes localized in one or another group of muscles. Such explosive outbursts of excitation in the hemispheres have a very pronounced after-effect upon their activity. In this respect one should distinguish changes which follow weak and rare attacks from changes following violent attacks or frequently recurring attacks of moderate strength.

We shall start by considering the effect of the former. On

observing conditioned reflexes from day to day it is very often possible to predict the approach of an attack of convulsions with accuracy. If, suddenly, without any obvious cause the conditioned reflexes diminish in strength and then disappear, it is an infallible sign of an approach of an attack of convulsions. Sometimes it is possible to notice a still earlier sign, consisting in the disappearance of differentiations, *i.e.* in a disturbance in the inhibitory process. After an attack has passed, the re-establishment of the conditioned reflexes occupies a variable length of time, requiring sometimes hours, and sometimes days. In some instances the re-establishment of conditioned reflexes assumes a complicated character. Immediately after the termination of the attack conditioned reflexes are present, but, some time after, they again disappear, now for a considerable length of time. This may possibly be explained by an initial irradiation of the outburst of excitation, followed subsequently by concentration and negative induction. So far as the effect of very strong or frequent attacks is concerned their after-effect is very variable. In one dog they were apparently the cause of an absolute deafness ; another dog, which after the operation behaved quite normally towards men and towards other dogs and food, began after a severe attack of convulsions to dodge and run away from other dogs and from men. Finally a fresh attack killed her. A third dog, after numerous and frequent attacks, showed quite peculiar symptoms. The dog will be described later in detail, but meanwhile I shall describe one of the symptoms. In this dog, after the attack, all the reflexes returned ; they had, however, to be used with practically simultaneous reinforcement. Even small delays (up to 5 seconds) quickly led on repetition to disappearance of the conditioned effect, with refusal of food and development of sleep. Obviously the dog suffered from a chronic state of *faiblesse irritable* such as was described in reference to another dog at the end of the preceding lecture. After each recurrence of the attack this peculiar symptom became more pronounced. It is natural to regard this change as due to a functional exhaustion of the cortical elements consequent on the convulsions ; the cortical elements now, under the action of external stimuli, rapidly undergo a transition into an inhibitory state, the connection of which with sleep has been discussed previously. In this dog the functional exhaustion, like the excitability producing it, affected the entire cortex. It is often, however, restricted to the particular analyser which was most directly affected by the surgical interference. Examples of this will be given later.

In some cases the effect of the scar manifests itself in a different manner, being limited to a hyper-excitability of analysers other than the motor one, and therefore not associated with convulsions. One dog after extirpation of the frontal lobes [experiments of Dr. Babkin] quickly recovered from the effects of the operation, but two months later it developed an extreme cutaneous hyperaesthesia which lasted for ten days : the animal would howl at the most gentle touch and even at its own movements, and after this would shrink down into a heap on the floor. Evidently the scar in the cutaneous analyser served as a source of irritation to the cortical area of localization connected with the receptors of injury (subjectively pain), if indeed such analyser exists in an independent localized form.

A still more interesting case was presented by another dog after a partial extirpation of the cortical part of the cutaneous analyser [experiments of Dr. Eroféeva]. One and a half months after the operation a vigorous attack of convulsions occurred. During this attack the animal was subjected to a further operation, the scar, which gave outgrowths considerably beyond the site of the original lesion, being carefully removed. The convulsions did not recur after the operation, but another form of disturbance developed which lasted at each recurrence for several days. When either experimenter or food came into the field of vision of the left eye (the animal being operated on the right side) it quickly turned away, and if free ran away, showing signs of extreme excitation. The same stimuli when applied from the right side of the animal produced no abnormal reaction. Often, free and on its own, the dog would suddenly glance to the left, quickly jump up and run madly away. This can all be interpreted if we assume that some remaining portions of the scar directly irritated the visual analyser on one side, thereby producing a distortion of the effect of the external stimuli falling on the retina and altering the significance of the visual object, which assumed in the dog's cortex unusual and extraordinary aspects to which the animal reacted as to any concrete and definite stimulus—exactly in the same manner as happens also with normal animals in response to any extraordinary visual stimulus. In short, the scar produced a phenomenon of illusion. Obviously a similar condition obtained in the dog previously mentioned, which after an attack of convulsions began to run away even from its usual attendant and from the food, exhibiting a violent general excitation. It is probable that the outburst of excitation resulting from the scar, after having freed the motor area of the cortex, was still retained for some time in the visual analyser. It is legitimate to regard these cases as the equivalent of epileptic disturbances of the motor analyser.

The foregoing observations led to our planning a detailed investigation of the effects of direct stimulation of the different cortical analysers. By permanently healing electrodes in different points of the hemispheres we are hoping to produce in our dogs by means of electrical stimulation definite changes in the reactions to our usual conditioned stimuli. The difficulties of technique have been overcome and the experiments are at present in progress.

It is unfortunate that the majority of our experiments with extirpation were performed in the earlier period of our research, when we had not definitely realized the peculiarities of the different individual types of the nervous system and had not yet any knowledge of the pathological effects arising under the influence of functional, *i.e.* non-surgical, disturbances.

After this preliminary review of the general effects of surgical interference with the cortex I shall describe in detail the results obtained by the fullest possible application of the method of conditioned reflexes to our operated animals with the object of determining the physiological significance of the entire cortex and of larger or smaller parts thereof.

In some of our animals a complete extirpation of the whole cortex was carried out (one animal survived the operation for $4\frac{1}{2}$ years). This operation had already first been introduced by Goltz, but it was undertaken in our experiments with the special object of determining by our method the relation of the cortex to the higher nervous activity of the dog [experiments of Dr. Zeliony]. The general behaviour of the animals after the complete extirpation of the cortex has been described in detail on several occasions by Dr. Zeliony himself. I shall therefore dwell only upon the relation of conditioned reflexes to the cortex. Since all the usual conditioned reflexes were definitely absent in these dogs after the extirpation, and neither old nor new reflexes could be obtained in spite of the most persistent reinforcing of artificial stimuli or testing for natural conditioned reflexes, we concentrated our attention upon one peculiar conditioned reflex, which, according to our previous experiments, in contrast to all other conditioned reflexes, was extremely stable. I refer to what we term " the water reflex "—a conditioned reflex in response to stimulation of the receptor surface of the mouth. If, by means of an apparatus which is placed in the dog's mouth, water is injected after a few preliminary injections of acid, the water which under normal conditions evokes hardly any salivary secretion (at most 1-2 drops) now causes a copious secretion. Evidently the stimulation by liquid of some receptor nerve-endings of the mucous membrane of the mouth, coinciding with the effect of the acidity, acquires conditioned properties determining this large salivary secretion together with a corresponding motor reaction typical of the reflex to acid. The conditioned water-reflex, as will be shown later, possesses all the properties of a conditioned reflex. In the dog which survived the removal of the hemispheres the longest time ($4\frac{1}{2}$ years), the water-reflex was established before the extirpation of the last portion of the hemispheres—the extirpation being performed in stages. The reflex measured 8-10 drops for injection of 5 c.c. of water. Beginning from the sixth day after complete extirpation of the hemispheres 5 c.c. of 0·25% solution of hydrochloric acid were repeatedly injected practically every day, over 500 injections being made in all. Only after seven months of this procedure did a salivary secretion to water appear, which gradually increased in strength until it measured 13 drops for injection of 5 c.cs. of water. Was this, however, a conditioned reflex ? Decidedly not. The reflex in this case differed fundamentally from the ordinary conditioned water-reflex. The most important difference was that it could not be made to undergo extinction, which occurs with extreme ease in the case of the real conditioned water-reflex in normal animals when water is injected several times in succession without the acid. In the decorticated animal the effect of repeated injection of water became constant. By observing the dog after the administration of water the true nature of this reflex was revealed. After injection of water the animal exhibited typical movements, which otherwise were observed only when the animal was hungry. It started walking to and fro with head bent low and twitching nostrils, as if reaching for something. On further investigation it became obvious that the contact of water with the mucous membrane of the mouth evoked in this dog a strong unconditioned alimentary reflex. This was corroborated by the fact that unconditioned reflexes, *e.g.* salivary reflexes, after removal of the cerebral cortex, become at first diminished, afterwards, however, gradually recovering their wonted strength and finally becoming very much increased above normal.

To present the final conclusion of these experiments with the utmost reserve, the cerebral cortex should be regarded as the essential organ for the maintenance and establishment of conditioned reflexes, possessing in this respect a function of nervous synthesis of a scope and exactness which is not found in any other part of the central nervous system.

Of the individual analysers most attention was paid to the acoustic, and I shall commence my description with this. An absolute deafness following extirpation of a part of the cerebral cortex was observed in three dogs. In two of these animals [experiments of

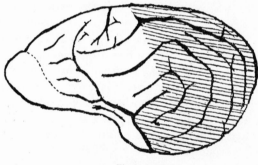

Fig. 9.

Dr. Koudrin] the cortical substance was removed posterior to a line starting from a point above and immediately behind the *gyrus sigmoideus*, stretching to the tip of the *gyrus sylviaticus* and then passing along the *fissura fossae sylvii* (Fig. 9). The operation was performed in two stages, first on one and then on the other side. Absolute deafness appeared immediately after the second operation. One of the dogs lived for nine months after the operation, the other for seven. In the third dog [experiments of Dr. Makovski] a bilateral extirpation was performed of the *gyri sylviaticus posterior, ectosylvius posterior* and *suprasylvius posterior*. On one side there were included also the middle and the frontal portions of these convolutions (Fig. 10). Absolute deafness occurred one and a half months after the operation. On the day previous to the deafness a weakening of the inhibitory processes was observed: this was probably followed during the night by an attack of convulsions. The animal lived after this, in apparently good health, for another month. During this period new conditioned reflexes were developed to stimuli belonging to the tactile, olfactory and visual analysers. The animal died during an attack of convulsions. Other animals, which were operated on in exactly the same manner as the last, continued to react to sound, though in some cases they survived the operation even longer.

How can we explain the absolute loss of all auditory reactions ? Since it must be regarded as definitely proved that after complete removal of the whole cortex dogs still continue to react to sound, it must be admitted that in the three cases of absolute deafness described above there must have been some damage of sub-cortical structures or a development of inhibition which spread into the sub-cortical areas. The latter possibility ought not to be excluded,

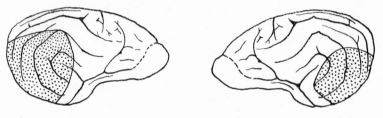

Fig. 10.

since on histological examination (unfortunately rather crude) no damage of sub-cortical structures could be observed ; further, in the first two dogs a general reaction to light, which at first entirely disappeared, returned two months after the operation, and a conditioned reflex to light even reached its pre-operative intensity ; finally, it is well known how extremely easily different impulses originating within the hemispheres inhibit reflexes of lower centres. If such an inhibitory effect is accepted as the cause of deafness in the third dog, we have to assume that this inhibition spread solely throughout the ramifications of the acoustic analyser, without involving any other analysers.

As a rule the general auditory motor reactions (pricking up the ears and lifting the head), after removal of the temporal lobes or of the whole posterior half of both hemispheres, return within a few hours, or a day or two at most ; in some cases they do not disappear at all. This general reaction to sound is an unconditioned investigatory reflex belonging to sub-cortical regions, since it remains present in dogs even after removal of the entire cerebral cortex. The rest of the auditory reactions must be attributed to the cortex, and these functions of the acoustic analyser at first entirely disappear after the limited operations described above, then return, never, however, recovering completely.

When, after bilateral removal of the temporal lobes, the investigatory reflex to sound has already returned, as well as conditioned reflexes to stimuli belonging to other analysers, all auditory conditioned reflexes are found still to be absent. Such a state may last for many days or even for several months, depending upon the extent of the operation. Moreover, it is of importance that both temporal lobes should be removed at one time, or in two operations shortly following one another, first on one side and then on the other. If the two operations are performed with a long interval between them the phase of complete disappearance of auditory conditioned reflexes may be absent. What does the temporary absence of auditory conditioned reflexes mean ? Several possible interpretations can be advanced. First, it is possible that the cells of the acoustic analyser still remaining after the operation are rendered incapable of developing a state of excitation, and under the influence of external stimuli pass directly into an inhibitory state, it may be on account of being weakened by the operation, or on account of being decreased in number, or on account of being previously kept in reserve and not involved as a general rule in the activity of the acoustic analyser before the operation. Second, it is possible that after the operation the analysing function of the cortical part of the acoustic analyser is so diminished that all the sounds now affecting the dog, both inside and outside the laboratory, acquire identical qualities and therefore, more frequently than not, fail to coincide with the unconditioned stimulus, with the result that the conditioned significance of the definite acoustic stimulus disappears on account of extinction. Finally, it is possible that under the influence of the operation the synthetic activity of the acoustic analyser, involved in the maintenance or establishment of conditioned reflexes, itself weakens or temporarily disappears. Special experiments were performed in order to test these suppositions [Dr. Krijanovsky].

In one test use was made of an auditory stimulus as a conditioned inhibitor. Two conditioned inhibitors of the same alimentary reflex to camphor were established in a dog ; one was a tactile stimulus, the other auditory (tone d', 288 d.v. of a pneumatic tuning fork).

Three days after bilateral removal of the temporal lobes (Fig. 11) the positive conditioned reflex to camphor had already reappeared. The conditioned inhibitors remained practically without any effect for several more days, but from the twelfth day on gave a full inhibition. It was noticed now that any other sounds had exactly the same inhibitory effect as the original conditioned inhibitor. All positive acoustic conditioned reflexes were absent at this stage ; neither the sound of splashing of acid nor the sound of cracking of biscuits, to both of which under normal conditions reflexes developed with extreme ease, could be made to evoke a conditioned response. The fact that any sound acted in the capacity of a real conditioned inhibitor and not as an agent of external

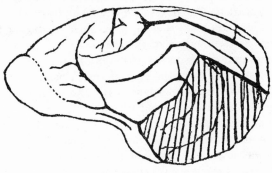

Fig. 11.

inhibition was proved by means of destruction of the conditioned inhibition by reinforcing the action of the inhibitory combination by the administration of food and then re-establishing it by discontinuing the reinforcement. In control experiments the same destruction and re-establishment was repeated with the tactile conditioned inhibitor. It follows from these experiments that the sounds acted as true conditioned inhibitors, and, therefore, that the analyser was capable of performing an inhibitory function while the function of excitation was still absent. In other words, the analysing function of the cortex was impaired. Only several days after the above experiments did the positive conditioned reflexes to sound begin to reappear.

In a second method of testing our suppositions, in particular the supposition of extreme generalization of sounds, we used long-trace reflexes in which, as is known, the stimuli are generalized beyond the limits of a single analyser (Lecture VII). In the case of long-trace reflexes perfectly neutral stimuli assume the character of accessory conditioned stimuli, which act in the same manner as the original trace stimulus, *i.e.* the secretion begins after the same latent period. Now it was determined to test whether these conditioned accessory reflexes to auditory stimuli in general would still be present at the time of absence of the specific reflexes to these stimuli. For this purpose the dog had a definite trace reflex established to a tactile stimulus in which the pause between the end of the conditioned stimulus and the beginning of the unconditioned stimulus was two minutes. Usually the conditioned secretion started during the second minute of the pause. Ten days after complete removal of the temporal lobes the trace reflex to the tactile stimulus reappeared. On the twelfth day an auditory stimulus gave 8 drops during 4 minutes, the secretion starting during the third minute after the termination of the stimulus. On the seventeenth day the same auditory stimulus gave 38 drops during 6 minutes, the secretion starting as in the case of the primary trace stimulus during the second minute of the pause. It was only on the thirty-fifth day that the conditioned reflexes to the actual isolated action of the conditioned auditory stimuli first began to appear. This experiment shows once more that the auditory stimuli had assumed an extremely generalized character, so that sound as a general stimulus still continued to act, although individual sounds had lost their specific conditioned significance. It is, moreover, evident that the function of synthesis was not lost, and after these experiments special testing of the third supposition was unnecessary.

The two types of experiment just described probably belonged to two different post-operative states of the acoustic analyser, the first an earlier, the second a later stage. This is the more probable since in other dogs which were subjected to a similar operation (Fig. 12) we also observed a generalization of auditory conditioned simultaneous and short-delayed stimuli [experiments of Dr. Babkin]. The following is one of these experiments :

A conditioned alimentary reflex had been established to a descending scale of four neighbouring tones, and this was completely differentiated from the same scale taken in the ascending direction. On the eighth day after removal of the temporal lobes the experiment proceeded as follows :

Experiment of 12th April, 1911.

Time	Conditioned stimulus during 30 seconds	Salivary Secretion in drops during 30 seconds	
11.13 a.m.	Descending scale of tones	7	Reinforced
11.25 ,,	Descending scale of tones	6	Reinforced
11.33 ,,	A subdued tone	2	
11.36 ,,	Tapping on a glass bottle	6	
11.39 ,,	Clapping the hands	1	Not reinforced
11.42 ,,	Whistling	3	
11.46 ,,	Tapping on a glass bottle	3	
11.49 ,,	Descending scale of tones	1	Reinforced
11.55 ,,	Tapping on a glass bottle	2	
11.58 ,,	Tapping on a glass bottle	1	Not reinforced
12.1 p.m.	Scratching on the table	0	
12.3 ,,	Descending scale of tones	2	Reinforced
12.15 ,,	Descending scale of tones	6	Reinforced
12.25 ,,	Tapping on a glass bottle	4	Not reinforced

All the stimuli, except the scale of tones, used in the above experiment were " neutral," *i.e.* had never been reinforced.

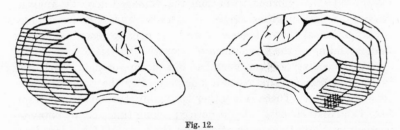

Fig. 12.

It is seen from this experiment that besides the previously established auditory conditioned stimulus many other sounds, which never previously had any conditioned significance, now acted sometimes as effectively as the descending scale of tones. When these extraneous sounds weakened in their effect on account of non-reinforcement, the conditioned stimulus also considerably diminished in its effect (11.49 ; 12.3). On reinforcing the conditioned stimulus the effect of the other sounds also became increased (12.25 p.m.). The sound in its capacity of a conditioned stimulus had become extremely generalized, and its analysis had become impaired so as to be practically negligible. When the power of analysis begins to reappear the improvement proceeds very often with extreme slowness. First of all musical tones are distinguished from other kinds of sound, like knocks and noises. The differentiation between different tones remains imperfect for a very long time; in these experiments of Dr. Babkin, for example, differentiation between single tones only began to return through gradual stages two months after the operation.

The absence or the diminished precision of the analysing function of the acoustic nervous apparatus described is obviously identical with what H. Munk terms " psychic deafness." It is impossible, however, not to see the fundamental difference between the purely physiological and the psychological interpretation of these facts. According to the definition of Munk " the animal hears but fails to understand," and experimentation becomes sterile in the interpretation of " understand." But the physiological point of view opens up a vast field for experimentally investigating the different stages of the re-establishment of functions in the damaged acoustic analyser. Under normal conditions sounds are differentiated according to their strength, duration, continuous or interrupted character, point of origin, and nature—whether tones, knocks, noises, etc. It must be expected—and in this respect it can be stated that we have definite proof—that in returning to normal the damaged acoustic analyser passes through different stages of activity, and only by detailed investigation of these stages can we hope ever to reach a complete understanding of the mechanism of acoustic analysis.

The foregoing does not complete our picture of the disturbances in the functions of the acoustic analyser after the removal of the temporal lobes. There is another, probably the most important, functional disturbance. It was noticed a long time ago, by many investigators, that after an operation upon the temporal lobes dogs cease to respond to their names. This was observed also in our experiments, and we believe that it can only be explained by a disappearance of the special analysis of conditioned auditory compound stimuli. In order to verify this point special experiments were performed by Dr. Babkin. Conditioned stimuli were established to different tones applied in different sequences or with different intervals between them. One definite sequence was used for a positive conditioned reflex, others for negative ones (differentiation). These differentiations, as mentioned in the eighth lecture, were much more difficult to establish than differentiations of single tones. Besides the differentiation of compound auditory stimuli, differentiations of single tones were also established. Both temporal lobes were then extirpated in these animals. The disturbances which followed the operation were exactly identical in the five dogs employed for the experiments. While the differentiation of single tones sooner or later became re-established with the same precision as before the operation (a differentiation of intervals of a single tone), there was never the slightest trace of any re-establishment of a differentiation of the successive compound stimuli, though most of the dogs were tested for 2-3 months after the operation, and one dog for nearly three years. In the latter dog [originally observed by Dr. Koudrin] the entire posterior part of the hemispheres was removed as in the two dogs previously described (see Fig. 9, p. 330). The final operation was performed on the 5th May, 1909. The experiments to be described were started towards the end of 1911. Alimentary conditioned reflexes were established to an ascending scale of tones of pneumatic tuning forks—290, 325, 370, and 413 d.v., and to a separate tone of a Stern's tone-variator—1200 d.v. The reflexes developed fairly quickly and a differentiation between the single tone of 1200 d.v. and a tone of 1066 d.v. was attempted through stages of differentiations from 600 and then 900 d.v. The final differentiation was successfully established. A differentiation of the descending scale, on the other hand, completely failed to be established in spite of 150 repetitions of the descending scale contrasted with 400 of the ascending scale. The reaction to calling the dog by name was also absent during the whole period of three years. The following example is taken from a late stage of these experiments (15th March, 1912).

Time	Conditioned stimulus during 30 seconds	Salivary Secretion during 30 seconds	
2.10 p.m.	Ascending scale of tones	7	Reinforced
2.29 ,,	,, ,, ,,	5	
2.44 ,,	,, ,, ,,	5	
2.53 ,,	Descending scale of tones	6	Not reinforced
2.58 ,,	,, ,, ,,	2	
3.2 ,,	,, ,, ,,	2	
3.7 ,,	,, ,, ,,	Traces	
3.12 ,,	Ascending scale of tones	Traces	Reinforced
3.20 ,,	,, ,, ,,	4	

To the same group of experiments probably belongs also the following, up to the present solitary, case [experiments of Dr. Eliason]. A conditioned alimentary reflex was established to a chord of tones of a harmonium 85-256-768 d.v. (F-c′-g″). When the reflex reached its maximum strength the different component tones were tried separately. They all produced a positive effect weaker than that of the chord but approximately equal in strength among themselves. The effect of intermediate tones was extremely small. After the removal of the anterior portions of the temporal lobes (Fig. 13) the relative effect of the different components underwent a considerable change. The effect of 768 d.v. and of the neighbouring tones disappeared altogether, though the reflex to the chord returned on the fifth day after the operation. The lower component of the chord—85 d.v.—when tested alone began to act with increased vigour, its effect often being equal to that of the whole chord. What can be the explanation of the extremely definite results of these experiments ? The first explanation that suggested itself was that

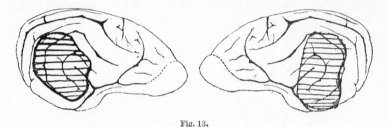

Fig. 13.

the reflexes to the higher musical tones had been selectively disrupted as a result of the operation. This, however, was absolutely disproved, since when the tone of 768 d.v. was reinforced independently of the chord it very quickly assumed independent and very definite properties as a strong conditioned stimulus. To our great regret this dog died before we could accomplish different modifications in the experiments. The absence of the effect of the higher tone before it was independently reinforced cannot be attributed to any difference in strength of the tones in the chord, since the highest tone was if anything stronger than the two lower ones. The observations are in accord with the theory of the existence of a special part of the acoustic analyser in which the synthesis and analysis of successive and simultaneous compound auditory stimuli is effected (the acoustic area of H. Munk). Such part of the acoustic analyser would provide a parallel with the undoubted projection of the retina upon a definite part of the visual analyser. According to this supposition such part of the acoustic analyser in the cortex must be regarded as a special receptive field which is connected with all the parts of the peripheral acoustic apparatus, so that on account of the specially favourable local structural peculiarities a facility is afforded for the formation of various and complicated connections, involving the establishment of reflexes to most complex compound auditory stimuli as well as their analysis. A partial destruction of this portion leads to a dropping out from the compounds of some of the individual components, and a complete destruction entirely eliminates the higher synthesis and analysis of compound stimuli. After complete removal of the temporal lobes auditory conditioned reflexes still continue to exist [Dr. Kalischer,[1] and our own experiments], and an elementary differentiation can still be effected, while after extirpation of the whole cortex all conditioned reflexes entirely and permanently disappear. Only one conclusion, therefore, can be drawn, namely, that in the cortex, besides the special part of the acoustic analyser, there must exist some extensions of the analyser dispersed more widely over the cortex, and maybe throughout its whole mass. These elements owing to their dispersion are not able to enter into complex interconnections, though they can still perform an elementary synthesis and analysis. It is possible also that the simplification or limitation of activity of different parts of the acoustic analyser increases with their distance from the cortical " nucleus " of the analyser.

The hypothesis of such a distribution of the cortical part of the acoustic, and probably of any other, analyser seems to me to conform best with the available facts, and to open also an unlimited field for further investigation. It would fit in with the wide dispersion, which will be proved later, of any one analyser between the other analysers, far beyond the limits of the hitherto accepted localizations. It would also agree with the existence of a special " nucleus " in each analyser in which, on account of the density and the exceptional concentration of the elemental units of the given analyser, the higher synthetic and analytic activity is rendered possible. Again, it could also without difficulty explain the gradual improvement by practice of the activity of the remnants of the analysers, the functions of which are so limited immediately after the lesion of its nucleus. Ultimately it should also determine the limits to which such an improvement could extend. In the dog last mentioned the elementary

[1] O. Kalischer. " Zur Funktion des Schläfenlappens des Grosshirns." Sitzungsber. der königl. preuss. Akademie der Wissensch. Physik. mathem. Kl. v. 10, p. 204. 1907.

analysis of tones had probably reached the maximal degree possible, the loss of the higher synthesis and analysis remaining permanent even after three years of practice.

The hypothesis suggested, of such a wide distribution of analysers in the cortex, naturally sets up further problems for experimentation which should be used to test its validity. In regard to the acoustic analyser, before a partial extirpation there should be developed as great a number as possible of positive elementary and compound stimuli, and various differentiations. The different general properties of the elementary stimuli should be determined for each dog, their threshold strength, the conditions under which positive stimuli acquire an inhibitory character, the mobility of the inhibitory process and the degree of its after-effect, and so on. Only such further experiments can demonstrate definitely the changes which occur as the result of an operation, how far these changes affect the general properties of the reflexes and what changes constitute the direct result of damaging different parts of the analyser. During the period of re-establishment of the acoustic function after the operation special attention must be paid, as was previously mentioned, to the determination of the different transition stages. It is obvious that in order to carry out such a plan a healthy and prolonged existence of the animal after the operation must be ensured. Unfortunately this cannot up to the present be satisfactorily attained.

LECTURE XX

THE pathological disturbances of the visual analyser, which will be discussed next, have not been studied in our laboratory to the same extent as those of the acoustic analyser, but such experiments as have been performed permit us to trace very similar relations in the activity of the two analysers after extirpation of corresponding parts of the cortex.

It was shown by Goltz with his decorticated animal, that the " investigatory reflex " to light can be brought about, in its most rudimentary form of a motor reaction, through sub-cortical areas alone, without any co-operation of the cortex. This, however, is all that could be deduced from Goltz's experiments. Neither is there any indication in the writings of subsequent authors as to the existence in such animals of any higher visual functions. In our decorticated dogs [experiments of Dr. Zeliony], even this elementary reaction was not sharply defined, so that it would seem unquestionable that the entire scope of the visual function beyond this very elementary and limited reaction belongs exclusively to the cerebral cortex, exactly as in the case of the analyser of the mouth (*e.g.* the water-reflex) and the acoustic analyser in the experiments previously described. It has been shown that even in the case of the primitive analyser of the mouth no conditioned connections could be established in absence of the cortex, although a certain rudimentary analysis was still possible (such dogs rejected many non-alimentary or irritating substances). In the case of the visual analyser there can be no question at all of any possible establishment of conditioned reflexes to visual stimuli exclusively through sub-cortical areas.

In common with all previous observers, including Minkovski, we obtained a very definite diminution of the visual field, either in the horizontal or the vertical direction, in one or both eyes, according to the site of the damage in the occipital lobe on one or upon both sides. Thus, objects which happen to fall within the intact parts of the visual field continue to evoke their corresponding reactions, while the same objects but slightly shifted in position fail to evoke any reaction on the part of the animal. Evidently the occipital lobes must contain the nucleus of the visual analyser, upon the integrity of which depends the existence of visual reflexes, involving the more complicated forms of synthesis and the finer shades of physiological analysis. After bilateral extirpation of the entire occipital lobes none of our dogs ever showed any sign of object vision during the whole time of survival after the operation (one animal survived three years). Neither men nor animals nor food were discriminated by these animals by sight. We would frequently lay upon the floor, or suspend on strings at different heights, pieces of food, but there was not a single dog after bilateral extirpation of the occipital lobes, which, however long it had been deprived of food, ever on one single occasion directed its movement by sight. The dogs directed themselves to the pieces of food obviously only by means of olfactory and tactile stimuli. The definite limitations of the visual field in the horizontal or vertical plane following damage of different regions of the occipital lobes show that the loss of object vision depends upon the absence of the higher synthesis and analysis of visual stimuli rather than upon disturbances in the accessory visual reactions—convergence and accommodation ; moreover, animals with removed occipital lobes equally fail to discriminate objects whether large or small, distant or near, in strong, medium or weak light.

Although the main nucleus of the visual analyser—the organ of the higher analysis and synthesis of visual stimuli—is located in the occipital lobes of the cortex, yet these do not constitute the entire analyser. The visual analyser is dispersed over a much wider area, and probably over the whole mass of the cortex. Even in the older days of the physiology of the cortex it was the teaching of several authorities that the frontal lobes also had a definite relation to vision. This conclusion was derived from the impairment of vision which appeared after extirpation of the frontal lobes—a form of negative evidence which cannot be accepted as sufficient proof, since the facts could be interpreted in terms of a protracted indirect inhibitory after-effect of the operation itself. At the present time, however, we are in a position to offer positive evidence for the view that a part of the analyser capable of performing a considerable visual analysis is situated in the anterior part of the cerebral cortex in front of a line beginning from a point above and immediately behind the *gyrus sigmoideus*, stretching obliquely downwards and laterally to the anterior angle of the *gyrus sylviaticus*, and then passing along the *fissura fossae sylvii* to the lower margin of the hemispheres (see Fig. 18, p. 363). We found in our dogs, after extirpation of the entire mass of the cortex behind this line, that stable conditioned reflexes could be established to changes in intensity of illumination, observations which are in complete agreement with the experiments of Kalischer. But, in addition to this, we found that a discrimination of tolerably fine gradations of the intensity of illumination could be definitely established. These observations give a simple and purely scientific interpretation of what has been called by H. Munk " psychic blindness." The visual analyser which is considerably damaged after removal of the occipital lobes can now establish conditioned connections only within the scope of a single limited function, namely, reactions to fluctuations in luminosity. On account of this the animal in an illuminated room is still able to avoid dark objects and to walk out through an open door guided by differences in luminosity. In view of these facts it would be more exact to reverse the psychological phrase " that the dog sees but does not understand," and to say " that the dog understands but does not see sufficiently well." Such formularization is, of course, impermissibly redundant, since the whole disturbance primarily consists in the limitation of the analysing activity. The scientific value of this objective point of view has been fully confirmed by our further investigation. In one of our dogs which retained the cortex only in front of the above-mentioned line, it was possible to establish conditioned reflexes involving a still higher function of the visual analyser than discrimination of differences in luminosity. This is the dog which was mentioned as having survived the operation for three years, and which was described at the end of the preceding lecture as having permanently lost the power of analysis of compound auditory stimuli. I shall describe our experiments upon this animal with the use of visual stimuli in detail [experiments by Dr. Koudrin]. The operation on the hemispheres was performed in two stages, with an interval of one month in between. The final operation took place on the 5th May, 1909. An alimentary conditioned reflex, established before the operation, to switching on a hundred candle-power lamp in a semi-darkened room, definitely returned on the fifth day after the final operation. On the eleventh day it reached an even greater intensity than in the pre-operative period. Experiments with the visual reflex were then abandoned, the work being continued with auditory stimuli as described in the previous lecture. On the 7th September of the same year we began to establish a conditioned reflex to a moving luminous cross projected upon a screen in a semi-darkened room. The reflex developed quickly, and in the course of a week became of a considerable magnitude. From the 28th September the luminous projection of the cross was held stationary. The reflex was still present although somewhat diminished in intensity. The development of a differentiation of the cross from a circle of equal area and equal luminosity was now begun. At the seventh and subsequent applications of the circle there was already a definite indication of a developing differentiation. The experiments were, however, interrupted and were not taken up again until after an intervening period of six months. After this interval the reflex to the cross was found still to be present. Its differentiation from the circle quickly developed and soon became constant. The following examples reveal a definite, though not yet absolute, differentiation.

Time	Conditioned stimulus during 30 seconds	Salivary Secretion	Remarks
		Experiment of 1st April, 1910.	
11.40 a.m.	Cross	8 drops during 30 seconds	Reinforced
11.50 ,,	Circle	6 drops during 60 seconds	Not reinforced
12.0 noon	Cross	6 drops during 30 seconds	Reinforced
		Experiment of 5th April, 1910.	
11.35 a.m.	Cross	6 drops during 30 seconds	Reinforced
11.45 ,,	Circle	1 drop during 60 seconds	Not reinforced
11.50 ,,	Cross	3 drops during 30 seconds	Reinforced

A post-mortem examination of the dog three years after the operation confirmed the completeness of the removal of the whole posterior part of the cortex.

There can be no doubt that in this dog the part of the visual analyser that was left in the anterior mass of the cortex was capable not only of establishing conditioned reflexes to changes in intensity of illumination, but also to different shapes of illuminated or shaded areas. At the same time, in this dog, as in all others after removal of the occipital lobes, no conditioned reflexes to separate concrete objects could at any time be established. The development of conditioned reflexes to differently shaped areas was successfully achieved so soon as four months after the operation, and could probably have been obtained even sooner. On the other hand, object vision was entirely absent for the whole post-operative period of the dog's life (3 years), and it is reasonable to suppose that this state of the visual analyser was final and irrevocable, at any rate towards the end of the life of the animal. In this connection it is of interest to inquire how it is that the dog could definitely discriminate areas of different shape during an experiment, and yet could not discriminate objects by their shapes when free. There is, of course, a vast difference between the environing conditions during the experiment and when the animal is set free amid a great number of different objects, each continually changing its aspect either in consequence of its own movement or the movement of the animal in relation to it. The sharpness of contour of the objects similarly never remains constant, depending on changes of illumination and upon the distance from the animal. During the experiment in the stand everything becomes much simpler as compared with the usual environment. Probably, therefore, a very gradual and prolonged practice would have been required for the surviving faculty of discriminating shapes to assume any sort of practical usefulness for the animal.

On the basis of our observations the results of damage of the visual and acoustic analysers may in the main be considered as comparable. A limitation of the visual field signifies a small damage of the visual analyser ; in the auditory analyser, if it is permissible to rely on the experiment upon a single dog, a dropping out of auditory compounds of elementary tones has an identical signification. A disappearance of discrimination of objects, *i.e.* disappearance of compounds made up of forms, shades, colours (in those exceptional dogs in which colour vision may be conjectured), in other words, a disappearance of the higher synthesis and analysis of visual stimuli, signifies a more extensive damage of the visual analyser. A comparable disturbance in the case of the acoustic analyser can be recognized in a disappearance of discrimination of compound stimuli, that is, a loss of higher synthesis and analysis of auditory stimuli. In the case of maximal disturbance of either of the two analysers—

apart from a total destruction—the only function which survives
is the discrimination of intensity of visual or auditory stimuli.
Between these extremes there are some intermediate stages, in which,
besides differences of intensity, differences in the configuration of
luminous areas can be discriminated in the case of the visual
analyser, and different types of sound—noises and musical tones—
in the case of the auditory analyser.

The next question we had to decide was whether the distribution
of the tactile analyser over the cortex is analogous to the distribution
of the acoustic and visual analysers ; in other words, whether besides
the special nucleus of the highest activity in this analyser there is
a wider dissemination of cortical tactile receptive cells with more
limited activities. Although we are not in a position to give a final
answer to this question we are yet disposed, on the basis of our experiments, to consider such a distribution as more than probable.
I shall give some of our old and also our recent material relative
to this question ; this material, besides its bearing on the distribution
of the analyser, also presents some other points of interest. Many
years ago it was observed that a removal of the anterior part of the
hemispheres led to a disappearance of tactile conditioned reflexes,
while reflexes to stimuli belonging to other analysers were retained
[experiments of Dr. Tihomirov]. In later experiments [by Dr.
Krasnogorsky] it was definitely established also that the motor area
is more or less clearly demarcated from the special nucleus of the
tactile analyser, and that definite parts of this special region represent
projections of different parts of the skin. One of the dogs had, besides
different reflexes belonging to other analysers, a tactile conditioned
reflex to acid, which had been experimentally generalized for the
whole surface of the skin. The *gyri coronarius* and *ectosylvius anterior*
were now removed on the left side (see Fig. 14). On the fourth day
after the operation conditioned reflexes belonging to the analysers
other than the tactile were present. The generalized conditioned
tactile reflex returned on the eighth day, but only to stimulation on
the left side of the animal, and soon reached its normal magnitude.
On the tenth day the tactile reflex returned on the right side of the
animal, but only to stimulation of the skin of the middle part of the
body. On the fore limb and hind limb, on the shoulder and pelvic
area it was entirely absent, the line of demarcation between those
areas which had regained, and those which had lost, the reflex to
tactile stimulation being very sharp. The loss of these reflexes

persisted up to the 90th day following operation, and after this they gradually became re-established, in order, from the shoulder and pelvis to the corresponding paw. These experiments, besides corroborating the localization given by H. Munk, present another interesting detail. During the period while the conditioned stimuli of the above-mentioned places of the skin had lost their positive effect they divulged a definite inhibitory effect, as has already been mentioned in the lecture dealing with sleep (p. 259). The seemingly ineffective stimulation of these different areas of the skin when used together with, or preceding, the stimulation of other cutaneous areas which continued to give a positive effect, or with, or preceding, conditioned stimuli belonging to other analysers, invariably diminished

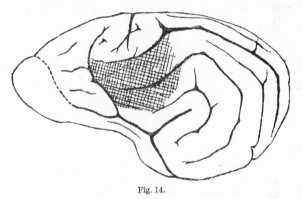

Fig. 14.

or even abolished such reflexes. Further, a repeated, and even more markedly a protracted, stimulation of these apparently ineffective places on the skin resulted in every experiment in a development of drowsiness and sleep, even in dogs which before the operation never showed any tendency to drowsiness in the stand. The sleep developed in these cases exclusively in connection with the tactile stimulation of these areas ; apart from their application the dog kept completely alert during the experiment.

These experiments were quite recently repeated, and with exactly the same results [Dr. Rosenkov]. In a dog in which the same convolutions were partially destroyed all the reflexes belonging to other analysers were present, but only so long as the areas of the skin disturbed by the operation were not stimulated. After stimulation of these areas the animal invariably became sleepy and all conditioned reflexes disappeared throughout the remainder of the experiment.

It was a problem of considerable interest to determine whether it would be possible by some means to disclose anything in the nature of a positive reaction to these tactile stimuli. We succeeded in demonstrating such an effect by the following modification of the experiments. The isolated stimulation of the refractory places of the skin was abbreviated from its usual duration of 30 seconds to 5 seconds. The abbreviated stimulus was now used several times in each experiment, and at the end of the experiment, in order to test the reflex, reinforcement was again delayed for 30 seconds. Under such conditions it was possible to observe the positive as well as the inhibitory effect of the stimulation. The positive effect appeared quickly, but was very small, and, what is important, disappeared while the conditioned stimulus was still acting, whereas the effect of all other conditioned stimuli increased, as usual, towards the end of their isolated action as the moment of reinforcement approached. The following is taken from an experiment by Dr. Rosenkov :

A metronome, a whistle, the light of an electric lamp, and a tactile cutaneous stimulation served as positive conditioned stimuli. After the cerebral operation the conditioned reflex to stimulation of the fore limb disappeared. The secretion of saliva was measured as usual by the graduated tube, five divisions of which correspond to one drop. The secretion before the operation in this dog was generally small. No attacks of convulsions had been observed following the operation. The tactile stimulation in the following table was always applied on the fore limb :

Time	Conditioned stimulus	Duration of the stimulus in seconds	Salivary Secretion in drops per 10 seconds during the isolated action of the conditioned stimulus
9.12 a.m.	Metronome	30	4, 6, 6
9.19 ,,	Tactile	5	– – –
9.27 ,,	Lamp	30	0, 1, 3
9.36 ,,	Tactile	5	– – –
9.46 ,,	Whistle	30	2, 4, 5
9.53 ,,	Tactile	5	– – –
10.2 ,,	Metronome	30	0, 3, 5
10.11 ,,	Tactile	30	**3, 2, 0**

A similar positive effect of stimulation of the usually ineffective places of the skin could be obtained also by some other devices—with the help of positive induction, by means of dis-inhibition, and by the use of caffeine. This animal obviously presents in respect of the affected cutaneous areas another instance of a maximal *faiblesse irritable*.

In all our experiments, including those which are being conducted at the present time [Dr. Fedorov], the refractory areas of the skin regain as a general rule, sooner or later after the cerebral operation, their normal positive effect, as has previously been observed by other workers. The question naturally arises as to the mechanism of such recovery. The first explanation to be thought of was a possible existence of direct nerve tracts which had successfully replaced the crossed ones. For the purpose of testing this possibility we now in some dogs extirpated the cortex completely on one side and studied the conditioned tactile reflexes from the skin of the opposite side of the body for the whole time that the animals survived (some of them living for over a year after the operation without attacks of convulsions). Up to the present such experiments have been completed on four dogs. Alimentary conditioned reflexes were employed in most cases ; sometimes, however, a defence reflex to acid or to a stimulus of an electric current was also used, the electric stimulus being applied to the skin on that side of the body which was not affected by the cortical lesion [experiments of Drs. Foursikov and Bikov]. The results in all these experiments, in spite of many different modifications, were absolutely negative, and in spite of increasing the cortical excitabliity by strychnine and caffeine the cutaneous reflexes never returned [experiments of Dr. Foursikov]. Experiments were also conducted to determine whether the tactile stimulation of the injured side of the body would exert any inhibitory influence upon other conditioned reflexes as it did after the partial destruction of the cutaneous analyser [experiments by Dr. Bikov]. In the cases of complete unilateral extirpation of the cortex no such inhibitory influence of the tactile stimuli of the affected side upon the various positive conditioned reflexes (including tactile reflexes from the normal side of the animal) could be observed, whether as an after-effect or during the actual administration of the stimuli ; similarly also these tactile stimuli did not induce sleep or drowsiness. These observations are the more important since the same places acquired strong inhibitory properties in those cases where there had been partial destruction of the cutaneous analyser. There was, of course, no question of revealing any positive effect of the stimuli by any of the methods which were successful in the case of partial extirpation. In the case of complete unilateral removal of the cortex, therefore, the tactile stimuli on the opposite side entirely lose their conditioned properties, both positive and negative. In other words, according to our experiments, there is no homolateral connection of the skin with the cortex. Vicariation in the case of partial destruction of the cutaneous analyser must therefore occur with the help of the outlying parts of the analyser in the hemisphere of the same side—a view which has already been advanced by other authors.

In order to study this question of vicariation more closely we resolved to produce an extirpation of as many of the frontal convolutions of one hemisphere as possible, so as to narrow the area from which the compensatory effect might be derived. In dogs operated in this manner the conditioned reflexes to tactile cutaneous stimuli, although they disappeared for a very long time, did nevertheless return. It was thought that the portions adjacent to the operated field might have taken over the function of the removed parts. However, additional destruction of these adjacent parts [experiments of Dr. Eurman] had practically no effect upon the re-established functions of the analyser. The vicariation of function, therefore, must be attributed to much more widely distributed cortical elements. This result made it important to test whether the method which we used for tactile stimulation of the skin was not contaminated by an auditory component so that the reflexes which we observed could be explained by the latter. An apparatus was therefore constructed which, at any rate to our own ear, was entirely without sound, and in order to make the control doubly sure we placed between the apparatus and the skin a medium which prevented the mechanical effect of the apparatus on the skin, without, however, abolishing any possible auditory component inaudible to us. Tactile conditioned reflexes could be developed without, but in no case with, the medium, in either normal or operated animals, proving, of course, that under ordinary conditions the reflexes were genuinely initiated purely by the tactile stimulation and not by any accessory auditory accompaniment.

We are inclined to think that, as in the case of the visual and acoustic analysers, the parts of the cutaneous analyser remaining after the first operation have only a limited function as compared with the function of the cortical elements situated in the extirpated nucleus of the analyser. We hope to test this theory by experiments with compound tactile conditioned stimuli and by using a differentiation of the direction of brushing the skin and testing this differentiation upon those places which have recovered from their temporary loss of conditioned reflexes after the extirpation of the frontal lobes. These experiments are in progress at the present time. All the experiments with respect to recovery of tactile reflexes after extirpation are, however, being vigorously repeated in view of their intrinsic importance and in view of the divergence of some results of recent experiments from one of our earlier observations (p. 362).

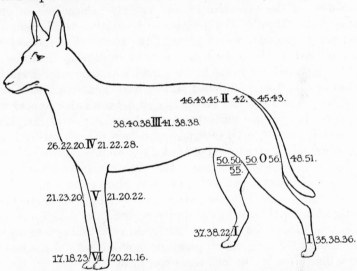

Fig. 15.—*O* and Roman figures:—Numbers of the places stimulated. Arabic figures:—Conditioned reflex in drops of saliva (1 drop = 0·01 c.c.). The figures to the right and left of the Roman figures were obtained by stimulation of the right and left sides of the animal respectively. The tactile reflex was established on the left side at place *O*. The fig. shows the spontaneous bilateral formation of accessory reflexes. Note that the strength of the reflexes at corresponding points is identical on both sides of the animal. The reflex which was established at place *O* was a short-trace reflex.

Besides studying, in the manner described, the relations of the tactile analyser in a single hemisphere, we have also investigated the interrelations of the analysers of the two sides. An observation has already been mentioned that tactile conditioned reflexes which were developed for different places on one side of the body reproduce themselves spontaneously with surprising accuracy on the symmetrical places of the other side of the body. This phenomenon has been especially carefully examined by Dr. Anrep, and its occurrence was demonstrated both for positive and negative reflexes to tactile stimuli (see Fig. 15). It was naturally expected that the development

of a differentiation of symmetrical places of the skin on opposite
sides of the body would turn out to be a matter of considerable
difficulty, and this actually was found to be the case [experiments
of Drs. Bikov and Grigorovich].

What is the mechanism of this curious phenomenon ? It was
only natural to consider first the commissural connections, and in
actual fact section of the corpus callosum completely abolished the
whole phenomenon. After the section conditioned reflexes to tactile
stimulation of the two sides became entirely independent of one
another [Dr. Bikov]. The positive and negative tactile reflexes
developed on one side now completely failed to reproduce themselves
spontaneously on the other side ; in order to develop conditioned
reflexes on the other side the tactile stimuli had to be independently
reinforced. Tactile conditioned stimuli were established with the
use of food, the use of the unconditioned defence reflex to acid, or
the use of the defence reflex to electrical stimulation of the skin.
The electric current in these experiments was of such strength as
to produce only a withdrawal of the leg and an investigatory reflex,
but no violent defence reaction. The experiments were varied in
many different ways, but the result was always the same. The
reflexes were confined to the side on which they were developed ;
reflexes on the other side had always to be developed independently.
There was also no longer any difficulty in establishing reflexes of
opposite sign for symmetrical places on opposite sides of the body.
This is illustrated by the following experiment :

After section of the corpus callosum a tactile stimulation of the
right thigh was given excitatory properties and of the left thigh
inhibitory properties ; and a tactile stimulation of the right shoulder
was given inhibitory properties and of the left shoulder excitatory
properties. The four reflexes had, of course, to be developed
independently.

Time	Conditioned tactile stimulus applied every 30 seconds	Salivary Secretion in drops during 30 seconds
4.25 p.m.	Right thigh	4
4.37 ,,	Right shoulder	0
4.46 ,,	Left shoulder	$4\frac{1}{2}$
4.58 ,,	Left thigh	0
5.12 ,,	Right thigh	3

In conformity with the above results all *extraneous* stimulations of the skin applied on one side of the animal, *e.g.* a thermal stimulus of 50° C., and a weak electric current, by evoking an investigatory reflex produced an inhibition only of the tactile reflexes on the same side of the body. These experiments were conducted on three animals.

Along with the experiments which were primarily designed for investigation of the tactile analyser, mention must be made of experiments with complete removal of the frontal lobes [experiments of Dr. Babkin]. The frontal lobes were removed upon both sides in front of *sulcus praecruciatus* and *sulcus praesylvius* down to the lower margin of the hemispheres, involving destruction of the olfactory

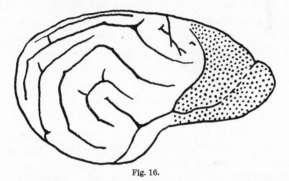

Fig. 16.

lobes (Fig. 16). Sometimes the knife during the operation, and in almost every case the subsequent pathological process (as shown by post-mortem examinations), involved part of the area behind the line indicated. The experiments were conducted on four dogs. In all cases the old visual and auditory conditioned reflexes returned and new ones could be established soon after the operation. Disturbances—and considerable ones—were noticed only in the tactile analyser and in the movements of the animal. The dogs lived for 1-6 months after the operation, death occurring in all cases on account of severe attacks of convulsions. During this time no positive tactile reflexes could be re-established for places on the body, but reflexes could be established in some cases for places on the extremities. Good negative reflexes, however, in which the tactile stimulus was used as a conditioned inhibitor, could be produced for any place of the skin. The animals suffered from a persistent cutaneous hyperaesthesia, so that some of them could not bear the loops round their legs during the experiments, and kept quiet only when the loops were discarded. Temporary disturbances in maintenance of posture and locomotion were observed. The animal would often assume an unnatural pose—drooping head and arched back, paresis of the extremities with twitchings. The motor disturbances were most pronounced in the movement of the mouth, the dog immediately after the operation being able to take food only with difficulty, and having to be fed by hand, especially in the case of solid food. The above were the only peculiarities of note.

In respect of the thermal cutaneous analyser only a small number of experiments have been performed. From these it appears that the thermal, does not entirely coincide with the tactile, analyser in cortical localization. In the case of extirpation of the *gyrus praecruciatus* [experiments of Dr. Shishlo] tactile conditioned reflexes for the hind limbs were re-established a few days after the operation, while the thermal reflexes (to cold and to a temperature of $47\frac{1}{2}°$ C.) conspicuously lagged behind, taking four weeks longer before they returned.

The method of conditioned reflexes was applied also for the verification of the statement made by some authors as to a definite relation of the *gyrus pyriformis* to the olfactory analyser. The experiments were performed on six dogs which had different " artificial " and " natural " secretory and motor reflexes [experiments of Dr. Zavadsky]. Different unconditioned reflexes were also carefully observed. The first of these reflexes to reappear after complete bilateral removal of the *gyri pyriformi* and the adjacent part of the *hippocampus* were the olfactory ones. Movements of the nostrils in response to olfactory stimuli were present so soon as the second or third day after the operation. On the third or fourth day the dogs could select accurately out of many paper bags those that contained meat or breakfast-sausage. On the sixth day the conditioned reflex to the smell of meat powder reappeared, while on the fourteenth day an artificial alimentary conditioned reflex to the odour of camphor became quite definite. The artificial conditioned olfactory reflexes had a positive effect in their first trial, evidence of a spontaneous recovery.

Finally we confronted the question as to the nature of the so-called motor area of the cortex. Is it in all its complexity and delicacy of activities a receptive field and analyser of stimuli initiated within the skeleto-motor apparatus of the organism ? In other words, is it comparable to other regions of the cortex which serve as receptive fields and analysers of stimuli falling upon the animal from the outside ? Or is it a region physiologically distinct from the remaining parts of the cortex ? Is it physiologically comparable to the posterior or to the anterior columns of the spinal cord ?

This question is nearly as old as the discovery of the motor area itself, but at the present time there are only a few observers who regard the motor area of the cortex as corresponding functionally to the posterior columns in the spinal cord. In the hope of procuring some fresh evidence we approached the study of this question from the point of view of conditioned reflexes, using some definite motor activity as a conditioned stimulus, and then experimentally determining the localization of this reflex in the cortex. The experiments performed bearing on the motor analyser of the cortex are rather more complicated than other experiments with conditioned reflexes in respect to technique. I have, therefore, no hesitation in giving these experiments in considerable detail, and illustrating my description by a large number of examples [experiments of Dr. Krasnogorski].

Passive flexion of the tibio-tarsal and the metatarso-phalangeal joints were used as conditioned stimuli. The flexion was performed in the following manner. For the passive flexion of the tibio-tarsal joint the thigh and the leg of the hind limb were fixed in a plaster cast attached to a metal frame which was screwed down to the table. In order to employ the metatarso-phalangeal joint the tarsus and metatarsus had also to be rigidly fixed in a special cast. Flexion of the joints was performed in the preliminary experiments by hand and later by a special mechanical device. When the reflex to flexion of the tibio-tarsal joint of the left leg became established the effect was tried of flexion of the same joint of the opposite leg. The reflex was found to be spontaneously present just as in the case of tactile conditioned reflexes. We now started to develop a differentiation of the flexion of the metatarso-phalangeal joint (toes) of the left leg from flexion of its tibio-tarsal joint (ankle). The differentiation became established after 42 reinforcements of the flexion of the toes contrasted with 74 flexions of the ankle. This differentiation spontaneously reproduced itself for the respective joints of the right side also. Since flexion of any joint invariably involves a mechanical stimulation of the skin, which by itself might have been responsible both for the conditioned reflexes and the differentiation, further experiments had to be performed in order to dissociate the cutaneous component from the actual flexion itself. For this purpose all sorts of mechanical stimulations of the skin were applied, touching, pressing, gripping, and rhythmic stretching of the skin on one side of the joint and folding on the opposite side in imitation of the natural stretching and folding in the case of flexion of the joint. The latter kind of stimulation produced the strongest effect. On repetition of these cutaneous stimuli, of course without any reinforcement, they finally became entirely ineffective while flexion itself, which was always reinforced, continued to act. It was realized, however, that all these precautions did not afford absolutely definite proof that flexion by itself acted in these experiments as the sole conditioned stimulus. It seemed quite possible that all our variations of mechanical stimulation of the skin did not entirely reproduce those accompanying flexion of the joint. It was essential to find a more conclusive proof that flexion itself became a conditioned stimulus. We expected to find such proof by completely excluding the cutaneous component by extirpating those cortical parts of the tactile analyser which were known to stand in relation to tactile stimuli from the areas involved, namely, the *gyri coronarius* and *ectosylvius* (see Fig. 14, p. 347). Previously to the operation additional alimentary conditioned reflexes were established to tactile stimulation of the hind limbs at five distinct places and to a tone of 500 vibrations. The operation was performed on the left side of the cortex. The tone was the first conditioned reflex to reappear, and this occurred on the seventh day. The first trial of the flexion on the damaged (right) side—on the eighth day after the operation—gave a negative result. The second trial—performed on the same day—gave a secretion of 2 drops during 30 seconds. The trial on the tenth day gave a secretion of 3 drops : on this day a simultaneous stimulation of the five tactile places on the same extremity remained entirely without effect. On the twelfth day the reflex to flexion reached 5 drops, while the stimulation of the five tactile places and folding and stretching of the skin still remained without effect. On the thirteenth day the folding and stretching of the skin over the joint exerted an inhibitory influence upon the effect of the tone applied simultaneously. Again, when on the fifteenth and sixteenth days the left (undamaged) hind extremity recovered from the inhibitory effect of the operation and the tactile stimulation of this limb gave already a considerable secretory effect, the same tactile stimulation applied simultaneously with folding and stretching of the skin over the right joint became ineffective. Thus, the folding and stretching of the skin over the right joint had now become, as an after-effect of the operation, inhibitory instead of excitatory. Nevertheless, flexion of the joint continued invariably to produce a salivary secretion. The following are the results of some of the individual experiments :

Intervals between the applications of the stimuli in mins.	Conditioned stimulus applied during 30 seconds	Salivary Secretion in drops during 30 seconds

Experiment on the eighth day after the operation.

—	Tone	2
10	Flexion of toes (right leg)	0
4	,, ,, ,,	2
7	Tactile stimulation of left planta	0
4	Flexion of toes (right leg)	2
7	,, ,, ,,	1

Experiment on the twelfth day after the operation.

—	Flexion of toes (right leg)	2
6	Tactile stimulation of 5 places on leg	0
12	,, ,, ,,	0
8	Tone	7
7	Flexion of toes (right leg)	5
6	Stretching and folding of the skin over right paw	0

Experiment on the fifteenth day after the operation.

—	Flexion of toes (right leg)	5
6	Stretching and folding of the skin over right paw	0
20	Flexion of toes (right leg)	1
6	,, ,, ,,	3
6	Tactile stimulation of left planta	4
6	Tactile stimulation of right planta	0
6	Tactile stimulation of right and left plantae	0
6	Tactile stimulation of left planta	2

Experiment on the sixteenth day after the operation.

—	Flexion of toes (right leg)	$4\frac{1}{2}$
7	Tactile stimulation of left planta	5
7	Tactile stimulation of left planta together with stretching and folding of the skin over the right paw	0
6	Tactile stimulation of left planta	4

The above experiments justify the two following conclusions. First, that a passive flexion of the joint by itself, *i.e.* independently of the involved cutaneous component, can serve as a conditioned stimulus. Second, that the stimuli arising from such movement and the associated cutaneous stimuli have different areas of representation in the cortex. The problem remains therefore to determine the localization of the cortical area of muscular proprioception. The problem was solved by the following experiment performed on a dog in which the *gyrus sigmoideus dexter* had been completely

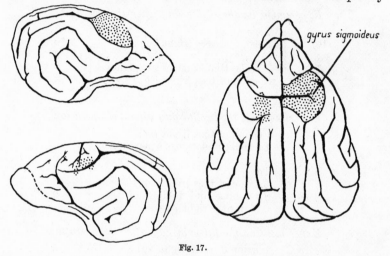

Fig. 17.

removed two months previously, since when obvious motor disorders had prevailed in both extremities of the left side. During the operation the *gyrus sigmoideus sinister* had also been very slightly damaged, but not sufficiently to produce any disturbing influence on the extremities of the right side. The tactile conditioned reflexes in this animal were normal over the whole surface of the skin. We began with the establishment of a conditioned reflex to flexion of the right (*i.e.* homolateral) metatarso-phalangeal joint. This reflex developed very quickly. We now began the differentiation of the flexion from its cutaneous component, using all the above-mentioned variations of mechanical stimulation of the skin and the joint, and never, of course, reinforcing the cutaneous stimuli. Within a month the differentiation was fairly well established (although it was not always absolute), showing that the right side was normal. The following is an example taken at random :

Time interval between stimuli	Conditioned stimuli applied during 30 seconds	Salivary Secretion in drops during 30 seconds
–	Flexion of the right joint	6
6	Stretching and folding of the skin over the right joint	3
2	Stretching and folding of the skin over the right joint	1
6	Flexion of the right joint	5
8	Stretching and folding of the skin over the right joint	0
3	Flexion of the right joint	6

We began now to test the reflexes on the left (*i.e.* heterolateral) side of the body. Stretching and folding the skin over the left hind paw was entirely ineffective right from the very start, in accordance with the symmetrical spontaneity of development of reflexes discussed before. In contrast with the right side, however, the reflex to the flexion itself was also absent. When the flexion on the left side was now reinforced, the corresponding mechanical tactile stimulation, when tested separately, was found also to have acquired secretory properties. On continuing these experiments, in spite of most persistent attempts at development of differentiation, it was found impossible to develop a conditioned reflex to flexion separately from the tactile cutaneous component. As soon as the effect of mechanical stimulation of the skin was extinguished the reflex to flexion invariably disappeared also. On reinforcing the flexion the cutaneous reflex also invariably returned. The result of these experiments must be interpreted as follows : pure flexion on the left side was by itself ineffective, but the reinforcement of the flexion of the joint produced a positive effect through the agency of the tactile component unavoidably accompanying flexion. In contrast with this, the differentiation between the flexion and the tactile stimulation on the right leg was constant and quite definite. The table shown on page 360 is an example.

The experiments show that the *gyrus sigmoideus* is the area of cortical representation of stimuli initiated in the skeleto-motor apparatus during the passive flexion.

Unfortunately we have not pursued this study further and have not employed any variations of the experiments other than those described. Before arriving at any final conclusion the experiments need to be repeated and more fully substantiated. If one bases conclusions on the experiments as they stand, the motor area of the cortex must be thought of as an analyser of the impulses from muscles and joints (proprioceptive), exactly as other areas are analysers of impulses from stimuli acting on the organism from the outside (exteroceptive). From this point of view the entire cortex represents

Number of minutes between stimuli	Conditioned stimuli applied during 30 seconds	Salivary Secretion during 30 seconds	
–	Flexion; right joint	8	Reinforced
7	Cutaneous; right joint	2	Not reinforced
$1\frac{1}{2}$	Cutaneous; right joint	1	
$1\frac{1}{2}$	Flexion; right joint	8	Reinforced
$1\frac{1}{2}$	Cutaneous; left joint	7	
$1\frac{1}{2}$	Cutaneous; left joint	6	
$1\frac{1}{2}$	Cutaneous; left joint	4	Not reinforced
$1\frac{1}{2}$	Cutaneous; left joint	3	
$1\frac{1}{2}$	Cutaneous; left joint	$1\frac{1}{2}$	
$1\frac{1}{2}$	Flexion; left joint	$\frac{1}{2}$	Reinforced
6	Cutaneous; left joint	4	
$1\frac{1}{2}$	Cutaneous; left joint	1	Not reinforced
$1\frac{1}{2}$	Cutaneous; left joint	1	
$1\frac{1}{2}$	Flexion; left joint	0	Reinforced

a complex system of analysers of the internal as well as of the external environment of the organism. Obviously, if one accepts this hypothesis in relation to the motor activity, there is good reason to extend it to the activity of most, if not all, other tissues of the organism. The important rôle played by auto-suggestion with all its extraordinary aspects, as, for example, imaginary pregnancy, and all sorts of imaginary diseases, can be understood from the physiological point of view only if we admit the existence of corresponding cortical analysers, even though they may be only little differentiated and indefinite.

LECTURE XXI

Pathological disturbances of the cortex, result of surgical interference (continued) : attempt to correlate the general post-operative behaviour of the animals with the disturbances in the activity of individual analysers.

It may be considered as firmly established that removal of the entire cerebral cortex converts the dog into a comparatively simple reflex machine. The animal retains the relatively limited number of unconditioned reflexes, but is completely deprived of the more complex and delicate co-ordination of its activities with the external world, since these adjustments are solely based upon innumerable conditioned reflexes established through the intermediation of the cerebral cortex. We possess also some knowledge as to the significance of different areas of the cortex—the cortical analysers, the united function of which determines the complete adjustment of the organism with its surroundings, or, in other words, determines the behaviour of the animal. A great deal can be learned of the physiological activity of the cortex as a whole by careful observation of the general state of the animal after extirpation of definite cortical areas, whether such extirpations are free from post-operative complications or are complicated by a further disintegration of the cortex through the growth of scar tissue or by other secondary effects of the operation. The present lecture will be devoted to the description of changes in the general behaviour of the animal, and an attempt will be made to correlate these changes with the different structural lesions of the cortex. We shall start our description with simpler, going on to more complicated, cases.

In one dog the upper part of the hemispheres was extirpated above the level of the *gyrus sylviaticus* [experiments by Dr. Orbeli]. The extirpation was made by means of a single incision on each side, the operation being performed in two stages with a long interval of time between. A fortnight after the operation upon the second hemisphere the general state of the animal became definitely constant,

361

remaining unchanged to the end of the experiments (4 months). As before, the animal was extremely lively, and when called reacted quickly, whipping round in the direction of the call. At a first glance its condition could not be distinguished from that of a normal dog. On closer observation, however, it was possible to observe a certain ataxy of the extremities, which on running were thrown up higher and brought down more vigorously than usual. Walking upon a smooth or wet floor the animal would very often slip ; moreover, on starting off it always performed some peculiar movements with its head. When walking in a definite direction the animal seldom ran into any obstacle, but as soon as it did encounter an obstacle a surprising abnormality in its behaviour appeared. It became entirely helpless if it ran even against the narrow leg of a table ; for a long time it would go on pressing forward, until slipping accidentally it would get by ; and this was the only way in which the animal could continue its progression. When placed with the front part of its body on a chair and then called, the dog started disorderly scrambling movements and fell off the chair sideways, or sometimes, moving forwards, it contrived to get its whole body on to the chair, where it remained, helplessly kicking its hind legs in the air. The foregoing is a brief sketch of the general abnormality of the dog.

Coming now to the study of its conditioned reflexes, it was found that all those which were present before the second operation became, with the exception of tactile and thermal reflexes, quickly restored, while new conditioned reflexes to olfactory and visual stimuli were easily established. Unconditioned reflexes to various tactile and thermal cutaneous stimuli were present—various " shaking," flexion and extension reflexes, responses by whining, howling and turning the head towards the point of application of the stimulus. I shall endeavour to correlate these deviations of the animal from normal with the disturbances of the functions of the different analysers. The activity of the olfactory and acoustic analysers was entirely unimpaired, and the activity of the visual analyser was only slightly disturbed. Remembering the peculiar movements of the head in locomotion, and taking into account that the animal was able to direct its movements by sight, it is obvious that a small portion of the lower part of the special nucleus of the visual analyser must have remained intact, allowing in certain positions of the head a higher synthesis and analysis of visual stimuli.

In contrast, the motor analyser was radically damaged : the general locomotor activity which is effected by sub-cortical parts remained, while the precise and delicate activity of the skeletal muscles, so far at any rate as determined by conditioned reflexes, had disappeared. As regards the extent of damage of the tactile analyser we are not yet quite clear. It is obvious that the loss of the dog's ability to direct its movements when it ran into an obstacle in its path could be entirely explained by the loss of conditioned signals arising in the skin. However, such a total loss of tactile conditioned reflexes in the case of this operation does not entirely fall into line with the results of some other experiments upon the localization of the cutaneous analyser (p. 347). The problem stands in need, therefore, of a thorough re-investigation. Excepting the inability to pass by any

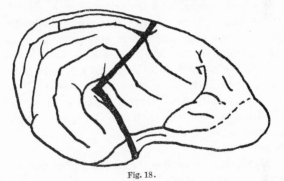

Fig. 18.

mechanical obstacles, the behaviour of this animal, both free and during the experiments, showed no further abnormality. Dogs operated on in this manner are well worth a more precise and detailed analysis of their condition than we were able to perform in the early period of our work.

In other dogs, some of which have already been mentioned, the whole posterior part of the cortex of both hemispheres was removed behind the line shown in Fig. 18. We shall consider now the more general aspects of the behaviour of these dogs. It will be remembered that the higher analysis of auditory and visual stimuli was absent, although the cruder analysis of different types of sounds, of the intensity of illumination and of different shapes was still present. Immediately after the final operation these animals kept sleeping almost continuously ; afterwards during their whole lives (one dog surviving for three years) they spent their time mainly in sleep, and therefore with ample food they quickly fattened up. The animals located food exclusively with the help of the cutaneous and olfactory analysers, and in general the co-ordination of the activities of these analysers became most astonishing. When the animal was placed amid small pieces of meat thrown about the floor or suspended on threads at different heights, the lightest touch of any part of its body against a piece was sufficient to evoke a most precise direction of its movements towards the piece of meat, which it took. Finally, the complete indifference of these animals to other dogs and to men, including their masters, should be especially noted. It is not difficult to understand the general passivity of these dogs (a characteristic already noticed by Goltz) and their great inclination to sleep, when one realizes how they lack to a large extent the activity of the main distance analysers—visual and acoustic ; hence also the extreme refinement of the activity of the analysers which are left, viz. the chemical analyser of smell, the cutaneous analyser, and the motor analyser. But the attention is startled by the general indifference of the animal to other dogs and men. It would be interesting to determine whether it was a result of their general diminution in reactiveness, or, as seems more probable, a result of a dropping out of compound visual and auditory stimuli as predominant stimuli, and the disappearance also of conditioned chain-reflexes.

I now pass on to the more complicated and at the same time the more instructive case—that of extirpation of the anterior part of the hemispheres in front of the line shown in Fig. 18. The behaviour of animals operated upon in this manner deviates extremely from normal, and the analysis of this behaviour presents great interest. We had two such animals, and both survived the operation for about a year. The operation was performed in two stages, the two sides being operated with an interval of several months. I shall describe the first dog in full [experiment by Dr. Demeedov], and shall then give the main points of difference of the other dog [experiments of Drs. Satournov and Kouraev].

After the final operation the animal kept sleeping almost continuously, awakening only before micturition and defaecation. Food was introduced into the stomach directly, through a gastric fistula which had been established previously to the second stage of the operation. It was only at the beginning of the third week after the final operation that the animal began to get up and stand on its legs unassisted, and then only for a very short time, swaying from side to side and finally sinking down again. Approximately a month after the operation the dog started to walk. The paws, however, often twisted out of their normal position and the limbs often mutually obstructed one another, getting crossed. In another month walking and running were practically normal, but, on whipping round suddenly, the dog could hardly preserve its balance. On meeting with obstacles the dog made disorderly scrambling movements, sometimes pushing forward and sometimes moving backwards or sideways ; in some cases it would chance to slip by the obstacle, but most often it had to be helped. The animal was quite incapable of performing two different locomotor actions at the same time. As a result of such attempts it would lose its balance and topple over. This peculiarity remained to the end of its life. Two weeks after the operation the animal began to lap milk, but only when the milk was brought in contact with its mouth. The whole time it lived, the animal would only start eating when the food touched the mucous membrane of lips, cheeks or tongue. Contact of the skin around the mouth with the food did not initiate eating. During the latter part of its life the animal when hungry became very excited, grabbing at everything it could reach with its mouth, and even biting its own legs and paws, which would make it howl. From the time when the animal began to eat, alimentary substances were easily discriminated from non-alimentary substances, such as sand, or food containing quinine or a large amount of acid or salt. The motor reactions to tactile stimuli appeared about two weeks after the operation, and after this the cutaneous sensibility progressively increased, so that, after two to three months, touching the animal to put it into or take it out of the stand, or even simply stroking the animal, evoked violent general excitation. The dog would struggle to get loose, would bare its teeth and bark. Similarly, when it came into contact with objects through moving about, and in the yard when its fur got ruffled by wind, or when drops of rain fell upon it, the same motor excitation would occur. It is interesting that during these periods of excitation a gentle stroking of the neck and head quieted the animal, which sometimes even fell asleep. On scratching definite places of the skin a scratch-reflex was invariably evoked, and it was often observed that a simultaneous administration of an auditory stimulus caused an intensification of the scratch-reflex when the scratching was weak—an example of the so-called " Bahnung-reflex." Motor reactions to sound, as expressed by pricking up and orientation of the ears, only reappeared 1½ months after the operation. The reactions gradually increased and sometimes were extraordinarily violent, so that even in response to comparatively weak sounds the animal showed pronounced general excitation. Under the influence of strong light the animal closed the eyes and turned the head away. Olfactory stimuli never produced any reaction, since the bulbus olfactorius and the olfactory tract were damaged on both sides. Sexual reflexes could never be detected under any conditions. No special relations either positive or negative to other animals or to men were ever observed. The animal sometimes had peculiar attacks lasting 1-8 minutes without any apparent cause—tremor of the whole body, clonic contractions of the jaws with a cramplike twisting of the head to one side, finishing up by ejection of urine and faeces. The convulsions were never observed in the body or extremities, and the animal did not fall down during the attacks. After an attack the animal became very excited, throwing itself about without any sense of direction, and barking; but finally it quieted down, got very drowsy and soon fell fast asleep.

The above general description of the animal seems to point to its having become entirely devoid of the higher nervous activity and transformed into a much simplified and inadequate reflex machine. Being similar in many respects to entirely decorticated animals, it was in many ways even less perfect in respect to locomotion. Indeed, animals after extirpation of the entire cortex begin to stand up much sooner after the operation, walk better and keep their balance better in different movements, than the dog just described. Judging by the state of the skeletal musculature, conditioned reflex activity appeared to be entirely lost. To determine whether this actually was the case we tried to analyse the condition of this dog by testing the reflex activity of the salivary gland.

The unconditioned salivary reflex had entirely disappeared immediately after the operation. It soon, however, returned, at first showing some deviations from normal which later righted themselves. Positive conditioned salivary reflexes, whether to visual, tactile, cutaneous or auditory stimuli, could not be established in spite of persistent attempts. In order to make doubly sure, even the dog's daily ration outside the experiments was now always accompanied by a sound of bubbling, but in spite of over five hundred repetitions no definite conditioned salivary reflex was ever obtained. After these failures stimulation was tried of that receptor surface which, as mentioned before, was generally found more resistant than any other in cases of extensive operations upon the cortex— namely, the mucous membrane of the mouth, the receptor for the water-reflex. These experiments will now be described in detail. It will be remembered from the previous description that water when introduced into the mouth does not produce any salivary secretion unless it has previously been reinforced by a simultaneous intro- duction of some substance which acts as an unconditioned stimulus, *e.g.* the administration of aqueous solutions of rejectable substances such as acid. After a very large number of administrations of acid to the dog now described, water first brought about a definite secretion a month after the operation, and systematic experiments with this reflex could be started fifty days after the operation. After the acid had been frequently administered in the course of several days, water, when administered as the first stimulus on an experimental day, produced a copious secretion (16 drops and more during one minute). This salivary secretion disappeared after repeated introduction of the stimulus of water alone, undergoing extinction just like any other conditioned reflex. The following are some examples of extinction :

Time	Stimulus	Salivary Secretion in drops during one minute

Experiment of 29th December, 1908 (the final stage of the operation was performed 23rd September, 1908).

Time	Stimulus	Salivary Secretion in drops during one minute
3.20 p.m.	Water	16
3.25 ,,	,,	16
3.30 ,,	,,	2
3.35 ,,	,,	4
3.38 ,,	0·25% aq. HCl	Copious secretion
3.41 ,,	,,	9
3.46 ,,	,,	6
3.54 ,,	0·25% aq. HCl	Copious secretion
4.0 ,,	,,	8
4.5 ,,	,,	9
4.10 ,,	,,	2
4.15 ,,	,,	2
4.20 ,,	,,	0

Time	Stimulus	Salivary Secretion in drops during one minute

Experiment of 1st January, 1909.

Time	Stimulus	Salivary Secretion
12.22 p.m.	Water	5
12.27 ,,	,,	2
12.32 ,,	,,	Traces
12.37 ,,	,,	0
12.42 ,,	0·25% aq. HCl	Copious secretion
12.50 ,,	,,	3
12.55 ,,	,,	3
1.0 ,,	,,	2
1.5 ,,	,,	0
1.10 ,,	0·25% aq. HCl	Copious secretion
1.16 ,,	,: ,,	,, ,,
1.24 ,,	Water	9

The conditioned water-reflex is as easily inhibited by different extraneous reflexes as are any other conditioned reflexes (external inhibition). The following are examples :

Time	Stimulus	Salivary Secretion in drops during one minute

Experiment of 1st January, 1909.

Time	Stimulus	Salivary Secretion
11.25 a.m.	Water	12
11.30 ,,	Water + loud tone	3
11.35 ,,	Water	16

Experiment of 25th April, 1909.

Time	Stimulus	Salivary Secretion
4.5 p.m.	Water	13
4.23 ,,	0·25% aq. HCl	Copious secretion
4.32 ,,	10% aq. sugar	,, ,,
4.36 ,,	Water	1
4.54 ,,	,,	10

Since this form of inhibition (external inhibition) is, however, not peculiar to conditioned reflexes, a similar effect being observed also upon unconditioned reflexes, we resolved to develop a conditioned inhibition for the water-reflex—*i.e.* to build up an actual inhibitory conditioned reflex (internal inhibition). It was expected that agencies belonging to other analysers, although incapable of acquiring positive conditioned properties, might nevertheless acquire the required negative conditioned properties, since examples of this had previously been observed (see p. 347). This expectation was fully justified, as it was found that both auditory and visual stimuli could serve successfully as conditioned inhibitors. Thus, administration of water simultaneously with sounding a definite tone became a constant inhibitory combination after 64 repetitions. The following are examples of experiments :

Time	Stimulus	Salivary Secretion in drops during one minute
Experiment of 2nd February, 1909.		
10.25 a.m.	0·25% aq. HCl	Copious secretion
10.34 ,,	,, ,,	,, 9 ,,
10.46 ,,	Water	9
10.55 ,,	0·25% aq. HCl	Copious secretion
11.4 ,,	,, ,,	,, 2 ,,
11.16 ,,	Water + tone	2
11.26 ,,	0·25% aq. HCl	Copious secretion
11.35 ,,	,, ,,	,, 10 ,,
11.48 ,,	Water	10
Experiment of 16th February, 1909.		
10.25 a.m.	0·25% aq. HCl	Copious secretion
10.36 ,,	,, ,,	,, 0 ,,
10.47 ,,	Water + tone	0
10.55 ,,	0·25% aq. HCl	Copious secretion
11.4 ,,	,, ,,	,, 6 ,,
11.16 ,,	Water	6
11.24 ,,	0·25% aq. HCl	Copious secretion
11.34 ,,	,, ,,	,, 0 ,,
11.45 ,,	Water + tone	0

Similar results were obtained when an increased illumination of the room was used as the conditioned inhibitor, the acid, of course, always being introduced into the mouth in dim light. The conditioned inhibition developed much more quickly in this case, and the experiment given below represents the 16th administration of water with increased illumination.

Experiment of 13*th March*, 1909.

Time	Stimulus	Salivary Secretion in drops during one minute
11.32 a.m.	Water	23
11.33 ,,	0·25% aq. HCl	Copious secretion
11.40 ,,	Water	26
11.41 ,,	0·25% aq. HCl	Copious secretion
11.48 ,,	,, ,,	,, ,,
11.57 ,,	Water + increased illumination	0
12.6 p.m.	0·25% aq. HCl	Copious secretion
12.14 ,,	Water + increased illumination	$\frac{1}{2}$

Finally, the effect of a dis-inhibition of the water-reflex after experimental extinction was tried, and this was plainly revealed under the appropriate conditions as shown by the following experiment performed in presence of a large audience at a meeting of the Medical Society in Petrograd.

Experiment of 19*th March*, 1909.

Time	Stimulus	Salivary Secretion in drops during one minute
8.9 p.m.	0·25% aq. HCl	Copious secretion
8.20 ,,	Water	12
8.24 ,,	,,	3
8.28 ,,	,,	$\frac{1}{2}$
8.32 ,,	Raw meat	Small secretion
8.36 ,,	Water	14
8.49 ,,	,,	$\frac{1}{2}$

Stimulation by raw meat produced a dis-inhibition of the extinguished water-reflex only during the early period of its after-effect. Later, the effect of extinction returned temporarily, in accordance with the general rules of conditioned reflexes.

We see, therefore, that in the first dog only an organ of a secondary physiological importance, with only a rudimentary relation to the external world, remained functionally intact, namely, the salivary gland; and even this sole surviving witness could attest the continued functioning of the cerebral cortex only in conjunction with the rudimentary analyser of the mouth.

We shall now turn our attention to the second dog, which had a slightly different extent of lesion. In removing the anterior part of the hemisphere the *bulbus* and *tractus olfactorius* were preserved with the utmost care, since we wished if possible to demonstrate the existence of conditioned reflexes to olfactory stimuli, as well as the water-reflex.

The result exceeded our expectations. In this dog, besides the water-reflex, the conditioned reflex to an odour of camphor became re-established. The natural olfactory conditioned reflexes to food were of course also present. The dog stretched out its head towards food—directed by smell, and occasionally grabbed food placed close enough to it. This was the only important difference between the two dogs. In relation to other animals and to men the second dog was also entirely indifferent. The helplessness amongst mechanical obstacles and the defects in locomotion were as pronounced as in the first dog. Generally speaking this second dog was as great an invalid and as incapable of continuing to exist without careful tending as the first. No positive conditioned reflexes to stimuli belonging to other analysers could be obtained.

The post-mortem examination revealed in both dogs an extreme atrophy of the remaining posterior part of the hemispheres.

I think that the general behaviour of these animals can be more or less clearly interpreted by correlating our observations upon their conditioned activity and the result of the post-mortem examination. All the cortical parts of the analysers, with the exception of the analyser of the mouth in both dogs, and in the second dog of the chemical analyser of smell in addition, either did not function at all or else only partially (inhibitory reflexes). The dogs, therefore, were deprived of innumerable signalling stimuli from the external world, stimuli which otherwise would determine their normal complicated activities. In the first dog the only analyser to remain intact was the one which is the most limited in its contact with the environment. In the second dog, besides this there remained also the activity of the distance analyser of smell, which is especially well developed in dogs. In this dog, however, the analyser of smell functioned neither so efficiently nor so constantly as in normal dogs. This may have been due to some damage of the analyser during the operation, or to its being constantly held under a certain inhibitory influence deriving from other analysers which had been damaged and which by themselves, although incapable of any positive activity, could yet respond to stimuli by the development and irradiation of an inhibition. The most important effector apparatus of the organism —its skeletal and motor system—was in both dogs incapable of performing its activities with the precision required for adjustment to changes in the external environment. Under normal conditions the activity of this system is determined by an associated action of two analysers, an external, cutaneous analyser—signalling in detail changes in the external mechanical relations of the animal to its environment—and an internal, motor analyser—performing a detailed analysis and complicated synthesis of corresponding movements. In the case of extensive disturbances of either, it is obvious that detailed motor reactions in response to changes in the external environment cannot be present. There is evidence, however, that in these two dogs some irregularly dispersed parts of the cutaneous and motor analysers still remained in the cortex, this being the probable explanation why stimulation of certain parts of the skin (stroking of the neck and head) undoubtedly evoked inhibitory (most probably conditioned) reflexes neutralizing the general excitation of the animal and leading to sleep, while stimulation of certain other parts evoked only unconditioned reflexes which are known to be the result of activity of the lower motor centres—various scratch reflexes and defence reflexes. The same consideration may explain also the differences between these two dogs and entirely decorticated animals, namely, that the latter begin much sooner after the operation to get on their feet, stand, walk about, and in general show much less disorder in their movements than the two dogs described. The presence of dispersed remnants of the motor analyser is also indicated by the epileptic attacks in these two dogs, occurring in the form of convulsions of the muscles of the head, neck and sometimes body, but never of the extremities. As regards the absence of the special " social " reflexes sufficient has already been said. It is most probable that their existence depends on exceedingly complex conditioned reflexes, which in these dogs, of course, could not have been present, since even elementary positive conditioned reflexes were absent in the majority of the analysers.

I shall now discuss another case, the analysis of which occupied a very long time. This dog showed a great deviation from the normal in its general reactions, not immediately after the operation and not on account of the surgical lesion of the cortex itself, but under the influence of a subsequent growth of scar tissue accompanied by frequent attacks of convulsions, which two years after the operation became so severe as finally to lead to the death of the animal. The dog was young, very lively, and with a well-balanced nervous system. The experiments were started before the operation and confined to the development of tactile and thermal cutaneous reflexes which, as mentioned before, have an exceptional tendency to induce an inhibitory state of the cortical elements, dogs soon becoming drowsy under their influence and falling asleep. This dog, however, remained wide awake in its stand during the whole time of an experiment. The operation on the cortex was performed in two stages, first on the one and then on the other side (9th March and 28th April, 1910), the *gyri postcruciati* being partially destroyed. It was now for some time observed that stimulation of the areas of the skin corresponding to the cortical field of the operation produced drowsiness of the animal. This, however, was overcome by the introduction of a new strong conditioned stimulus (buzzer). After a short period of time all the small defects which developed after the operation almost completely disappeared and the dog behaved generally as normal. On the 11th May, 1910, it had a first attack of convulsions. Since the work that had been planned originally was at this time already completed, the dog was kept for a considerable time without observation. During the following summer the attacks of convulsions recurred, and in the autumn and winter the attendant looking after the animal reported that it had developed extremely peculiar behaviour and on being touched now entered into a state of extreme excitation, snarling, barking and baring the teeth in a manner which had never been observed before in this animal. In the beginning of January 1911 the dog was given over to Dr. Satournov. Its general behaviour was now as follows : Taken out of the kennel and placed on the floor it became wildly excited, soon, however, quieting down, after which it remained standing in the same place upwards of an hour at a time, only moving the head and sniffing the air. It would then make some forward or circular movement preliminary to defaecation or micturition, which quickly followed. Then it would continue standing in the same place. With the approach of the usual feeding time the dog would begin to walk about sniffing the air. A dish of food placed in front of it would make it stretch out its head after the food and even follow if the dish were removed. The act of eating was normal, the standing posture quite firm and without swaying, but as the dog walked the front legs would splay out, and when it turned quickly on a smooth floor the front legs would slip, but the animal would seldom fall. Sometimes the animal walked into obstacles, sometimes went round them. Sexual reflexes in spite of careful observations were never observed. The animal never answered to calling, and generally did not exhibit any reactions to other dogs or to men. If the hair on any part of the skin, especially of the neck and head, were touched however slightly by hand, other animals, wind, drops of rain, or any object with which the dog might come into contact, an extraordinary outburst of excitation followed, expressed by growling, barking, baring of the teeth and hostile movements generally. Usually the animal lifted up its head into the air and practically never turned it towards the point of origin of the touch. At the same time a continuous pressure upon the skin—for example, by apparatuses attached to the skin during experiments, or by the loops of the stand—left the dog quiet.

As was previously mentioned, the whole time the animal survived general attacks of convulsions recurred from which it usually recovered comparatively quickly. The conditioned reflex activity of this strange animal was studied in order to elucidate if possible the reason for its behaviour. An old conditioned alimentary reflex to a buzzer was easily and quickly re-established. A new conditioned reflex to a tone of an organ pipe of 300 d.v. was established, as was also a new reflex to an odour of camphor as well as a differentiation of the sound of another organ pipe three tones higher, and a conditioned inhibition of the reflex to camphor in conjunction with a metronome. The experimenter [Dr. Satournov] did not succeed in re-establishing any of the tactile conditioned reflexes which were present before the pathological condition developed. He observed, however, that positive conditioned stimuli were in general very apt to develop inhibitory properties, and that the inhibitory process was extremely inert, exhibiting a very prolonged after-effect upon positive reflexes.

The next investigator who worked on this dog [Dr. Kouraev], realizing the peculiarity just mentioned, worked mainly with short-delayed reflexes, and succeeded without difficulty in re-establishing the reflexes to tactile stimuli. The tendency of the nervous system to inhibition continued to increase, as did also the occurrence and severity of the attacks of convulsions, until on the 19th May, 1912, vigorous attacks continuing with only short intermissions during twelve hours finally killed the animal. The post-mortem examination revealed, after removal of the scar, that the defect in the substance of the cortex involved the following convolutions—the posterior part of the *gyrus postcruciatus*, the anterior parts of the *gyri supra-splenialis, entolateralis* and *ectolateralis*, the *gyrus suprasylvius medius*, the upper half of *gyrus coronarius*, and to some extent the *gyrus ectosylvius medius*. The occipital and temporal lobes were very definitely atrophied, the mass of the cortex in these two areas being diminished and the convolutions flattened out. The frontal lobes remained apparently entirely intact.

The post-mortem examination showed that the actual destruction involved in the main the posterior part of the cortex, the anterior part being affected to a much smaller extent. Naturally therefore the behaviour of this dog, as shown by observation of its conditioned reflexes, resembled that of animals in which the posterior part of the cerebral cortex had been extirpated. The animal was, unfortunately, not subjected to analysis of reflexes to compound auditory and visual stimuli. The absence of such reflexes could, however, be inferred from the fact that the dog did not react to calling and did not exhibit any social relations with other animals or with men, indicating an absence of chain, and probably all complex, reflexes. Certain irregularities in walking obviously depended upon a small damage of the motor analyser. It is difficult, however, to find an adequate explanation for the prolonged standing of the dog in one place and the exaggerated reactions to touching the skin. So far as the former is concerned it is impossible to decide whether it is an expression of a dominance of inhibition in the cortex subsequent to the periods of violent excitations (convulsions), or whether it should be regarded as a result of a partial damage of the cutaneous analyser. The latter explanation would seem to find support in the retention of the usual mobility of the head and neck. The exaggerated reaction to touching the skin might be of cortical origin or a reflex through subcortical centres. Since, however, tactile conditioned reflexes were present, the latter seems improbable. It is also difficult to reconcile the extreme excitability of the cutaneous analyser with the hypothesis of a predominance of the inhibitory process in the cortex. To solve these problems it would have been necessary to perform further variations of the experiments, and these were not at that time practicable.

In describing the cases in the present lecture, I do not make the slightest pretence to have given a satisfactory explanation of the entire nervous mechanism underlying the deviations from normal in the general behaviour of the dogs after surgical damage of the cortex. My aim has been simply to show that problems as to this mechanism are the legitimate province of physiology, and to demonstrate that a reasonable possibility of studying them is given even by present-day methods.

On the whole the experiments upon conditioned reflexes brought forward in the last three lectures confirm the observations of old and recent authors upon the same problem, though we have also been able to add some new facts and to formulate some new problems. But what our experiments do most emphatically refute is the doctrine of special "association" centres, or, more generally, of the existence in the hemispheres of some special area on which the higher functions of the nervous system depend—a doctrine which has already been strenuously opposed by H. Munk.

LECTURE XXII

The general characteristics of the present investigation and its special difficulties —Discovery of certain errors necessitating the modification of some earlier interpretations.

A SCIENTIFIC investigation of biological phenomena can be conducted along several different lines each of which would treat the problem from a different point of view. For instance, one may have in view the purely physico-chemical aspect, analysing the elements of life by the methods of physics and chemistry. Again, keeping in view the fact of evolution of living matter one can try to elucidate the functions of complex biological structures by studying the functions of individual cells and of elementary organisms. Finally, one can make an attempt to elucidate the activities of complex structures in their fullest range directly, seeking for rigid laws governing this activity, or, in other words, trying to define all those conditions which determine the form this activity takes at every instant and in all its variations. The line of inquiry which has been adopted in the present investigation obviously belongs to the third point of view. In this research we were not concerned with the ultimate nature of excitation and inhibition as such. We took them as two fundamental properties, the two most important manifestations of activity, of the living nervous elements. Nor was it our aim to interpret the activity of the hemispheres in terms of elementary functions of the nervous system, as has been done, for example, in the physiology of the nerve fibres. We intentionally neglected also the controversial problem of the actual localization of these two fundamental processes, and did not attempt to assign them to either of the two elements of the nervous structure, namely, the nerve cell and the synaptic junction or fibrillary connection between two individual nerve cells. The acceptance of the more general conception of the two processes of inhibition and excitation as the basic functions of the nervous cellular structures was sufficient for the purposes of our research, the study of conditioned reflexes being of the nature of a general investigation of the functions of the cellular structures of the cortex as exhibited in various reactions of the organism to a multitude of separate stimuli which originate from within or from without the organism—stimuli for the reception of which there is such an unbounded number of separate cortical cells and which after extirpation of the cortex lose their significance for the organism. It is highly probable that excitation and inhibition, the two functions of the nerve cell which are so intimately interwoven and which so constantly supersede each other, may, fundamentally, represent only different phases of one and the same physico-chemical process. The primary aim of our research was the accurate determination and tabulation of different phases of the cortical activity— the absence or presence of an inhibitory or excitatory phase, the exact conditions under which the intensity of the excitatory or inhibitory process varied, and the mutual interrelation between these processes. It is obvious that in its intrinsic nature our work is closely allied to the work of Sherrington and his co-workers upon the spinal cord, and it is impossible not to notice in how many points the different aspects of the nervous activity of the cortex correspond with those described in the physiology of the spinal cord ; a fact which seems strong evidence of a similarity of the fundamental laws governing the nervous activity in the two cases.

Research upon the activity of the cortex along these lines must unavoidably present exceptional difficulties. The extraordinary reactivity of the cortex, on the one hand, and the unbounded volume of stimuli continually pouring into it, on the other hand, are responsible for the two fundamental peculiarities of the cortical activity— namely, first, that it is determined in every minutest detail, and second, that it is in a state of perpetual flux, changing so rapidly that it becomes practically impossible to observe any aspect of it in an entirely pure and uncontaminated form and to appraise and control all the determining conditions. The minutest changes in the environment or inside the organism itself—changes which may be imperceptible to us and unsuspected—have a profound effect upon the cortical activities. It is obvious that these special peculiarities of the research are in many instances the cause of fallacies, especially since it is so tempting to adhere to different fancied analogies and plausible generalizations—a tendency which cannot be too much guarded against in the present state of the research. The mind, so to speak, often fails to keep pace with the tremendous variety of interrelations, and this is why our interpretations were often too limited and led to errors which have had to be constantly corrected. Indeed I have no doubt that the presentation of the subject-matter attempted in these lectures will in the future still be corrected in many details. Errors in interpretation, and errors sometimes in the methods of observation, are naturally to be expected in a study of such astounding complexity. These special peculiarities of our subject is the reason why I thought it advisable to delay a systematic presentation of our prolonged researches until now : new problems are perpetually arising, and at the same time an equally large number of questions are still left unsettled. We often feel compelled to turn our attention from problems which directly confront us to some unexpected new phenomena which introduce fresh problems or which necessitate a revision of old points of view. This general aspect of the investigation into the cortical activity I want particularly to emphasize in the present lecture, taking for my examples some fresh observations which have not been discussed in the preceding lectures.

The surprising minuteness of detail in which the cortical activity is determined by external and internal agencies, and the extraordinary precision and delicacy of the responsiveness of the cortex to even the minutest changes in these agencies, are clearly illustrated by the two following observations, which are both taken from the later period of our work.

The dog used in the first of these experiments has already been referred to in the preceding lectures. It passed through the experience of the great flood in Petrograd, and afterwards served for an investigation of a functional disturbance of the acoustic analyser (p. 316). In the course of a month in which the animal behaved again normally a differentiation of pitch was developed. During the isolated action of the conditioned stimulus (10 seconds) the secretory effect was as much as 5 drops ; the difference between the effects of strong and weak stimuli was very definite, and the food given in reinforcement was always taken with avidity. In the stand the animal stood quietly. We now introduced an apparently very small modification in the experiment, the isolated action of the conditioned stimulus being prolonged a further 5 seconds. As a result of this the entire conditioned activity was immediately disturbed. The following are illustrative experiments taken from the two periods of the research :

Experiment of 19*th June,* 1926 (*normal experiment*).

Time	Conditioned stimulus during 10 seconds	Salivary Secretion in drops during 10 seconds	Remarks
10.33 a.m.	Tone, 250 d.v.	4½	The animal stands quietly
10.38 „	Tone, 150 d.v. (inhibitory)	0	and exhibits a definite alimentary motor re-
10.48 „	Bubbling sound	5	action to conditioned
10.52 „	Lamp	3½	stimuli ; takes the food
10.59 „	Bubbling sound	5	at once

Experiment of 24*th June,* 1926 (*experiment after prolongation of the isolated action of the conditioned stimulus*).

Time	Conditioned stimulus during 15 seconds	Salivary Secretion in drops during 15 seconds	Remarks
10.28 a.m.	Tone, 250 d.v.	7	Alimentary reaction ; takes the food During the interval the animal is very excited
10.34 „	Lamp	2	Weak alimentary re- action ; takes the food During the interval the animal is again very excited
10.49 „	Buzzer	0	The dog turns away, but takes the food 15 secs. after presentation
10.54 „	Lamp	1½	Alimentary reaction ; takes the food at once
11.1 „	Buzzer	0	Turns away ; does not take the food

The first application of the conditioned stimulus in the experiment of 24th June produced a greater secretory effect than usual, for the obvious reason that the isolated action of the conditioned stimulus had been protracted for a further 5 seconds. The alimentary motor reaction in response to the stimulus was lively, the food being consumed at once ; everything promised a normal experiment, and there were so far no indications of any special deviation from normal. However, already during the interval between the first and second stimuli the animal showed an unusual state of excitation. This was followed later on by an obvious paradoxical phase : a strong stimulus (buzzer) failed to elicit the secretory reaction while the motor reflex considerably diminished. The animal on the first application of the buzzer (10.49 a.m.) accepted the food after some delay, and on the second application (11.1 a.m.) did not touch the food at all. A weak stimulus (lamp) nevertheless continued to evoke a secretion (although a diminished one) and to evoke a motor alimentary response. We returned to the usual length of isolated action of the conditioned stimulus (10 seconds) on the following day. The disturbance, however, became still more pronounced, the secretory effect being absent throughout the experiment, while the animal turned to the food only after weak stimuli and would not touch it after strong ones. On the third day all reflexes returned to normal, except that the tone which had been the first stimulus employed on the day (24th June) when the isolated action of the stimuli was prolonged, still gave a diminished secretory effect (only a half of its usual secretion during 10 seconds). A further experiment with a temporary prolongation of the isolated action of the conditioned stimuli produced exactly the same pathological state (paradoxical phase) of the animal. These observations provide a brilliant example of the exquisite delicacy in the reactivity of the cortex, showing how considerable may be the effect of such minute changes in the conditions of an experiment.

The second dog, also previously mentioned,—" Brains "—was of an extremely inhibitable type, and the same change in the experimental conditions led to exactly opposite results. This dog when left in the stand without application of any stimuli quickly became drowsy, with the result that not only conditioned reflexes disappeared but also reflexes in response to the actual administration of food. For the purpose of overcoming this drowsiness we had used the usual method of abbreviating the isolated action of the conditioned stimulus to $\frac{1}{2}$-1 second. After three weeks of this practice the drowsiness disappeared, and the dog now took the food immediately on presentation and consumed it with avidity. A prolongation of the isolated action of the conditioned stimulus to 5 seconds revealed the presence of a conditioned secretory reflex. On continuation of the experiments with the isolated action of 5 seconds the reflex maintained its strength for several days. After this the reflex again diminished and the animal once more succumbed to drowsiness. However, it was now sufficient to prolong the conditioned stimulus to 10 seconds for the animal to become again alert ; the secretory effect returned after several repetitions of the prolonged stimulus, and, what is important, it appeared within the first 5 seconds of the isolated action of the conditioned stimulus. On continuation of the experiments with the isolated action of 10 seconds the animal again became drowsy and the secretory conditioned reflex again disappeared. A further prolongation of the conditioned stimulus to 15 seconds produced a similar effect to that of the first prolongation to 10 seconds, *i.e.* a temporary return of the alert state and a considerable conditioned secretion starting well within the first 5 seconds. The same sequence of events was repeated yet twice more on prolongation of the conditioned stimulus to 20 and 25 seconds. The following is an example of an experiment :

Experiment of 28th February, 1925.

Time	Conditioned stimulus applied during 15 seconds	Latency of salivary secretion	Salivary Secretion in drops during 15 seconds
8.53 a.m.	Metronome	7	1
9.3 ,,	Tactile	–	0
9.18 ,,	Whistle	–	0

On the next day the isolated action of the conditioned stimuli was prolonged to 20 seconds. The following is an experiment after two days' practice with the longer interval :

Experiment of 3rd March, 1925.

Time	Conditioned stimulus applied during 20 seconds	Latency of salivary secretion	Salivary Secretion in drops during 20 seconds
9.2 a.m.	Metronome	4	5
9.12 ,,	Whistle	2	8
9.24 ,,	Tactile	10	$3\frac{1}{2}$

Thus every small prolongation of the isolated action of the conditioned stimulus evoked after a few repetitions a temporary state of excitation of the dog : the drowsiness disappeared, and the secretory reaction reappeared, starting soon after the beginning of the conditioned stimulus and well within the period in which there was no secretion during the shorter isolated action of the stimulus.

The latter fact shows that the enhanced secretion was not merely due to the prolongation of the period of observation but was the genuine result of a cortical excitation.

We thus see that one and the same change led to opposite effects in the two dogs : in the first it resulted in inhibition, in the second it abolished inhibition. Most probably the difference in the effects was dependent on the fact that the first animal was alert during the experiments (i.e. in a state of cortical excitation), while the other dog was drowsy (i.e. in a state of cortical inhibition).

We are constantly confronted by cases in which pathological changes in the state of the animal are brought about by some unknown secondary conditions. It has repeatedly been mentioned in the preceding lectures that conditioned reflexes to stimuli belonging to different analysers are normally of different magnitude. Remembering that the nervous process is considered by present-day physiologists to be identical in all nerve fibres, and having somehow conceived the idea that the difference in our perception of light, sound, etc., must have some physical basis in differences of corresponding cortical elements, we were for a considerable time inclined to attribute the difference in the magnitude of the conditioned effect to individual peculiarities of the cells of the different analysers. Reinvestigation of the whole question, as has been mentioned already, showed that the differences in the magnitude of the conditioned reactions to stimuli belonging to different analysers, depend fundamentally upon the intensity of the stimuli themselves (p. 269). This conclusion, it will be remembered, was arrived at in the following manner. We knew for a long time that in a conditioned compound stimulus made up of two agencies belonging to different analysers one of the stimuli almost invariably overshadows the other, as can easily be revealed by testing the individual components separately. In such a compound our usual auditory stimuli, in the majority of dogs, overshadowed visual, tactile and thermal components, but in a compound made up of a weakened auditory stimulus and a strong visual one the relations were entirely reversed. This observation proved the difference in response to be due not to fundamental differences in the cellular structure of the various analysers, but to the relative intensity of the individual stimuli. Now, although the above holds good in the majority of cases, in some few animals the difference in the magnitude of the conditioned response to different agencies was found to be entirely absent. We have already directed considerable attention to the study of this deviation, but we are not yet in a position to state definitely under what special conditions it occurs. Some of the determining conditions are, however, known. These special cases depend to some extent upon the general type of the nervous system of the animal—excitable or inhibitable. In the inhibitable type the usual relation between intensity of stimulus and magnitude of effect is especially obvious, occurring practically without exception otherwise than in extreme pathological states. It is true that if the period of isolated action is short there may not be any apparent difference between the effects of strong and weak stimuli, since in the initial stage the effect is practically the same in both cases ; but with a prolongation of the stimulus the secretion augments rapidly in the case of strong stimuli and only slowly in the case of weak stimuli. In the case of excitable and very greedy dogs it is, on the contrary, the abbreviation of the conditioned stimulus which helps to disclose the usual relation between the magnitudes of the effects of weak and of strong stimuli, a relation which may not be apparent when the stimuli are more prolonged.

On account of the immense number of different conditions determining the different states of activity of the cortex I feel that even now the physiological analysis of many seemingly simple and well-known facts is very often far from perfect. I will describe, for example, the observations upon one of our recently acquired animals [experiments of Drs. Podkopaev and Virjikovsky]. In this case the conditioned reflexes to different agencies were developed with the following important variation in the usual method. The first agent to which conditioned properties were to be given was applied alternately with and without reinforcement by food. The conditioned reflex developed comparatively quickly (by the 20th application). In the case of the next stimulus the reinforcement was given at every third application. The reflex developed even quicker than before (by the 7th application). The animal became, however, extremely excited. Finally a third agent was reinforced only at every fourth application, and in this case the conditioned reflex failed to develop and the animal became somewhat drowsy. The last stimulus was applied a total of 240 times (60 times in conjunction with food).

Let us, having recourse to all our previous knowledge, endeavour to interpret these facts. Why, in the last case, did the conditioned reflex fail to develop ? or, at any rate, why was it for so long delayed, if, indeed, it would have developed at all ? The fundamental mechanism of development of a conditioned reflex depends upon excitation of some definite point in the cortex coincidently with a more intense excitation of some other point, probably also of the cortex, which leads to a connection being formed between these two points ; and reversely, if such a coincident stimulation of these points is not repeated for a long time the path becomes obliterated and the connection disrupted. But when once such a path has been firmly established it remains intact without further practice, for months and years. It is obvious that under suitable conditions a new connection must be formed at the very first occurrence of the simultaneous excitation and become strengthened by every repetition. In ordinary experiments with normal dogs about twenty reinforced repetitions are required to establish the first of any conditioned reflexes experimentally produced, and this number sufficed in the first variation (alternate reinforcement) described above. In the establishment of subsequent reflexes under normal conditions only three to five repetitions are necessary, and yet in the case now under discussion (reinforcement of every fourth application) sixty repetitions produced no result. The first possible explanation is the prolongation of the interval between the separate reinforcements, but this cannot be the reason in our case since with the same intervals of time, but omitting the non-reinforced applications during the intervals, the conditioned reflex invariably and quickly develops. It is obvious, therefore, that the frequent repetition of the non-reinforced agent must oppose a powerful resistance to the development of a conditioned reflex. We know already that every new stimulus which evokes the investigatory reflex ceases on repetition to have any effect unless the stimulus has been followed up with some other reflex. Such a disappearance of the effect is known to be due to a development of inhibition in those cortical elements upon which the stimulus acts. Consequently, in the third variation of the experiment such an inhibition might have developed on account of the application of three non-reinforced stimuli, the cortical elements never acquiring with the fourth, reinforced stimulus a sufficient state of excitation for a connection to be formed with the excited alimentary nervous elements. But although such an interpretation seemed highly plausible it failed when subjected to the following experimental test. When the stimulus had been repeated 240 times (60 times with reinforcement) a pre-established conditioned stimulus was applied 30 seconds after the ineffective stimulus. No inhibitory after-effect was ever observed. Obviously, therefore, the ineffective agent could not have produced any widespread inhibition. It was still possible, however, that on account of prolonged practice the inhibitory effect had become extremely concentrated in a narrow region ; but neither was this explanation supported by our experiments, for when we now began to reinforce the agent at each successive application the conditioned secretory effect was already considerable at the third reinforcement, showing that the rate of development of the new conditioned reflex was maximal. We cannot, therefore, regard the stimulus as having had any definite inhibitory properties. Several further possible explanations have also been tested experimentally, but we have hitherto failed to disclose the nature of this phenomenon. So far, our experiments simply show that we have not yet gained command over all the conditions which determine the development of conditioned reflexes. The conditions enumerated in the second lecture, however sufficient they may be as regards the development of all those reflexes with which we have been accustomed to deal, nevertheless do not finally exhaust the subject, since having had all of them in our mind we have still failed to understand the results of the experiments described above. There must exist some further condition which has up to the present been overlooked. This failure only serves to demonstrate once more the surprising extent to which, in every detail, the cortical activity is determined, and the astonishing reactivity of the cortical elements.

It was, of course, obvious from the start that there was no immediate possibility of attacking the complex activity of the cortex from its physico-chemical aspect. Neither did there appear to be any real hope of approaching an understanding of the cortical activity through the study of the elementary properties of the nervous tissue. We have come now to see that we do not possess even yet a full descriptive knowledge of the various aspects of this activity. Our chief task in studying the cortical activity at the present time must therefore consist in reducing the tremendous mass of various separate observations to terms of a progressively diminishing number of general and more fundamental units. This we have fully realized, and in some cases we seem to be approaching our goal, but in other cases we find ourselves confronting some entirely new aspects of the cortical activity, which sometimes are within, and at other times beyond the range, of our present powers of analysis.

In the beginning of the present research, on the basis of very definite but purely external signs, we distinguished three types of inhibition—external inhibition, internal inhibition, and sleep. Accumulation of further observations permitted us to fuse the last two types by showing that the apparent differences are only secondary. Sleep and the various forms of internal inhibition are aspects of one and the same process, which in the one set of cases is fragmented and localized, in the other case diffused. When in the course of our further investigation of conditioned reflexes we met with the phenomenon of mutual induction, it was natural that we should perceive the similarity between negative induction and external inhibition. Hence a fundamental identity of all the three types of inhibition appeared very probable, and special efforts were directed to the collection of further evidence on the point. Some of this evidence has been given before, and fresh evidence will be added in the present lecture. In the lecture upon induction an experiment was described in which a conditioned defence reflex to a tactile stimulation of a place on the skin exerted an inhibitory after-effect upon a conditioned alimentary reflex to tactile stimulation of other places. We found reason to believe that this inhibition was in part cortical (p. 202). In the lecture upon different transition phases between the alert state and sleep it was shown that some of these phases can be observed not only during the after-effect of internal (differential) inhibition, but also under the influence of external inhibition (p. 276). I am now in a position to add some further considerations in favour of the identity of internal and external inhibition. We are inclined to regard the frequently mentioned fact of overshadowing in a compound conditioned stimulus of the weaker by the stronger component as based upon external inhibition. The cortical elements belonging to the strong stimulus inhibit those of the weak stimulus, and the latter, therefore, can establish only a weak connection with the unconditioned centre. This theory is substantiated by the fact that the strengths of newly established conditioned connections depend on the relative strengths of the conditioned stimuli. This consideration obviously approximates still more the phenomenon of external inhibition to negative induction, in which the application of the positive conditioned stimulus reinforces, or even re-establishes, the inhibitory state of the nervous elements acted upon by the inhibitory stimulus. Many of my collaborators [Drs. Mishtovt, Krjishkovsky and Leporsky] noticed that for a quick and complete establishment of a conditioned inhibitor it is of considerable importance to choose a stimulus which is not much weaker in strength than the positive component of the combination. Recent experiments performed in this connection by Dr. Foursikov not only corroborate these observations, but bring out the important fact that the external inhibition which on account of the investigatory reflex is produced at the first application of the new stimulus, often gradually and almost imperceptibly undergoes transition into the permanent conditioned inhibition. In spite of the cumulative effect of the foregoing evidence it is by no means conclusive, and I feel entitled to advance the view, that external and internal inhibition are fundamentally the same, only as a strong probability.

It was noticed in the nineteenth lecture that three different types of external stimuli lead to an inhibitory state of the cortex, namely, very weak stimuli, very strong stimuli, and unusual stimuli, and an attempt was made to give a general biological interpretation of this effect. The physiological mechanism of the effect of these stimuli is as yet obscure, neither do I find it possible to discuss the problem of inhibition in its entire range. The experimental material, although considerable, is not yet sufficient to establish any general and definite conception of the nature of inhibition and its relation to excitation. Explanations which seem to fit some one group of phenomena fail when applied to other groups. Many observations do not fit in with any of the theories, and our conception of the mechanism involved has had to be changed many times in the course of our research, never entirely satisfactorily. Here again, as in the whole of our research, we can only collect and systematize facts. The fact that very powerful and very weak stimuli have a stronger tendency than medium stimuli to produce inhibition belongs to the category of unsolved problems along with the mechanism of disinhibition, the positive effect of negative stimuli in the " ultraparadoxical phase " and the negative effect of positive stimuli in the case of damage to the cortex. In many instances we fail even to see which of the phenomena are closely related to each other and which are isolated and radically different. To illustrate the difficulty of such cases I shall attempt to deal with the question of the production of inhibition by new events or a rearrangement in the grouping of old events. We change, for example, the manner in which the conditioned stimulus is reinforced by food. Instead of a plate automatically moving with food from behind a screen, a measured amount of food is now delivered mechanically into a stationary plate. Many dogs after this change persistently decline the food, and all conditioned reflexes disappear. This, of course, is a case of inhibition, but what explanation can be suggested as to its mechanism ? It may be compared with an observation discussed in the thirteenth lecture where a change in the sequence of a series of conditioned stimuli led in some animals to a more or less profound inhibition of the entire conditioned activity—an inhibition which lasted for several days, notwithstanding that a return was made to the previous order of stimulation. What happens here with a small number of conditioned stimuli can well be imagined to take place in respect to the entire environment. Constant repetitions of external events in a stereotyped order may lead to a definite stereotyped pattern of activity in the cortex, each new distribution of the stimuli now producing a disturbance in the pattern of the cortical activity, leading to inhibition in exactly the same manner as in our experiments with alteration in the sequence of the conditioned stimuli. This comparison does not, however, explain the mechanism of the development of inhibition in this particular case. Was it a result of the investigatory reflex due to the change in environment, or are the investigatory reflex and this very prolonged inhibition two independent phenomena ? In favour of the first supposition the fact can be advanced that in very inhibitable dogs the investigatory reflex exercises an extraordinarily prolonged inhibitory after-effect.

The whole subject of conditioned reflexes has, of course, been continuously growing and expanding during the twenty-five years of its existence. The present lecture should show to the reader the exceptional difficulties we still meet with. Many similar difficulties, though some of them now seem trivial, confronted us throughout ; even in our comparatively early material we still find scope for revision, and for the correction of different, sometimes important, errors. I shall discuss one of these which was discovered and corrected in repeating some old experiments during the preparation of these lectures, and another which is still beng investigated.

In the fourth lecture three different modes of re-establishment of extinguished conditioned reflexes were described. In the first, spontaneous recovery occurred after a longer or shorter interval of rest ; such recovery was slow in developing, but stable. In the second, quick recovery was brought about with the help of reinforcement by the underlying unconditioned reflex. In the third, quick recovery was effected through the introduction of some extraneous reflex. The recoveries in the last two cases were described as fundamentally differing from one another, since the former was not only rapid, but also stable, whereas the latter, though equally quick, was only temporary—vanishing with the disappearance of the extraneous reflex and its after-effect, when the inhibition would again acquire its full intensity and maintain itself until the final recovery occurred spontaneously, just as if no extraneous stimulus had ever intervened. The term " dis-inhibition " was therefore applied only to the latter case. The difficulty of interpreting the mechanism of this difference was immediately recognized. Recently during experiments upon some new aspects of the relation between the conditioned and the unconditioned stimulus these old observations were repeated, and found to be inaccurate [experiments of Dr. Podkopaev].

The recovery of an extinguished conditioned reflex is found in both cases to be temporary—in the case of the special reinforcing agent as well as under the influence of an extraneous reflex. In both cases the extinguished conditioned stimulus recovers its positive effect only for a time, then the positive effect again disappears, recovery occurring spontaneously. When the extinguished conditioned reflex is alimentary while the extraneous one is a defence reflex based on acid, the extent and duration of the disinhibition can be seen with great ease and regularity to be identical whichever method of restoration is employed. These experiments were conducted on two dogs, and they entirely corroborated one another. I shall describe the experiments on one of the dogs in detail. On extinguishing the conditioned alimentary reflex to a metronome it was found that the reflex remained at zero for 20 minutes counting from the last non-reinforced application of the conditioned stimulus. Then spontaneously the reflex began slowly to recover, reaching at the thirtieth minute 40% of its original value. After a fresh extinction to the first zero the conditioned stimulus was immediately reinforced, but it was again found twenty minutes later to give a zero effect. When, however, in another experiment it was tested 10 minutes after a similar reinforcement a positive effect was exhibited. Exactly similar results were obtained when acid instead of food was administered at the first zero, the reflex being again tested at the previously mentioned intervals of time. The following are the actual figures of some of the experiments : The conditioned stimulus on its first application on a particular day gave 6 drops in twenty seconds ; the stimulus was reinforced immediately after complete extinction ; tested after 10 minutes it gave 3 drops in twenty seconds. On the following day the experiment was repeated under precisely similar conditions. The stimulus gave, to start with, 7 drops during 20 seconds, and tested twenty minutes after reinforcement at the first zero of extinction gave no trace of any secretory effect. The experiments were now performed with administration of acid after the extinction of the alimentary conditioned reflex to its first zero. In the first experiment the reflex measured at the start 5 drops in twenty seconds. Tested 10 minutes after administration of acid following the first zero it gave 2 drops. On the following day the conditioned stimulus again gave 5 drops at first, but tested twenty minutes after administration of acid following the first zero it remained without any secretory effect. The maximum of the disinhibiting effect in both cases was reached, of course, much earlier than ten minutes from the administration of food or acid following the first zero. The error in our older experiments was due to an obvious fallacy. The comparison of the rate of recovery in the two cases had been made between the effect of the special reinforcing agent and the effect of the much weaker extraneous reflexes evoked by different auditory, visual, tactile and other stimuli which generally have only a short after-effect, while the comparison should have been made with the dis-inhibiting effect of other extraneous agencies, e.g. chemical ones, which have as long an after-effect as has food. The error was facilitated by the fallacious conception that the unconditioned stimulus underlying the conditioned one must stand in some special relation to the latter, conferring special powers of re-establishment after extinction. The result of these recent experiments inclines us more and more to believe that the inhibitory process arises in the nerve cells themselves and not in the connecting path between those cells excited by the conditioned stimulus and those excited by the special unconditioned stimulus employed. Otherwise it is difficult to reconcile the fact of the identical restorative action of the acid and food.

The second probable error I wish to describe is still undergoing investigation, but I permit myself to discuss it now, on the one hand on account of the extreme importance of the point involved, and on the other hand because it illustrates once more the exceptional difficulties presented in this research to the establishment of exact facts. It will be remembered that in the second lecture we discussed the essentials necessary for the establishment of conditioned reflexes. After establishing that the action of the originally neutral but potentially conditioned stimulus must overlap that of the unconditioned stimulus, we insisted also that the former must precede, by however short a time, the commencement of the latter. When the unconditioned stimulus was applied 5-10 seconds before the neutral stimulus it was found impossible to develop a conditioned reflex even by 300-400 repetitions, whereas by the usual method any conditioned reflex can be established in the average dog by so few as 3-20 repetitions. It was natural to suppose that the strong unconditioned stimulus acting on some part of the cortex evoked in virtue of external inhibition such a profound inhibitory state in the rest of the cortex that all stimuli reaching these parts became ineffective. Such a state may be compared with that of a man preoccupied with some definite activity, who remains " deaf " and " blind " to anything occurring round about him—a familiar psychical phenomenon which is accepted from a physiological point of view as undoubtedly corresponding with an objective reality. The plausibility of the above reasoning made us confident of its validity until recently, when our point of view changed. The question was raised as to the mechanism by means of which an early reinforcement of the conditioned stimulus, *i.e.* a shortening of its isolated action, obstructs the development of inhibition in the cortical cells acted upon by the conditioned stimulus. In investigating this problem with a modification of the experiments we came unexpectedly on a new fact, viz. that if the unconditioned stimulus is administered *before the pre-established* conditioned stimulus the conditioned reflex becomes inhibited. Our attention naturally became directed to the exactly comparable case where, instead of a pre-established conditioned stimulus, we deal with a neutral agent which is intended for the development of a conditioned reflex. The effect of the unconditioned stimulus on both is precisely the same, since it exhibits in either case the properties of an external inhibitor. In contrast with these observations an introduction of a small modification in these time relations between the unconditioned stimulus and either of the other two causes the hitherto neutral agent to acquire conditioned properties and the conditioned stimulus to be strengthened in its pre-established ones. This contrast reminds us of another set of facts—the relation between the development of a secondary conditioned reflex and the development of conditioned inhibition, the case in which under identical external conditions, but with a small change in the time relations between the two stimuli, there develops in the one case a process of excitation, in the other case a process of inhibition. All these observations concerning the action of the unconditioned stimulus point to the view (which involves a considerable modification of our original conception), that the mechanism of development of a conditioned reflex and the mechanism of external inhibition are somehow similar, and that the process of external inhibition bears some relation to the development of new connections between different cortical elements. If the analogy between external inhibition and the development of conditioned reflexes holds good, it should be expected that in the case where the unconditioned stimulus slightly precedes the action of the neutral agent there would in the very beginning be an opportunity for formation of a link between their respective cortical points, leading to the formation of an unstable conditioned reflex. This reflex would, however, rapidly undergo inhibition on repetition of the superimposed stimulation. The first preliminary experiments have fully confirmed our supposition. We had already noticed that administration of the unconditioned stimulus immediately preceding the pre-established conditioned one led only gradually to a definite diminution of the reflex, a diminution which was the more rapid and the more profound the smaller the intensity of the conditioned stimulus. Remembering this, we applied the similar combination of the unconditioned stimulus with the hitherto neutral stimulus, but repeated this combination only a very few times, to avoid the development of the inhibitory process. In many cases the expected result was obtained. The hitherto neutral stimulus when now tested alone revealed undoubted conditioned properties [experiments of Mlle. Pavlova and Drs. Kreps, Podkopaev, Prorokov and Koupalov]. Considering now after these preliminary experiments the results obtained in the much earlier experiments by Dr. Krestovnikov (p. 27), we found that the neutral stimuli were tested by him for a conditioned effect only after a very large number of repetitions of the unconditioned stimulus slightly preceding the neutral agent; moreover, even under these circumstances the stronger neutral stimuli when tested singly had at the first test some secretory effect. This secretory effect, however, was explained as a casual and not a true conditioned effect—a brilliant illustration of the danger of too hasty generalizations. We imagined that if it were a true conditioned reflex it would increase in intensity on repetition of the combination, and not diminish and finally vanish, as happens in these experiments. It is possible also that we were misled by the absence of a definite conditioned motor reaction.

As before remarked, the problem here dealt with is being worked out in all its implications, under the strictest control and with the help of the knowledge which has been gained in the last few years. If the preliminary experiments described above should be fully upheld, an important fact in the physiology of the cortex will be disclosed—namely, that new connections can be established in the cortex, not only in the areas of optimal excitability, but also in those areas which are in one or another phase of inhibition.

In the present lecture it has been my aim not so much to dwell on the details of the different experiments as to lay the strongest emphasis upon the fundamental peculiarities of the method of conditioned reflexes. I believe that the wealth of facts discussed in all the preceding lectures is in itself a sufficient indication that the whole problem is worthy of an intense scientific research, which should result in accumulation of a great number of valuable data. I have not, therefore, hesitated to expose in the present lecture some of the weaknesses in our own scientific venture. Full realization of the difficulties seems to me preferable to disregarding them. Moreover, it has been my desire to forewarn future workers in this field of the extraordinary complexity and the difficulties which they are bound to encounter.

On the whole, looking back upon this new field of physiological research I find it full of fascination, especially since it satisfies two of the fundamental cravings of the human intellect—striving to realize ever new and new truths, and to protest against the pretension of finality in truth we have already gained. In this domain there will for long remain an immense breadth of uncharted ocean compared with the small patches of the known.

LECTURE XXIII

The experimental results obtained with animals in their application to man.

In applying to man the results of investigation of the functions of the heart, digestive tract and other organs in the higher animals, allied as these organs are to the human in structure, great reserve must be exercised and the validity of comparisons must be verified at every step. Obviously even greater caution must be used in attempting similarly to apply our recently acquired knowledge concerning the higher nervous activity in the dog—the more so, since the incomparably greater development of the cerebral cortex in man is pre-eminently that factor which has raised man to his dominant position in the animal world. It would be the height of presumption to regard these first steps in elucidating the physiology of the cortex as solving the intricate problems of the higher psychic activities in man, when in fact at the present stage of our work no detailed application of its results to man is yet permissible.

Nevertheless, inasmuch as the higher nervous activity exhibited by the cortex rests, undoubtedly, on the same foundation in man as in the higher animals, some very general and tentative inferences can even now be drawn from the latter to the former. In the future it may confidently be expected that a full and detailed knowledge of at least the elementary facts of this activity will be obtained as regards both normal and pathological states. The similarities between the manifestations of this activity in man and animal being more obvious under normal conditions, I shall dismiss these briefly, discussing in more detail certain pathological cases.

It is obvious that the different kinds of habits based on training, education and discipline of any sort are nothing but a long chain of conditioned reflexes. We all know how associations, once established and acquired between definite stimuli and our responses, are persistently and, so to speak, automatically reproduced, sometimes even although we fight against them. For instance, in the case of games and various acts of skill, it is as difficult to abolish all sorts of superfluous movements as to acquire the necessary movements ;

and it is equally difficult to overcome established negative reflexes, *i.e.* inhibitions. Again, experience has taught us that a difficult task should be approached by gradual stages. We know also how different extra stimuli inhibit and discoordinate a well-established routine of activity, and how a change in a pre-established order dislocates and renders difficult our movements, activities and the whole routine of life. Again, we know how weak and monotonous stimuli render us languid and drowsy, and very often lead to sleep. We are also well acquainted with different cases of partial alertness in the case of normal sleep, for example a sleeping mother next to her sick child. All these phenomena are analogous to those constantly met with in our animals as described in the preceding lectures, and there is no point in further discussing them in the present lecture. The discussion of pathological cases, however, will prove instructive.

Contemporary medicine distinguishes " nervous " and " psychic " disturbances—neuroses and psychoses, but this distinction is, of course, only arbitrary. No real line of demarcation can be drawn between these two groups : it is impossible to imagine a deviation of higher activities from normal without a functional or structural disturbance of the cortex. The distinction between " nervous " and " psychic " affections is a distinction made on grounds of greater or smaller complexity and subtlety in the disturbance of the nervous activity. Our experiments definitely show the validity of such a distinction. So long as we deal with animals in which the patho-logical disturbance results from functional interferences including violent changes in the conditions of life (such as our dogs experienced in the great flood in Petrograd), or on account of small operations on the cortex, we can grasp the mechanism of these disturbances more or less satisfactorily and express it in terms of neuro-physiology. Such disturbances would come under the classification of " neuroses." But if the disturbances are the results of extirpation or destruction by scar of large parts of the cortex we encounter great difficulty in picturing the mechanism of the resulting disturbance in the nervous activity, and we depend more largely upon various suppositions which still remain to be verified and controlled. Such disturbances would be classified as " psychoses." Obviously this difference in our attitude is due entirely to the much greater complexity of the disturbance in the latter cases, and to the inadequacy of present-day physiological analysis. We shall not discuss any conjectured subjective sphere of our animals, but shall consider both cases simply as disturbances in the normal cortical activity—smaller and more elementary in the former and more extensive and more complicated in the latter cases.

In the dog two conditions were found to produce pathological disturbances by functional interference, namely, an unusually acute clashing of the excitatory and inhibitory processes, and the influence of strong and extraordinary stimuli. In man precisely similar conditions constitute the usual causes of nervous and psychic disturbances. Different conditions productive of extreme excitation, such as intense grief or bitter insults, often lead, when the natural reactions are inhibited by the necessary restraint, to profound and prolonged loss of balance in nervous and psychic activity. So, too, neuroses and psychoses may develop as a result of different powerful stimuli, e.g. extreme danger to oneself or to near friends, or even the spectacle of some frightful event not affecting one directly. At the same time we know that the same influence may produce a profound disturbance in some individuals and show no trace of effect on others, according to the power of resistance of the nervous system in each case. Exactly the same difference is observed also in dogs, which show a great variation in regard to the production of pathological disturbances. We had dogs in which one of the most efficacious methods of evoking nervous disturbances, namely, a direct transition from an inhibitory to an excitatory rate of stimulation of the same place of the skin, failed to produce the slightest effect after a great number of repetitions on many days. In others disturbance occurred eventually after many repetitions, while in some it was produced by a single juxtaposition of the stimuli. In the same manner the great flood, which, as was mentioned previously, led to a profound disturbance, obviously analogous to traumatic neurosis in man, produced this effect only in some of the dogs, namely, those of an extremely inhibitable type.

It has been seen that the above-mentioned method may lead to different forms of disturbance, depending on the type of nervous system of the animal. In dogs with the more resistant nervous system it leads to a predominance of excitation ; in dogs with the less resistant nervous system, to a predominance of inhibition. So far as can be judged on the basis of casual observation I believe that these two variations in the pathological disturbance of the cortical activity in animals are comparable to the two forms of neurosis in man—in the pre-Freudian terminology *neurasthenia* and *hysteria*—

the first with exaggeration of the excitatory and weakness of the inhibitory process, the second with a predominance of the inhibitory and weakness of the excitatory process. There are grounds for considering the first type as having a more resistant nervous system which (at least in some cases) is able to perform a large amount of coordinated activity, while the weaker type of nervous system is quite incapable of adaptation to the ordinary conditions of life. The first type also goes through periods of weakness, and this can easily be understood, since for the most part such individuals are continuously excited, active, profligate of nervous activity—and the nervous exhaustion must, of course, be made good. This type may be regarded as having a longer period in the sequence of activity and rest of the nervous system as compared with the normally balanced brain, the periods of excitation and inhibition being more accentuated. Though the second type may exhibit violent attacks of excitation this does not imply greater vigour of their nervous system : the excitation is generally without aim and without result—so to speak, crudely mechanical. In the observations made on dogs we obtained, I believe, some indication as to the origin and character of this excitation. We had one dog [experiments of Dr. Frolov] of a very inhibitable type, or, as it would be more commonly described, a very cowardly and submissive animal. This animal served for experiments upon gastric secretion, and in the course of the experiments it had to remain in the stand for many hours in succession. It never went to sleep while in the stand : though remaining very quiet it preserved a fully alert posture, only moving slightly and sometimes carefully shifting its legs. This state of the animal was not semi-cataleptic, since it invariably responded to the call of its name. When it was taken from the stand and freed from the loops and leash, this dog invariably entered into astonishing fits of excitation, howling, throwing itself vigorously about, sometimes upsetting the stand and falling off the table. This excitation (which by the way was not caused by desire for micturition or defaecation) could not be stopped in any way, whether by shouting, petting or by striking the animal, which became absolutely unrecognizable. A few minutes of exercise in the yard restored it to its normal state, the animal leading the way of itself into the experimental room, jumping up on the stand and again standing motionless. The same behaviour was sometimes observed in other dogs, but never in so exaggerated a form. These wild attacks of excitation may possibly be regarded as a brief outburst of positive induction following a prolonged and intense inhibition. A similar explanation may also be suggested for the fits of excitation in neurosis of the second type in which the inhibitory tendency prevails. The possible participation of another cause also is suggested by experiments [by Dr. Podkopaev] on another dog. This dog was a quiet animal with a well-balanced nervous system, not very alert, which did not jump into the stand of itself, but when placed in the stand stood quietly and never slept. The positive and negative conditioned reflexes were very constant and precise. The dog had several conditioned reflexes established to stimulation of places along one side of the body, a stimulus on a definite place on the hind leg being a positive alimentary stimulus and all the rest negative. All these reflexes had developed rapidly and were very precise. During the application of the tactile stimuli the animal had always remained quiet, not making any local or general movements ; even the positive motor alimentary reaction was very weak, and the dog was slow in taking the food. The development of the negative reflexes had been begun at the front paw—the most remote from the positive place. Suddenly and quite unexpectedly the stimulation of the front paw began to be accompanied by a motor reaction in the form of rapid twitching of the stimulated extremity. Sometimes the twitching assumed the rhythm of the tactile stimulus. Such local motor reactions began now to appear on the successive stimulation of other inhibitory places in closer and closer proximity to the place of positive significance, the reaction at the same time becoming more vigorous, more extensive and involving all extremities. The head and neck, however, remained motionless, not participating in the activity of the extremities. Salivary secretion was of course absent. When, however, the place on the thigh nearest to the positive one was now also made positive the motor reaction to the stimulation of this place vanished entirely. The same happened also to the motor reaction for other places when they were transformed from negative into positive ones —with the exception only of the two most remote places which, though acquiring the positive secretory effect, continued to evoke the local motor reaction in a much weakened form. The fact that this phenomenon made its appearance not during the establishment, but only after the complete development, of the differentiation—this and its localized form make it probable that the disturbance was of spinal origin, occurring on account of a partial functional disconnection of the cortical cutaneous analyser from the lower centres. A similar explanation may be advanced for analogous cases in man.

We have a number of further observations which recall some more or less well-known forms of nervous disturbance in man. I shall remind you of the dog [experiments of Dr. Rickman (p. 302)] which was brought into a state in which it could not withstand any strong conditioned stimuli—immediately entering into an inhibitory state so that a conditioned activity could be elicited only by the use of very weak stimuli. It is permissible to draw a parallel, of course only as regards the mechanism, between the case of this dog and the cases of many years of sleep in human patients—for example, of a young girl described by Pierre Janet and of an adult man as observed in one of the Petrograd hospitals for nervous disorders. The patients in both cases were lying in a continuous sleep, entirely motionless, did not speak a word and had to be fed artificially and kept clean. Only during the stillness of the night, when the daily bustle of life with its strong and varied stimuli quieted down, had the patients a chance of exhibiting some activity. The patient of Pierre Janet was observed to eat and even write during the night. It was reported of the Petrograd case that sometimes during the night he got out of bed. When this patient, at the age of 60, after nearly twenty years of continuous sleep, began to improve and could speak, he recounted that he often heard and saw everything occurring around him, but had no strength either to move or to speak. Both these cases obviously presented an extreme weakening of the nervous system— especially of the cortex—which quickly led under the influence of any strong stimuli to a development of complete inhibition, i.e. sleep.

In the same dog we observed also another symptom of pathological nervous activity which has often been described, in the neuro-pathological literature, for man. This dog had a narrowly localized chronic functional lesion of the cortical part of the acoustic analyser, any stimulation of the deranged part of the analyser by an appropriate agent leading to inhibition of the entire cortex. We are aware of many states of the nervous system in man in which a perfectly normal activity can be maintained only so long as the man is not affected by any, sometimes almost a negligible, component—even the remotest hint—of those strong stimuli which originally evoked the nervous disturbance.

Finally, I want to remind you of the case, described in the nineteenth lecture, of periodical visual illusion in one of our dogs (p. 327).

This was probably due to distortion of the effect upon the cortex of the external visual stimuli by local, internal stimuli originating in the extending scar. Many similar cases of illusions in man are probably due to the interference of similar cortical stimuli of internal local origin.

Though our research abounds in cases of pathological disturbances which are comparable to those observed in man, I do not feel either safe or justified in proceeding in my comparison beyond the above observations, and these should not be taken as in any sense explaining the incalculably complex symptoms observed in man, but only as showing that a comparison of a general nature can even now be made. Similar comparisons between experimental animals and man can be made also in respect to therapeutic measures—general and pharmacological. It has been stated already that rest and interruption of experiments in many cases helped in the restoration of normal conditions. Several interesting details must, however, be described. One of our dogs was brought into an extremely excitable state by a clash of the inhibitory with the excitatory process [experiments of Dr. Petrova]. All forms of inhibition were disturbed, all negative conditioned stimuli acquiring positive properties. On application of any of the conditioned stimuli—those formerly positive as well as those formerly negative—the animal entered into a state of pronounced excitation which, as generally happens, was accompanied by severe hyperpnoea. The disuse of negative conditioned reflexes did not improve the condition of the animal. Hyperpnoea continued and the positive reflexes remained excessive. It was then resolved to use only those of the positive stimuli which were physiologically weak, *i.e.* the visual and tactile, and to discard the auditory, which as a rule in our experiments were strong. The beneficial result of this treatment was immediate. The animal became quiet, hyperpnoea disappeared and the magnitude of the salivary effect returned to normal. After some time it became possible gradually to introduce again the stronger positive stimuli without upsetting the result of the treatment. Furthermore, after several days a pre-established differentiation of the tactile stimuli according to place (one of the easiest forms of internal inhibition) spontaneously reappeared in full vigour, and this without any signs of excitation on the part of the animal. This is an instructive case, showing how a diminution in the strength of stimuli affecting the hemispheres led to a diminution of the excessive excitability of the cortical elements. Of course, in the treatment of neurotic conditions in the human subject similar therapeutic measures are very widely adopted.

I shall describe also another case which seems to me very instructive from the point of view of therapy. In this instance we are concerned with a dog which was entirely out of the ordinary run and which had an obviously abnormal reaction to cutaneous stimuli, a reaction associated with a strong excitation of the cortex [experiments of Dr. Prorokov (p. 183)]. On application of the usual tactile stimulus to the skin of the thigh the animal immediately began to wriggle its hind quarters, stamp its hind legs, throw up its head in a peculiar manner and make peculiar little noises, sometimes yawning. On administration of food and while it was being eaten the reaction disappeared. Contrary to our expectation the presence of this reaction did not in any way interfere with the development of a conditioned reflex to the tactile stimulus, a phenomenon which usually occurs in the presence of some extraneous motor reactions in animals, e.g. retraction of the extremities or local twitching of the platysma muscle. In the case under discussion, however, a conditioned reflex developed very quickly, and, what was quite exceptional, this tactile cutaneous salivary conditioned reflex was even stronger in intensity than the reflexes to the most powerful auditory stimuli. Similarly, the motor alimentary reaction—which usually replaced the peculiar special reaction somewhere towards the middle of the isolated action of the cutaneous conditioned stimulus—was considerably stronger than the motor reaction observed with any other conditioned stimulus. Furthermore, the usual period of " alimentary " excitation observed as an after-effect following reinforcement with food was the most intense and the most prolonged in the case of the tactile cutaneous stimulus. In the experiments in which the tactile stimulus was used the dog showed signs of a general excitation : at the slightest sound from the experimenter's room the animal immediately responded by the peculiar motor reaction. Obviously the tactile cutaneous stimulation in this dog brought about a vigorous and widely irradiated excitation in the cortex. The nature of this excitation remained, however, unknown. It did not seem to be associated with any sexual reflexes since it was not accompanied by erection of the penis. It seemed to be something like the common reaction to tickling. At any rate it was a sufficiently interesting nervous phenomenon to study, and we determined to overcome it. For this purpose we began to develop internal inhibition in the form of differentiation of tactile stimuli according to their place of application. On account of initial generalization the application of the tactile stimulus to the shoulder gave some conditioned secretion, and this also was accompanied by the special motor reaction. On repetition of the stimulus without reinforcement the motor and the salivary components of the conditioned reflex disappeared (8 repetitions), and this was followed by the disappearance of the special motor reaction (40 repetitions). The stimulation of the place on the thigh continued, however, to evoke the special motor, and the alimentary motor, reaction in succession. A differentiation was now developed to stimulation of a place on the side of the animal nearer to the thigh. The different stages repeated themselves in the same way as for stimulation on the shoulder, but again the special reaction to stimulation of the thigh did not diminish. Finally a differentiation was developed to a tactile stimulation on the hind paw, and now the special motor reaction in response to the stimulation on the thigh first began to weaken, and then disappeared altogether. At the same time the strength of the salivary reflex to the tactile stimulus took up its usual position in the series of conditioned reflexes as regards the relative strengths of the stimuli producing them, falling from its predominant place to a position below the conditioned reflexes to auditory stimuli.

In this manner we see that the development of several inhibitory areas in the cortical part of the cutaneous analyser abolished the special cutaneous reflex, at the same time preserving, and even rendering normal, the alimentary cutaneous conditioned reflex.

This example and other observations suggest that a gradual development of internal inhibition in the cortex should be used for re-establishment of the balance of normal conditions in cases of an unbalanced nervous system. The method is being used at present on the dog, described in the eighteenth lecture, which had a narrowly localized functional injury of the acoustic analyser. Since this region was specially related to the beating of a metronome we resolved to develop a differential inhibition of other auditory stimuli related to normal areas of the acoustic analyser. We hope that irradiation of the inhibition to the defective metronome-point will have a beneficial effect, restoring this point to its normal excitability and normal activity. I do not know whether similar therapeutic measures (not counting of course general sedatives such as hot baths) are applied in human neurotherapy.

We shall now attempt a discussion of borderline states of the nervous system in our dogs, states merging from a normal into a pathological character which, on the analogy of corresponding human states, should in some instances be described as psycho-pathological. These are different hypnotic phases, such as the transition phases between the alert state and sleep, and the passive defence reflex. We have seen in the sixteenth lecture that the transition of animals from the alert state into sleep is based upon the development in the brain of an inhibitory process which, under the influence of definite stimuli, is initiated in the cortex and reaches different stages of intensity and extensity during the different phases of the developing sleep. Undoubtedly, even at present, the observations made upon animals allow in part of a physiological interpretation of the fundamental aspects of hypnotism in the human subject.

We shall consider first the conditions under which hypnotic states develop. In animals, as we already know, they appear, as the result of monotonous stimuli of a small and medium intensity repeated for a long time (the most common case in our experiments), more or less gradually, while in the case of stimuli of a considerably greater intensity they appear quickly—a form of animal hypnotism which has been known for a very long time. The stimuli directly initiating these states, both weak and strong, can also be signalled by any other stimuli which have conditioned properties in respect to the first. In this connection the special mode of formation of conditioned reflexes described in the sixth lecture will be remembered where the neutral stimulus repeated several times in conjunction with the pre-established inhibitory stimulus acquired inhibitory properties of its own [experiments by Dr. Volborth (p. 106)]. The method of inducing hypnosis in man involves conditions entirely analogous to those which produced it in our dogs. The classical method consisted in the performance of so-called " passes "—weak, monotonously repeated tactile and visual stimuli, just as in our experiments upon animals. At present the more usual method consists in the repetition of some form of words, describing sleep, articulated in a flat and monotonous tone of voice. Such words are, of course, conditioned stimuli which have become associated with the state of sleep. In this manner any stimulus which has coincided several times with the development of sleep can now by itself initiate sleep or a hypnotic state. The mechanism is analogous to the inhibitory chain reflexes, which are similar to the positive conditioned chain reflexes, *i.e.* reflexes of different orders which have been described in the third lecture [experiments of Dr. Volborth]. Finally, hypnosis in the case of hysteria (in the sense of Charcot) can be obtained by the application of strong and unexpected stimuli, as in the old method of initiating hypnosis in animals. It is obvious that in this respect physiologically weak stimuli may act in the same manner if, on account of a coincidence in time, they have acquired signalling properties in respect to the strong ones. Most of the procedures producing hypnosis become more and more effective the more frequently they are repeated.

One of the first expressions of hypnosis in man is the loss of so-called voluntary movements and the development of a cataleptic state, *i.e.* maintenance by different parts of the body of the position given to them by external forces. This may best be regarded as an isolated inhibition of the motor analyser which has not descended to the sub-cortical motor centres. Other areas of the cortex may continue to function quite normally. A man in a state of hypnosis may understand what we tell him, may realize what kind of unnatural posture we have given him and may attempt to change it, but is incapable of doing so. The outward signs of the hypnotic state are similar in men and animals. It has already been described in the sixteenth lecture how some animals retain their alert posture while all conditioned reflex activity disappears—obviously a case of inhibition of the entire cortex without descent of the inhibition into sub-cortical regions. Other dogs continue to react to all the conditioned stimuli by the secretory component of the reflex only, exhibiting no motor reaction and not touching the food—obviously a case of an isolated inhibition of the motor analyser. Finally, in animals hypnotized by the old method it could often be observed that the body and extremities remained motionless while the animal yet continued to follow everything with its eyes, and even accepted the food. This is obviously a case of a still more localized inhibition within the motor analyser. The local " tonic " (*i.e.* spinal flexor and extensor) reflexes, which are observed in man and animals in some cases, become understandable only if we postulate complete inhibition of the motor analyser of the cortex.

When we come to deal with more complicated forms of the hypnotic state, it obviously becomes, for several reasons, difficult, or even impossible, to draw a parallel between man and animals. As already stated, we know only a few of the phases of the hypnotic state, especially as regards their relative intensity, and we have no definite idea as to the sequence of their development. We are not familiar with the manner in which these phases manifest themselves under natural conditions of life in animals, since the transition phases were observed not in the natural individual and social sphere of life, but only in the restricted sphere of a laboratory environment. In man, however, we become familiar with these phenomena under more normal conditions of life and we can evoke and investigate them with the help of the most valuable signalling medium—speech. Of course, on account of the extraordinary complexity of the behaviour of man as compared with the higher animals, the latter may not exhibit some of the phases of the hypnotic state seen in man at all. It is, therefore, only those crude and elementary results obtained in the animal which can be used for an attempt at a physiological interpretation of the different hypnotic phases in man. Let us consider the automatism of the hypnotized subject who repeats in a stereotyped fashion the movements of the hypnotist, being able to perform even difficult movements such as balancing along a difficult path. Obviously we deal with a certain degree of inhibition of some parts of the cortex—a state in which the more complicated forms of normal activity are excluded and replaced by responsiveness to immediate stimuli. This partial inhibition allows of or even favours the establishment and reinforcement of the physiological connections between certain stimuli and certain activities, e.g. movements. In this manner, in hypnosis all activities based on "imitation" are accentuated and we see revealed the long-submerged reflex which in all of us in childhood forms and develops the complicated individual and social behaviour. Similarly, some change in the environment, which in former days had repeatedly evoked certain movements affecting certain analysers, in hypnosis calls forth without fail and in a stereotyped manner the old response. It is a common occurrence that, being predominantly preoccupied with some one activity, we can simultaneously perform some other activity which has long been practised, i.e. those parts of the cortex involved in this older response, although in a state of partial inhibition through negative induction, still continue to function in a normal manner. That this interpretation is somewhere near the mark I become more and more convinced, through observing the diminution in the reactivity of my own brain through my advancing age (my diminished memory of recent events). Moreover, with time I progressively lose the faculty, when busy with one activity, of performing correctly another also. Apparently the concentrated excitation of some definite point induces, on account of diminished excitability of the cortex, such a strong inhibition of the rest of the cortex that even the conditioned stimuli of the old firmly established reflexes are now below the threshold for excitation. The above described phase of hypnosis in the human subject may perhaps be compared with what I have termed the narcotic phase of transition in dogs, when strong and old reflexes persist while the more recent ones disappear.

Among the various aspects of the hypnotic state in man attention may be drawn to " suggestion " so-called and its physiological interpretation. Obviously for man speech provides conditioned stimuli which are just as real as any other stimuli. At the same time speech provides stimuli which exceed in richness and many-sidedness any of the others, allowing comparison neither qualitatively nor quantitatively with any conditioned stimuli which are possible in animals. Speech, on account of the whole preceding life of the adult, is connected up with all the internal and external stimuli which can reach the cortex, signalling all of them and replacing all of them, and therefore it can call forth all those reactions of the organism which are normally determined by the actual stimuli themselves. We can, therefore, regard " suggestion " as the most simple form of a typical conditioned reflex in man. The command of the hypnotist, in correspondence with the general law, concentrates the excitation in the cortex of the subject (which is in a condition of partial inhibition) in some definite narrow region, at the same time intensifying (by negative induction) the inhibition in the rest of the cortex and so abolishing all competing effects of contemporary stimuli and of traces left by previously received ones. This accounts for the large and practically insurmountable influence of suggestion as a stimulus during hypnosis as well as shortly after it. The command retains its effect after the termination of hypnosis, remaining independent of other stimuli, being impermeable to them, since at the time of primary introduction of the stimulus into the cortex it was prevented from establishing any connection with the rest of the cortex. The great number of stimuli which speech can replace explains the fact that we can suggest to a hypnotized subject so many different activities, and influence and direct the activities of his brain. It could be questioned why does suggestion carry in itself such a commanding influence as compared with dreams, which are usually forgotten and only have a very small vital significance ? But dreams are due to traces, generally of very old stimuli, while suggestion is a powerful and immediate stimulus. Moreover, hypnosis depends upon a smaller intensity of inhibition than sleep. Suggestion, therefore, is doubly effective. Still further, suggestion as a stimulus is brief, isolated and complete, and therefore vigorous, while dreams are generally linked up into chains of various, sometimes inconsistent or antagonistic, traces of stimuli. The fact that it is possible to suggest to a hypnotized subject almost anything, however little it may correspond to the physical reality, and to evoke a reaction in opposition to the actual reality—for example, the reaction appropriate to a bitter taste when the reality is a sweet taste—this fact, I believe, can be compared with the fact observed in the paradoxical phase of transition in the dog, that weak stimuli have a greater effect than strong ones. The real stimulus from the sweet substance going directly to the corresponding cortical cells should be expected to be much stronger than the substituted verbal stimulus of " bitter," which goes through auditory cells to the chemical analyser of taste for bitter—just as a conditioned stimulus of the first order is always stronger than one of the second order. The significance of the paradoxical phase is not limited to pathological states such as those previously observed, and it is highly probable that it plays an important part in normal men too, who often are apt to be much more influenced by words than by the actual facts of the surrounding reality. I hope to be able to produce a phenomenon in animals analogous to " suggestion " in man during hypnosis.

The fact that certain phases of the hypnotic state in man remain more or less stationary repeats itself in dogs. Similarly, under certain conditions and in dependence on the individual condition of the nervous system the hypnotic state in man, as in animals, passes more or less quickly into complete sleep.

The passive defence reflex stands in a definite connection with the hypnotic state. As I suggested previously (p. 312) the old form of hypnosis in animals may be regarded with reason as a reaction of passive self-preservation, occurring when the animal meets with some very powerful or extraordinary external stimulus, and consisting in a more or less profound immobilization of the animal by means of an inhibition, beginning in the cortical cells representative of all the skeletal muscles (motor analyser). This reflex was often observed in our experimental animals, of course in different degrees of intensity and in somewhat different forms, always, however, retaining its fundamental inhibitory character. The variations consisted in a smaller or greater diminution of the movements, in a smaller or greater weakening, or in the disappearance, of conditioned reflexes. The passive defence reflex was usually evoked by relatively unfamiliar and powerful external stimuli. The relative strength of a stimulus will of course depend on the state of the given nervous system, on its inherent properties, the state of health or disease, and on different periods of life. Animals which have been employed many times in front of a large audience remain quite normal under such conditions, while those which are exposed for the first time enter into a state of powerful inhibition. The exceptional dog described before (p. 402) behaved towards even the slightest changes in the environment as if to strong stimuli, and its activities became deeply inhibited. Some of the dogs which passed through the extraordinary stimulus of the flood entered into a chronic pathological state and now became inhibited under the influence of strong conditioned stimuli, which previously had produced a specific conditioned effect. Finally, some other dogs become as easily inhibited but only in some definite phases of hypnosis. The following is a particularly striking case. A dog which under the conditions of our experiments remains fully alert accepts the food following the conditioned stimuli quickly and with avidity. By repeated application of weak conditioned stimuli a certain stage of hypnosis is induced in the animal, which soon becomes practically motionless. When a strong conditioned stimulus is now applied the animal first turns in the direction from which the food is administered, then turns away without touching it. To a casual observer the animal looks frightened. A weak conditioned stimulus is now applied and the animal immediately approaches the plate and quietly takes the food. On dispersing the hypnotic state all the conditioned stimuli again give their normal effect. Obviously in the special phase of hypnosis of the animal the old and usual stimuli now produce the effect of very strong ones, evoking an inhibitory reflex. In a similar manner, in our exceedingly inhibitable dog " Brains " as soon as the pitch of the excitability of the cortex was raised by the special method described on page 381, there was observed a considerable weakening of the otherwise almost continuous reflex of passive self-preservation.

In all the cases which have just been described what is most striking is the extremely characteristic passive self-protective postures of the animal. When I recall a large number of experiments performed one after another and year after year it is hardly possible not to conclude that at least in most cases what is known in psychology under the names of " fear," " cowardice " or " caution " has a physiological substrate in a state of inhibition of the nervous system, which varies in intensity and so produces different intensities of the reflex of passive self-protection. Developing these conceptions further we are bound to regard the obsession of fear, and different phobias as natural symptoms of inhibition in a pathological and weakened nervous system. There are, of course, certain forms of fear and cowardice, as for instance flight and panic, and certain postures of servility, which apparently do not conform with the idea of an underlying inhibitory process, having a much more active aspect. These types must, of course, be subjected to experimental analysis, but it is perhaps not impermissible to regard them provisionally as developing in co-operation with, and as a result of, inhibition of the cortex. We have even now a few observations which conform with this point of view.

I would like to turn briefly to the experiments described at the end of the preceding lecture. If on repeating them in different variations the preliminary results should find full confirmation, these results will throw some light upon one of the darkest points of our subjective self—namely, upon the relations between the conscious and the unconscious. The experiments if confirmed will have demonstrated that such an important cortical function as synthesis (" association ") may take place even in those cortical areas which are in a state of inhibition on account of the existence at that moment of a predominant focus of strong excitation. Though the actual synthesizing activity may not enter our field of consciousness the synthesis may nevertheless take place, and under favourable conditions it may enter the field of consciousness as a link already formed, seeming to originate spontaneously.

In concluding this series of lectures I want to repeat that all the experiments, those of other workers as well as our own, which have set as their object a purely physiological interpretation of the activity of the higher nervous system, I regard as being in the nature only of a preliminary inquiry, which has however, I fully believe, entirely justified its inception. We have indisputably the right to claim that our investigation of this extraordinarily complex field has followed the right direction, and that, although not a near, nevertheless a complete, success awaits it. So far as we ourselves are concerned we can only say that at present we are confronted with many more problems than ever before. At first, not to lose sight of the main issue, we were compelled to simplify, and, so to speak, schematize the subject. At present, after having acquired some knowledge of its general principles, we feel surrounded, nay crushed, by the mass of details, all calling for elucidation.

BIBLIOGRAPHY

THE following bibliography comprises all the published researches upon the physiology of conditioned reflexes performed in my own laboratories in Petrograd. The first paper giving a more or less systematic description of "natural" conditioned reflexes—then called "psychic reflexes"—was published by Dr. Wolfson in the form of a thesis entitled *Observations upon Salivary Secretion* (Petrograd, 1899). The term "conditioned reflex" was first used in print by Dr. Tolochinov, who completed his experiments in 1901 and communicated the results at the Congress of Natural Sciences in Helsingfors in 1903.

The bibliography is divided into twenty-three sections. This division has been made for the convenience of those who wish to obtain a preliminary acquaintance with one or another aspect of the subject. The titles of papers quoted in more than one section are given in full in that section to which their main part belongs. Since the papers referred to in one section treat also of other aspects, a detailed knowledge can be achieved only by reading the main bulk of the literature. In each section the literature is set down in chronological order. Many of the experiments quoted in these lectures were taken from researches which have only recently been completed and are not yet published, or which are still in progress. These could not, therefore, be included in the bibliography.

I. GENERAL

(1) *Pavlov, I. P.* " Twenty years of objective study of the higher nervous activity (behaviour) of animals." State publication, 3rd edition, 1925. *Articles*, Nos. 1, 2, 3, 4, 7, 9, 10, 11, 13, 17, 20, 21, 23, 26, 29, 31, 33, 35.

II. METHODS

(1) *Pavlov, I. P.* "Twenty years of objective study of the higher nervous activity of animals." *Article*, No. 12.

(2) *Hanike, E. A.* "The construction of sound-proof chambers." *Bulletin of the Scientific Institute of Lesgaft*, vol. v. 1922.

(3) *Hanike, E. A.* " Upon the production of pure tones." *Archive of Biological Sciences,* vol. xxiii. Nos. 4-5, 1924.

(4) *Podkopaev, N. A.* " The technical methods employed in the study of conditioned reflexes." Petrograd, 1926.

III. EXTERNAL INHIBITION

(1) *Babkin, B. P.* See section IVa (3) chapter vii.

(2) *Vassiliev, P. N.* " The action of extraneous stimuli upon established conditioned reflexes." *Proc. Russian Med. Soc. in Petrograd,* vol. 73, 1906.

(3) *Mishtovt, G. V.* " Development of inhibition of an artificial conditioned reflex (auditory) by means of different stimuli." *Thesis,* Petrograd, 1907 ; Preliminary communication in the *Proc. Russian Med. Soc. in Petrograd,* vol. 74, 1907.

(4) *Perelzweig, I. J.* See section IVa (4) chapter iv.

(5) *Kasherininova, N. A.* See section X (1).

(6) *Nikiforovsky, P. M.* " An interesting form of dis-inhibition of conditioned reflexes." *Proc. Russian Med. Soc. in Petrograd,* vol. 76, 1909.

(7) *Bilina, A. S.* " The simple inhibition of conditioned reflexes." *Thesis, Petrograd,* 1910.

(8) *Egorov, J. E.* " The influence of different alimentary conditioned reflexes one upon another." *Thesis, Petrograd,* 1911.

(9) *Savich, A. A.* " Further contributions to the study of the influence of conditioned reflexes one upon another." *Thesis, Petrograd,* 1913.

(10) *Rosova, L. V.* " Interaction between different forms of external inhibition of conditioned reflexes." *Thesis, Petrograd,* 1914.

(11) *Foursikov, D. S.* " Effect of external inhibition upon the development of differentiation and of a conditioned inhibitor." *Russian Journal of Physiology,* vol. iv. 1922.

(12) *Foursikov, D. S.* " Effect of the investigatory reaction upon the development of a conditioned inhibitor and of differentiation." *Russian Journal of Physiology,* vol. iv. 1922.

IV. INTERNAL INHIBITION

(a) Extinction

(1) *Tolochinov, I. E.* " Contributions à l'étude de la physiologie et de la psychologie des glandes salivaires." *Forhändlingar vid Nordiska Naturforskare och Läkaremötet.* Helsingfors, 1903.

(2) *Boldirev, P. N.* " The development of artificial conditioned reflexes and their properties." *Proc. Russian Med. Soc. in Petrograd,* 1905-1906.

(3) *Babkin, B. P.* "A systematic investigation of the higher nervous (psychic) functions in the dog." *Thesis, Petrograd,* 1904.

(4) *Perelzweig, I. J.* "Contributions to the study of conditioned reflexes." *Thesis, Petrograd,* 1907.

(5) *Zeliony, G. P.* See section VIII (1).

(6) *Kasherininova, N. A.* See X (1) chapter 8.

(7) *Eliason, M. M.* "Restoration of extinguished reflexes by the use of unconditioned stimuli." *Proc. Russian Med. Soc. in Petrograd,* vol. 74, 1907.

(8) *Zavadsky, I. V.* See IVc (2).

(9) *Volborth, G. V.* See XX (4).

(10) *Gorn, E. L.* See IVb (5).

(11) *Potehin, S. I.* "Contributions to the physiology of internal inhibition of conditioned reflexes." *Thesis, Petrograd,* 1911 ; Preliminary communication, *Proc. Russian Med. Soc. in Petrograd,* vol. 78, 1911.

(12) *Degtiareva, V. A.* See IVd (7).

(13) *Kogan, B. A.* See V (4).

(14) *Chebotareva, O. V.* See IVd (5).

(15) *Ten-Cate, J. J.* "Contributions to the study of irradiation and concentration of extinctive inhibition." *Bulletin of the Institute of Lesgaft,* vol. 3, 1921.

(16) *Podkopaev, N. A.* See V (11) and (12).

(17) *Frolov, G. P.,* and *Vindelband, O. A.* "A special case of extinction of an artificial conditioned reflex." Commun. at 38th meeting of Petrograd Physiol. Soc., 1923.

(18) *Popov, N. A.* "Extinction of the investigatory reflex in the dog." *Russian Jour. Physiol.,* vol. iii. 1923.

(19) *Neitz, E. A.* "Mutual interaction of conditioned reflexes." *Bulletin of Military Med. Acad.,* 1908 ; Preliminary Commun. *Proc. Russian Med. Soc. in Petrograd,* vol. 74, 1907.

(20) *Pimenov, P. P.* See IVe (7) chapter 2.

(21) *Makovsky, I. S.* See XII (4).

(22) *Valkov, A. V.* "A special case of irradiation of extinctive inhibition." Commun. at 60th meeting of Petrograd Physiol. Soc., 1924.

(23) *Popov, N. A.* "Extinction of the investigatory reflex in the dog." *Russian Jour. Physiol.,* vol. iii. 1923.

(24) *Frolov, G. P.,* and *Windelband, O. A.* "A special case of extinction of an artificial conditioned reflex." *Archive of Biological Sciences,* vol. xxv. Nos. 4 and 5, 1926.

(b) Differentiation

(1) *Zeliony, G. P.* " Contribution to the problem of the reaction of dogs to auditory stimuli." *Thesis, Petrograd,* 1907 ; Prelim. Commun. *Russian Med. Soc. in Petrograd,* vol. 73, 1906.

(2) *Beliakov, V. V.* " Contributions to the physiology of differentiation of external stimuli." *Thesis, Petrograd,* 1911.

(3) *Snegirev, G. V.* " Contributions to the study of conditioned reflexes : Specialization of auditory conditioned reflexes in the dog." *Clinical Monographs of Practical Medicine,* Petrograd, 1911.

(4) *Potehin, S. I.* See IVA (11).

(5) *Gorn, E. L.* " Contributions to the physiology of internal inhibition of conditioned reflexes." *Thesis, Petrograd,* 1912 ; Preliminary Commun. *Proc. Russian Med. Soc. in Petrograd,* vol. 79, 1912.

(6) *Friedman, S. S.* " Further contributions to the physiology of differentiation of external stimuli." *Thesis, Petrograd,* 1913.

(7) *Ponizovsky, N. P.* " Inhibitory after-effect of differential, and of conditioned inhibition upon heterogeneous conditioned reflexes." *Thesis, Petrograd,* 1912.

(8) *Koupalov, P. S.* " Initial generalization and subsequent specialization of conditioned reflexes." *Archive of Biological Sciences,* vol. xix. No. 1, 1915.

(9) *Goubergritz, M. M.* " An improved method of developing differentiation of external stimuli." *Thesis, Petrograd,* 1917.

(10) *Foursikov, D. S.* " Differentiation of interrupted auditory stimuli by the dog." *Bulletin of the Institute of Lesgaft,* vol. ii. 1920.

(11) *Anrep, G. V.* " Pitch discrimination in the dog." *Jour. Physiol.* liii. 1920.

(12) *Shenger-Krestovnikova, N. R.* " Contributions to the physiology of differentiation of visual stimuli, and determination of limit of differentiation by the visual analyser of the dog." *Bulletin of Institute of Lesgaft,* vol. iii. 1921.

(13) *Foursikov, D. S.* See III (11).

(14) *Foursikov, D. S.* See III (12).

(15) *Frolov, G. P.* " Differentiation of conditioned trace-stimuli and of trace-inhibitors." *Russian Jour. of Physiol.,* vol. vi. Nos. 4-6, 1924.

(16) *Valkov, A. V.* " The ultimate fate of the internal inhibition of differentiation." *Bulletin of Petrograd Agricultural Institute,* vol. i. 1924 (abstract in *Physiol. Abstracts,* vol. 8, 1924).

(17) *Rosenthal, I. S.* " Upon the specialization of conditioned reflexes." *Archive of Biol. Sciences,* vol. xxiii. Nos. 4-5, 1924.

(18) *Pavlov, I. P.* " Twenty years of objective study of the higher nervous activity of animals." *Article,* No. 16.

(19) *Rosenthal, I. C.* "The mutual interactions of the excitatory and inhibitory processes (a new type of differentiation of tactile conditioned stimuli)." *Collected Papers of the Physiol. Lab. of I. P. Pavlov*, vol. i. Nos. 2-3, 1926.

(c) Delayed Reflexes

(1) *Potehin, S. I.* See IVA (11).
(2) *Zavadsky, I. V.* "Inhibition and dis-inhibition of conditioned reflexes." *Thesis, Petrograd*, 1908 ; Prelim. Commun. *Russian Med. Soc. in Petrograd*, vol. 75, 1908.
(3) *Kreps, E. M.* "The effect of prolongation of delay upon the excitability of the cortex." *Archive of Biol. Sciences*, vol. xxv. Nos. 4-5, 1926.

(d) Conditioned Inhibition

(1) *Perelzweig, I. J.* See IVA (4) chapter 8.
(2) *Krjishkovsky, K. N.* "A contribution to the problem of conditioned inhibition." *Proc. Russian Med. Soc. in Petrograd*, vol. 76, 1909.
(3) *Nikolaev, P. N.* "A contribution to the problem of conditioned inhibition." *Thesis, Petrograd*, 1910.
(4) *Leporsky, N. I.* "A contribution to the problem of conditioned inhibition." *Thesis, Petrograd*, 1911.
(5) *Chebotareva, O. M.* "Further contributions to the physiology of conditioned inhibition." *Thesis, Petrograd*, 1912 ; Preliminary Commun. *Russian Med. Soc.*, vol. 80, 1913.
(6) *Ponizovsky, N. P.* See IVA (7).
(7) *Degtiareva, V. A.* "Contributions to the physiology of internal inhibition." *Thesis, Petrograd*, 1914.
(8) *Pavlova, A. M.* "Contributions to the physiology of conditioned inhibition." *Thesis, Petrograd*, 1915.
(9) *Anrep, G. V.* "Irradiation of conditioned inhibition." *Russian Jour. Physiol.*, vol. i. Nos. 1-2, 1917.
(10) *Foursikov, D. S.* See III (11).
(11) *Foursikov, D. S.* See III (12).
(12) *Anrep, G. V.* "Irradiation of conditioned reflexes." *Proc. Royal Soc.*, vol. B. 94, 1923.

(e) Trace Reflexes

(1) *Pimenov, P. P.* "A special type of conditioned reflexes." *Thesis, Petrograd*, 1907.
(2) *Grossman, F. S.* "Contributions to the physiology of conditioned trace reflexes." *Thesis, Petrograd*, 1909 ; Prelim. Commun. *Russian Med. Soc. in Petrograd*, vol. 77, 1910.

(3) *Dobrovolsky, V. M.* " Alimentary trace reflexes." *Thesis, Petrograd,* 1911.

(4) *Pavlova, V. I.* " Conditioned trace reflexes." *Proc. Russian Med. Soc. in Petrograd,* vol. 80, 1913.

(5) *Belitz, M. F.* " Conditioned trace reflexes." *Thesis, Petrograd,* 1917.

(6) *Frolov, G. P.* See IVb (15).

(7) *Frolov, G. P.* " Transformation of conditioned trace stimuli and trace conditioned inhibitors into non-trace stimuli." *Collected Papers of Physiol. Lab. of I. P. Pavlov,* vol. i. Nos. 2-3, 1926.

(f) Sleep as Internal Inhibition

(1) *Solomonov, O. S.,* and *Shishlo, A. A.* " Conditioned reflexes and sleep." *Proc. Russian Med. Soc. in Petrograd,* vol. 77, 1910.

(2) *Solomonov, O. S.* " Thermal and tactile conditioned reflexes leading to sleep." *Thesis, Petrograd,* 1910.

(3) *Rojansky, N. A.* " Contributions to the physiology of sleep." *Thesis, Petrograd,* 1913 ; Prelim. Commun. *Russian Med. Soc. in Petrograd,* vol. 79, 1912.

(4) *Rosenthal, I. S.* " Transition of internal inhibition into sleep in extinction of the investigatory reflex." *Communication Petrograd Physiol. Soc.,* May, 1923.

(5) *Pavlov, I. P.* " Twenty years of objective study of the higher nervous activity of animals." *Articles,* 14, 24, 30.

(6) *Bierman, B. N.* " Experimental sleep." *State Publication,* 1925.

V. Irradiation and Concentration of Excitation and Inhibition

(1) *Krasnogorsky, N. I.* " Studies upon central inhibition and upon the localization of the tactile and motor analysers in the cortex of the dog." *Thesis, Petrograd,* 1911.

(2) *Ponizovsky, N. P.* See IVb (7).

(3) *Petrova, M. K.* " Investigations upon irradiation of excitation and inhibition." *Thesis, Petrograd,* 1914 ; Prelim. Commun. *Russian Med. Soc. in Petrograd,* vol. 80, 1913.

(4) *Kogan, B. A.* " Irradiation and concentration of extinctive inhibition." *Thesis, Petrograd,* 1914.

(5) *Manouilov, T. M.* " Contribution to the physiology of inhibition and excitation." *Thesis, Petrograd,* 1917.

(6) *Anrep, G. V.* " Interaction between two different types of internal inhibition." *Archive of Biol. Sciences,* xx. No. 4, 1917.

(7) *Anrep, G. V.* " A static state of irradiation of excitation." *Archive of Biol. Sciences,* xx. No. 4, 1917.

(8) *Anrep, G. V.* " Irradiation of conditioned inhibition." *Russian Jour. Physiol.* vol. i. Nos. 1-2, 1917.

(9) *Ten-Cate, J. J.* See IVA (15).

(10) *Anrep, G. V.* " Irradiation of conditioned reflexes." *Proc. Royal Soc.* vol. B. 93, 1923.

(11) *Foursikov, D. S.* " A static state of irradiation of inhibition." *Archive of Biol. Sciences,* vol. xxiii. Nos. 1-3, 1923 ; Prelim. Commun. *Russian Jour. Physiol.* vol. iv. 1922.

(12) *Siriatsky, V. M.* " A method for disclosure of residual inhibition after concentration of the inhibitory process." Commun. at 48th meeting of Petrograd Physiol. Soc., 1923.

(13) *Rosenthal, I. S.* " A static state of irradiation of excitation." *Archive of Biol. Sciences,* vol. xxiii. Nos. 1-3, 1923.

(14) *Kreps, E. M.* " The after-effect of differentiated stimuli." Commun. at 36th meeting of Petrograd Physiol Soc., 1923.

(15) *Valkov, A. V.* See IVA (22).

(16) *Podkopaev, N. A.* " The mobility of the inhibitory process." *Collected Papers of Physiol. Lab. of I. P. Pavlov,* vol. vii. No. 1, 1924 (abstract in *Physiol. Abstracts,* vol. viii. 1924).

(17) *Podkopaev, N. A.* " Determination of the exact moment at which irradiation of inhibition begins." *I. P. Pavlov Jubilee Volume,* 1924 (abstract in *Physiol. Abstracts,* vol. viii. 1924).

(18) *Siriatsky, V. N.* " The cerebral cortex as a mosaic." Commun. at 2nd Congress of Psycho-neurologists in Petrograd, January, 1924.

(19) *Archangelsky, V. M.* " Comparative intensities of different types of internal inhibition." *Collected Papers of Physiol. Lab. of I. P. Pavlov,* vol. i. No. 1, 1924.

(20) *Pavlov, I. P.* " Twenty years of objective study of the higher nervous activity of animals." *Articles,* 14, 19, 22, 32.

(21) *Ivanov-Smolensky, A. G.* " Irradiation of extinctive inhibition in the acoustic analyser of the dog." *Collected Papers of the Physiol. Lab. of I. P. Pavlov,* vol. i. Nos. 2-3, 1925 ; also *Pavlov Jubilee Vol.,* 1925.

(22) *Bikov, K. M.* " Mutual interaction of excitation and inhibition in the cerebral cortex." Commun. at the 58th meeting of Petrograd Physiol. Soc., January, 1925.

(23) *Kreps, E. M.* " Positive induction and irradiation of inhibition in the cortex." *Pavlov Jubilee Vol.,* 1925.

VI. OLFACTORY ANALYSER (normal conditions)

(1) *Zavadsky, I. V.* " Gyrus pyriformis in its relation to the sense of smell in the dog." *Proc. Russian Med. Soc. in Petrograd,* vol. 76, 1909 ; *Archive of Biol. Sciences,* vol. xv. Nos. 3-5, 1910.

VII. Visual Analyser (normal conditions)

(1) *Orbeli, L. A.* " Visual conditioned reflexes in the dog." *Thesis,* *Petrograd,* 1908 ; Prelim. Commun. *Russian Med. Soc. in Petrograd,* vol. 74, 1907.

(2) *Orbeli, L. A.* " The question of discrimination of colour in the dog." *Problems of Medical Science,* vol. i. 1913.

(3) *Frolov. G. P.* " Reactions of the central nervous system to changes in intensity of illumination." *Proc. Petrograd Soc. for Natural Sciences,* vol. 69, No. 1, 1918.

VIII. Acoustic Analyser (normal conditions)

(1) *Zeliony, G. P.* " The reactions of the dog to auditory stimuli." *Thesis, Petrograd,* 1907 ; Prelim. Commun. *Med. Soc. in Petrograd,* vol. 73, 1906.

(2) *Zeliony, G. P.* " A conditioned reflex to an interruption of a sound." *Proc. of Russian Med. Soc. in Petrograd,* vol. 74, 1907 ; also *Karkov Med. Jour.,* 1908.

(3) *Eliason, M. M.* " Investigation upon the acoustic functions of the dog under normal conditions and after bilateral partial extirpation of the auditory area." *Thesis, Petrograd,* 1908.

(4) *Zeliony, G. P.* " Über der Reaktion der Katze auf Tonreiz." *Zentralblatt für Physiologie,* Bd. xxiii. 1909.

(5) *Bourmakin, V. A.* " Generalization of conditioned auditory reflexes in the dog." *Thesis, Petrograd,* 1909.

(6) *Zeliony, G. P.* " Upon the ability of the dog to discriminate auditory stimuli applied in succession, according to different numbers of their repetition." *Proc. Russian Med. Soc. in Petrograd,* vol. 77, 1910.

(7) *Babkin, B. P.* " Contributions to the study of the acoustic analyser." *Proc. Russian Med. Soc. in Petrograd,* vol. 77, 1910.

(8) *Ousiévich, M. A.* " Further contributions to the study of the acoustic analyser." *Proc. Russian Med. Soc. in Petrograd,* vol. 78, 1911.

(9) *Babkin, B. P.* " The so-called psychic deafness as analysed by the objective method." *Roussky Vrach,* No. 51, 1911.

(10) *Babkin, B. P.* " Further studies upon the normal and the injured acoustic analyser in the dog." *Proc. Russian Med. Soc. in Petrograd,* vol. 78, 1911.

(11) *Anrep, G. V.* " Pitch discrimination in the dog." *Jour. Physiol.* vol. 53, 1920.

(12) *Andréev, A. A.* " The resonance theory of Helmholtz in the light of new observations upon the function of the peripheral end of the acoustic analyser in the dog." *Pavlov Jubilee Vol.,* 1925.

(13) *Ivanov-Smolensky, A. G.* " Irradiation of extinctive inhibition in the acoustic analyser of the dog." *Pavlov Jubilee Vol.*, 1925 ; also *Collected Papers of Physiol. Lab. of I. P. Pavlov*, vol. i. Nos. 2-3, 1926.

IX. THERMAL ANALYSER (normal conditions)

(1) *Voskoboinikova-Granstrem, E. E.* " Temperature of 50° C. as a new artificial conditioned stimulus." *Proc. Russian Med. Soc.*, vol. 73, 1906.

(2) *Babkin, B. P.* " Contributions to the physiology of the frontal lobes of the cortex in the dog." *Bulletin Milit. Med. Acad.*, 1909.

(3) *Shishlo, A. A.* " Thermal centres in the cortex of the hemispheres ; sleep as a reflex." *Thesis, Petrograd*, 1910 ; Prelim. Commun. *Russian Med. Soc. in Petrograd*, vol. 77, 1910.

(4) *Solomonov, O. S.* " Thermal conditioned stimuli." *Proc. Russian Med. Soc. in Petrograd*, vol. 77, 1910.

(5) *Solomonov, O. S.* " Thermal conditioned reflexes and the reflex of sleep in the dog." *Thesis, Petrograd*, 1910.

(6) *Vasiliev, P. N.* " Differentiation of thermal stimuli by the dog." *Thesis, Petrograd*, 1912.

X. TACTILE ANALYSER (normal conditions)

(1) *Kasherininova, N. A.* " Contributions to the study of salivary conditioned reflexes in response to tactile stimuli in the dog." *Thesis, Petrograd*, 1908 ; Prelim. Commun. *Proc. Russian Med. Soc. in Petrograd*, vol. 73, 1906.

(1) *Kasherininova, N. A.* " Tactile stimuli as conditioned salivary stimuli." *Proc. Russian Med. Soc. in Petrograd*, 73, 1926.

(3) *Krasnogorsky, N. I.* See V (1).

(4) *Archangelsky, V. M.* " Peculiarities of tactile conditioned reflexes in the case of partial destruction of the cutaneous analyser." *Proc. Russian Med. Soc. in Petrograd*, vol. 80, 1913.

(5) *Archangelsky, V. M.* " Contributions to the physiology of the cutaneous analyser." *Archive Biol. Sciences*, vol. xxii. No. 1, 1922.

XI. THE MOTOR ANALYSER (normal conditions)

(1) *Krasnogorsky, N. I.* See V (1).

(2) *Archangelsky, V. M.* " Contributions to the physiology of the motor analyser." *Archive of Biol. Sciences*, vol. xxii. No. 1, 1922.

XII. The effects upon conditioned reflexes of extirpation of different parts of the cerebral cortex

(1) *Tihomirov, N. P.* " An investigation of the functions of the hemispheres in the dog by an objective method." *Thesis, Petrograd,* 1906.

(2) *Toropov, N. K.* " Visual conditioned reflexes in the dog after extirpation of the occipital lobes." *Thesis, Petrograd,* 1908 ; Prelim. Commun. *Proc. Russian Med. Soc. in Petrograd,* vol. 75, 1908.

(3) *Orbeli, L. A.* " Contributions to the question of localization of conditioned reflexes in the central nervous system." *Proc. Russian Med. Soc. in Petrograd,* vol. 75, 1908.

(4) *Makovsky, I. S.* " Auditory reflexes after extirpation of the temporal lobes." *Thesis, Petrograd,* 1908 ; Preliminary Communication, *Proc. Russian Med. Soc. in Petrograd,* vol. 75, 1908.

(5) *Eliason, M. M.* See VIII (3).

(6) *Sasonova, A.* " Matériaux pour servir à l'étude des réflexes conditionées." *Thesis, Lausanne,* 1909.

(7) *Babkin, B. P.* See IX (2).

(8) *Krijanovsky, I. I.* " Acoustic conditioned reflexes after extirpation of the temporal lobes in the dog." *Thesis, Petrograd,* 1909.

(9) *Demeedov, V. A.* " Conditioned reflexes after extirpation of the anterior halves of the hemispheres in the dog." *Thesis, Petrograd,* 1909.

(10) *Satournov, N. M.* " Further contributions to the study of conditioned salivary reflexes in a dog with the anterior halves of the hemispheres removed." *Thesis, Petrograd,* 1911.

(11) *Kourdrin, A. N.* " Conditioned reflexes in the dog after extirpation of the posterior halves of the hemispheres." *Thesis, Petrograd,* 1911.

(12) *Kouraev, S. P.* " Observations at a remote post-operative stage upon a dog with damaged anterior lobes." *Thesis, Petrograd,* 1912.

(13) *Babkin, B. P.* " The fundamental characteristics of the functions of the acoustic analyser in a dog after removal of the posterior halves of the hemispheres." *Proc. of Russian Med. Soc. in Petrograd,* vol. 79, 1912.

(14) *Zeliony, G. P.* " Observations upon dogs after complete removal of the cerebral cortex." *Proc. Russian Med. Soc. in Petrograd,* vol. 79, 1912 ; also a second commun. in same volume.

(15) *Archangelsky, V. M.* See X (3).

(16) *Rosenkov, I. P.* " Contributions to the question of correlation of excitation and inhibition in a dog after homolateral extirpation

of gyri coronarius and ectosylvius sin." *Archive Biol. Sciences,* vol. xxiii. Nos. 4-5, 1924.

(17) *Rosenkov, I. P.* "Contributions to the question of correlation of excitation and inhibition in a dog after bilateral extirpation of gyri coronarius and ectosylvius." *Collected Papers of Laboratories of I. P. Pavlov,* vol. i. Nos. 2-3, 1925.

(18) *Pavlov, I. P.* "Twenty years of objective study of the higher nervous activity of animals." *Articles,* 5, 15, 18.

(19) *Foursikov, D. S.* "The effect of extirpation of the cortex of one hemisphere in the dog." *Russian Jour. Physiol.* viii. 1-2, 1925.

(20) *Foursikov, D. S.,* and *Eurman, M. N.* "The effect of extirpation of the cortex of one hemisphere." *Russian Jour. Physiol.* viii. 1-2, 1925.

(21) *Foursikov, D. S.* "The effect of extirpation of the cortex of one hemisphere (third communication). Generalization and the development of conditioned reflexes to tactile stimuli." *Russian Jour. Physiol.* viii. 5-6, 1925.

(22) *Foursikov, D. S.,* and *Eurman, M. N.* "Conditioned reflexes in dogs after removal of one hemisphere." *Archive Biol. Sciences,* vol. xxv. Nos. 4-5, 1926.

XIII. The Synthesizing Activity

(1) *Perelzweig, I. J.* See IVa (4).

(2) *Zeliony, G. P.* "A special type of conditioned reflexes." *Archive Biol. Sciences,* vol. xiv. No. 5, 1909.

(3) *Zeliony, G. P.* "Analysis of complex conditioned stimuli." *Proc. Russian Med. Soc. in Petrograd,* vol. 77, 1910.

(4) *Nikolaev, P. N.* "Analysis of complex conditioned reflexes." *Archive Biol. Sciences,* vol. xvi. No. 5, 1911.

(5) *Pavlov, I. P.* "Twenty years of objective study of the higher nervous activity of animals." *Article,* 8.

(6) *Stroganov, V. V.* "Development of a conditioned reflex to, and differentiation of, compound stimuli." *Pavlov Jubilee Vol.,* 1925.

(7) *Bikov, K. M.* "The properties of different components of compound stimuli." *Collected Papers of Physiol. Laboratories of I. P. Pavlov,* vol. i. Nos. 2-3, 1926.

XIV. The Strength of Conditioned Stimuli

(1) *Palladin, A. V.* "Development of artificial conditioned reflex to a sum of two stimuli." *Proc. Russian Med. Soc. in Petrograd,* vol. 73, 1906.

(2) *Tihomirov, N. P.* "The intensity of stimulus as an independent conditioned stimulus." *Proc. Russian Med. Soc. in Petrograd,* vol. 77, 1910.

(3) *Babkin, B. P.* "Contributions to the problem of the relative strengths of conditioned stimuli." *Proc. Russian Med. Soc. in Petrograd,* vol. 78, 1911.

XV. INDUCTION

(1) *Foursikov, D. S.* "Interrelations between excitation and inhibition." *Collected Papers of Physiol. Labs. of I. P. Pavlov,* vol. i. No. 1, 1924 ; Prelim. Commun. *Russian Jour. Physiol.,* vol. iii. 1-5, 1921, and vol. iv. 1922.

(2) *Foursikov, D. S.* "Mutual induction in the cerebral cortex." *Archive Biol. Sciences,* vol. xxiii. 1-3, 1923 (abstract in *Physiol. Abstracts,* vol. 8, 1923.)

(3) *Kalmikov, M. P.* "The positive phase of mutual induction as observed in one and the same group of nervous elements of the cortex." *Collected Papers, Physiol. Labs. I. P. Pavlov,* vol. i. 2-3, 1926.

(4) *Stroganov, V. V.* "The positive and negative phase of mutual induction in the hemispheres of the dog." *Collected Papers, Physiol. Labs. I. P. Pavlov,* vol. i. 2-3, 1926.

(5) *Kreps, E. M.* See V (23).

XVI. INDIVIDUAL CHARACTER OF ANIMALS

(1) *Besbokaia, M. J.* "Contributions to the physiology of conditioned reflexes." *Thesis, Petrograd,* 1913.

(2) *Frolov, G. P.* "The passive defence reflex and its influence upon conditioned reflexes." *Pavlov Jubilee Vol.,* 1925.

(3) *Kreps, E. M.* "An attempt to establish a classification of experimental animals according to types." *Collected Papers, Physiol. Labs. I. P. Pavlov,* vol. i. 1924.

XVII. TIME AS A CONDITIONED STIMULUS

(1) *Feokritova, J. P.* "Time as a conditioned stimulus to salivary secretion." *Thesis, Petrograd,* 1912.

(2) *Stoukova, M. M.* "Further contributions to the study of the significance of time as a conditioned stimulus." *Thesis, Petrograd,* 1914.

(3) *Deriabin, V. S.* "Further contributions to the study of the significance of time as a conditioned stimulus." *Thesis, Petrograd,* 1916.

(4) *Frolov, G. P.* " The physiology of the so-called sense of time." Commun. at 2nd Congress of Psycho-neurologists, Petrograd, January, 1924.

XVIII. Pharmacology of Conditioned Reflexes

(1) *Zavadsky, I. V.* " An application of the method of conditioned reflexes to pharmacology." *Proc. Russian Med. Soc. in Petrograd,* vol. 75, 1908.

(2) *Nikiforovsky, M. P.* " Pharmacological methods in application to conditioned reflexes." *Thesis, Petrograd,* 1910.

(3) *Potehin, S. I.* " The pharmacology of conditioned reflexes." *Proc. Russian Med. Soc. in Petrograd,* vol. 78, 1911.

(4) *Krilov, V. A.* " Development of conditioned reflexes to stimuli acting through the blood (automatic stimuli)." *Pavlov Jubilee Vol.,* 1925.

(5) *Podkopaev, N. A.* " Development of a conditioned reflex to an automatic (direct) stimulus." *Collected Papers of Physiol. Labs. I. P. Pavlov,* vol. i. 2-3, 1926 (abstract, *Zentralblatt für die gesammte Neurologie und Psychiatrie,* Bd. xxxix. 1925).

XIX. Bilateral Synergetic Activity of the Hemispheres

(1) *Anrep, G. V.* See V (7).

(2) *Anrep, G. V.* See V (8).

(3) *Anrep, G. V.* See V (10).

(4) *Podkopaev, N. A.,* and *Grigorovich, L. S.* " The development of symmetrical positive and negative reflexes." *Vrashebnoe Delo,* Nos. 1-2, 3-4, 1924.

(5) *Pavlov, I. P.* " Twenty years of objective study of the higher nervous activity in animals." *Article,* 34.

(6) *Bikov, K. M.* " Contributions to the question of the symmetrical reproduction of function of the hemispheres." *Pavlov Jubilee Vol.,* 1925.

(7) *Bikov, K. M.* and *Speransky, A. D.* " Observations upon dogs after section of the corpus callosum." *Collected Papers, Physiol. Labs. of I. P. Pavlov,* vol. i. No. 1, 1924 (abstract in *Zentralblatt für die gesammte Neurologie und Psychiatrie,* Bd. xxxix. 1925).

XX. The Significance of the Alimentary Centre

(1) *Pimenov, B. P.* " Development of conditioned reflexes in the case of application of the stimulus before or after the administration of the unconditioned stimulus." *Proc. Russian Med. Soc. in Petrograd,* vol. 73, 1906.

(2) *Boldirev, V. N.* "Conditioned reflexes and the experimental modification of their intensity." *Karkov Med. Jour.*, 1917.

(3) *Hasen, S. B.* "Relative magnitudes of conditioned and unconditioned salivary reflexes." *Thesis, Petrograd*, 1908.

(4) *Volborth, G. V.* "Contributions to the physiology of conditioned reflexes." *Proc. Russian Med. Soc. in Petrograd*, vol. 75, 1908.

(5) *Perelzweig, I. J.* See IVA (4).

(6) *Krestovnikov, A. N.* "An important stipulation in the development of conditioned reflexes." *Proc. Russian Med. Soc. in Petrograd*, vol. 80, 1913.

(7) *Krestovnikov, A. N.* "An important stipulation in the development of conditioned reflexes." *Bulletin of the Institute of Lesgaft*, vol. 3, 1921.

(8) *Frolov, G. P.* "The influence of abrupt changes in the composition of the food upon some aspects of the higher nervous activity in animals." *Archive of Biol. Sciences*, xxi. 3-5, 1922.

(9) *Rosenthal, I. S.* See IVF (4).

(10) *Popov, N. A.* See IVA (23).

(11) *Foursikov, D. S.* "Water as a stimulus." *Russian Jour. Physiol.*, vol. 3, Nos. 1-5, 1921 ; also *Pavlov Jubilee Vol.*, 1925.

XXI. The Investigatory Reflex

(1) *Foursikov, D. S.* See III (12).

(2) *Rasenkov, I. P.* See XII (17).

(3) *Chechoulin, S. I.* "New observations upon extinction of the investigatory reflex." *Archive Biol. Sciences*, xxiii. 3-5, 1923.

XXII. The Higher Nervous Activity (conditioned reflexes) in some special conditions of the central nervous system

(1) *Krjishkovsky, N.* "Die Veränderungen in der Function der oberen Abschnitte des Nervensystems bei der Hündin während der Brunst." *Zentralblatt für Physiologie*, Bd. xxiv. No. 11, 1909.

(2) *Shenger-Krestovnikova, N. R.* See IVB (11).

(3) *Foursikov, D. S.* "The effect of pregnancy upon conditioned reflexes." *Archive Biol. Sciences*, xxi. Nos. 3-5, 1922.

(4) *Rosenthal, I. S.* "The effect of pregnancy upon conditioned reflexes." *Russian Jour. Physiol.*, vol. v. 1922.

(5) *Rosenthal, I. S.* "The effect of inanition upon conditioned reflexes." *Archive Biol. Sciences*, xxi. Nos. 3-5, 1922.

(6) *Kreps, E. M.* "On the influence of heat in a bitch upon its higher nervous activity." *Physiol. Abstracts*, vol. 5, 1923.

(7) *Andréev, L. A.* " Observations upon the functions of the senile central nervous system." *Collected Papers, Physiol. Labs. I. P. Pavlov*, vol. i. No. 1, 1924.

(2) *Rasenkov, I. P.* " Modifications of the excitatory process in the cortex under some complex conditions." *Collected Papers, Physiol. Labs. I. P. Pavlov*, vol. i. No. 1, 1924.

(9) *Pavlov, I. P.* " Twenty years of objective study of the higher nervous activity of animals." *Articles*, 25 and 36.

(10) *Prorokov, I. P.* " A peculiar motor reaction in the dog and its suppression." *Collected Papers, Physiol. Labs. I. P. Pavlov*, vol. i. Nos. 2-3, 1925.

(11) *Petrova, M. K.* " Pathological deviations of the inhibitory and excitatory process in a case of their clashing." *Collected Papers, Physiol. Labs. I. P. Pavlov*, vol. i. Nos. 2-3, 1925.

(12) *Petrova, M. K.* " The combatting of sleep : the mutual counterbalancing of the excitatory and inhibitory processes." *Pavlov Jubilee Vol.*, 1925.

(13) *Valkov, A. V.* " Observations on the higher nervous activity in thyroidectomized puppies." *Pavlov Jubilee Vol.*, 1925.

(14) *Podkopaev, N. A.* " A peculiar motor reaction in the dog in conjunction with a development of inhibition in the cortex." *Collected Papers, Physiol. Labs. I. P. Pavlov*, vol. i. Nos. 2-3, 1925.

(15) *Petrova, M. K.* " The therapy of experimental neuroses in dogs." *Archive Biol. Sciences*, vol. xxv. Nos. 1-3, 1925.

(16) *Siriatsky, V. V.* " Pathological deviations in the activity of the central nervous system in the case of clashing of excitation and inhibition." *Russian Jour. Physiol.*, vol. viii. Nos. 3-4, 1925.

XXIII. Papers not included in the preceding sections

(1) *Parfenov, O.* " A special case of the activity of salivary glands in the dog." *Proc. Russian Med. Soc. in Petrograd*, 73, 1906.

(2) *Volborth, G. V.* " Inhibitory conditioned reflexes." *Thesis, Petrograd*, 1912 ; Prelim. Commun. *Proc. Russian Med. Soc. in Petrograd*, vol. 77, 1910.

(3) *Zitovich, I. S.* " The origin of the natural conditioned reflexes." *Thesis, Petrograd*, 1910 ; Prelim. Commun. *Proc. Russian Med. Soc. in Petrograd*, vol. 77, 1910.

(4) *Eroféeva, M. N.* " Electrical stimulation of the skin of the dog as a conditioned salivary stimulus." *Thesis, Petrograd*, 1912 ; Prelim. Commun. *Proc. Russian Med. Soc. in Petrograd*, vol. 79, 1912.

(5) *Eroféeva, M. N.* " Contribution to the physiology of conditioned reflexes to injurious stimuli." *Proc. Russian Med. Soc. in Petrograd,* vol. 80, 1913.

(6) *Eroféeva, M. N.* " Further observations upon conditioned reflexes to nocuous stimuli." *Bulletin of Institute of Lesgaft,* vol. iii. 1921.

(7) *Foursikov, D. S.* " Conditioned chain reflexes and the pathology of the higher nervous activity." Commun. to 2nd Congress of Psycho-neurologists in Petrograd, January, 1924 ; Prelim. Commun. *Russian Jour. Physiol.,* vol. iv. 1922.

(8) *Pavlov, I. P.* " Twenty years of objective study of the higher nervous activity of animals." *Articles,* 27 and 28.

(9) *Koupalov, P. S.* " Periodical fluctuations in the rate of conditioned salivary secretion." *Archive Biol. Sciences,* vol. xxv. No. 45, 1926.

INDEX

429

A CATALOGUE OF SELECTED DOVER BOOKS
IN ALL FIELDS OF INTEREST

A CATALOGUE OF SELECTED DOVER BOOKS
IN ALL FIELDS OF INTEREST

LEATHER TOOLING AND CARVING, Chris H. Groneman. One of few books concentrating on tooling and carving, with complete instructions and grid designs for 39 projects ranging from bookmarks to bags. 148 illustrations. 111pp. 7⅞ x 10.
23061-9 Pa. $2.50

THE CODEX NUTTALL, A PICTURE MANUSCRIPT FROM ANCIENT MEXICO, as first edited by Zelia Nuttall. Only inexpensive edition, in full color, of a pre-Columbian Mexican (Mixtec) book. 88 color plates show kings, gods, heroes, temples, sacrifices. New explanatory, historical introduction by Arthur G. Miller. 96pp. 11⅜ x 8½.
23168-2 Pa. $7.50

AMERICAN PRIMITIVE PAINTING, Jean Lipman. Classic collection of an enduring American tradition. 109 plates, 8 in full color—portraits, landscapes, Biblical and historical scenes, etc., showing family groups, farm life, and so on. 80pp. of lucid text. 8⅜ x 11¼.
22815-0 Pa. $5.00

WILL BRADLEY: HIS GRAPHIC ART, edited by Clarence P. Hornung. Striking collection of work by foremost practitioner of Art Nouveau in America: posters, cover designs, sample pages, advertisements, other illustrations. 97 plates, including 8 in full color and 19 in two colors. 97pp. 9⅜ x 12¼.
20701-3 Pa. $4.00
22120-2 Clothbd. $10.00

AN ATLAS OF ANATOMY FOR ARTISTS, Fritz Schider. Finest text, working book. Full text, plus anatomical illustrations; plates by great artists showing anatomy. 593 illustrations. 192pp. 7⅞ x 10¾.
20241-0 Clothbd. $6.95

THE GIBSON GIRL AND HER AMERICA, Charles Dana Gibson. 155 finest drawings of effervescent world of 1900-1910: the Gibson Girl and her loves, amusements, adventures, Mr. Pipp, etc. Selected by E. Gillon; introduction by Henry Pitz. 144pp. 8¼ x 11⅜.
21986-0 Pa. $3.50

STAINED GLASS CRAFT, J.A.F. Divine, G. Blachford. One of the very few books that tell the beginner exactly what he needs to know: planning cuts, making shapes, avoiding design weaknesses, fitting glass, etc. 93 illustrations. 115pp.
22812-6 Pa. $1.75

CREATIVE LITHOGRAPHY AND HOW TO DO IT, Grant Arnold. Lithography as art form: working directly on stone, transfer of drawings, lithotint, mezzotint, color printing; also metal plates. Detailed, thorough. 27 illustrations. 214pp.
21208-4 Pa. $3.50

DESIGN MOTIFS OF ANCIENT MEXICO, Jorge Enciso. Vigorous, powerful ceramic stamp impressions — Maya, Aztec, Toltec, Olmec. Serpents, gods, priests, dancers, etc. 153pp. 6⅛ x 9¼.
20084-1 Pa. $2.50

AMERICAN INDIAN DESIGN AND DECORATION, Leroy Appleton. Full text, plus more than 700 precise drawings of Inca, Maya, Aztec, Pueblo, Plains, NW Coast basketry, sculpture, painting, pottery, sand paintings, metal, etc. 4 plates in color. 279pp. 8⅜ x 11¼.
22704-9 Pa. $5.00

CHINESE LATTICE DESIGNS, Daniel S. Dye. Incredibly beautiful geometric designs: circles, voluted, simple dissections, etc. Inexhaustible source of ideas, motifs. 1239 illustrations. 469pp. 6⅛ x 9¼.
23096-1 Pa. $5.00

JAPANESE DESIGN MOTIFS, Matsuya Co. Mon, or heraldic designs. Over 4000 typical, beautiful designs: birds, animals, flowers, swords, fans, geometric; all beautifully stylized. 213pp. 11⅜ x 8¼.
22874-6 Pa. $5.00

PERSPECTIVE, Jan Vredeman de Vries. 73 perspective plates from 1604 edition; buildings, townscapes, stairways, fantastic scenes. Remarkable for beauty, surrealistic atmosphere; real eye-catchers. Introduction by Adolf Placzek. 74pp. 11⅜ x 8¼.
20186-4 Pa. $2.75

EARLY AMERICAN DESIGN MOTIFS, Suzanne E. Chapman. 497 motifs, designs, from painting on wood, ceramics, appliqué, glassware, samplers, metal work, etc. Florals, landscapes, birds and animals, geometrics, letters, etc. Inexhaustible. Enlarged edition. 138pp. 8⅜ x 11¼.
22985-8 Pa. $3.50
23084-8 Clothbd. $7.95

VICTORIAN STENCILS FOR DESIGN AND DECORATION, edited by E.V. Gillon, Jr. 113 wonderful ornate Victorian pieces from German sources; florals, geometrics; borders, corner pieces; bird motifs, etc. 64pp. 9⅜ x 12¼.
21995-X Pa. $3.00

ART NOUVEAU: AN ANTHOLOGY OF DESIGN AND ILLUSTRATION FROM THE STUDIO, edited by E.V. Gillon, Jr. Graphic arts: book jackets, posters, engravings, illustrations, decorations; Crane, Beardsley, Bradley and many others. Inexhaustible. 92pp. 8⅛ x 11.
22388-4 Pa. $2.50

ORIGINAL ART DECO DESIGNS, William Rowe. First-rate, highly imaginative modern Art Deco frames, borders, compositions, alphabets, florals, insectals, Wurlitzer-types, etc. Much finest modern Art Deco. 80 plates, 8 in color. 8⅜ x 11¼.
22567-4 Pa. $3.50

HANDBOOK OF DESIGNS AND DEVICES, Clarence P. Hornung. Over 1800 basic geometric designs based on circle, triangle, square, scroll, cross, etc. Largest such collection in existence. 261pp.
20125-2 Pa. $2.75

150 MASTERPIECES OF DRAWING, edited by Anthony Toney. 150 plates, early 15th century to end of 18th century; Rembrandt, Michelangelo, Dürer, Fragonard, Watteau, Wouwerman, many others. 150pp. 8⅜ x 11¼.   21032-4 Pa. $4.00

THE GOLDEN AGE OF THE POSTER, Hayward and Blanche Cirker. 70 extraordinary posters in full colors, from Maîtres de l'Affiche, Mucha, Lautrec, Bradley, Cheret, Beardsley, many others. 9⅜ x 12¼.   22753-7 Pa. $5.95
                                                                                        21718-3 Clothbd. $7.95

SIMPLICISSIMUS, selection, translations and text by Stanley Appelbaum. 180 satirical drawings, 16 in full color, from the famous German weekly magazine in the years 1896 to 1926. 24 artists included: Grosz, Kley, Pascin, Kubin, Kollwitz, plus Heine, Thöny, Bruno Paul, others. 172pp. 8½ x 12¼.   23098-8 Pa. $5.00
                                                                                        23099-6 Clothbd. $10.00

THE EARLY WORK OF AUBREY BEARDSLEY, Aubrey Beardsley. 157 plates, 2 in color: Manon Lescaut, Madame Bovary, Morte d'Arthur, Salome, other. Introduction by H. Marillier. 175pp. 8½ x 11.   21816-3 Pa. $4.00

THE LATER WORK OF AUBREY BEARDSLEY, Aubrey Beardsley. Exotic masterpieces of full maturity: Venus and Tannhäuser, Lysistrata, Rape of the Lock, Volpone, Savoy material, etc. 174 plates, 2 in color. 176pp. 8½ x 11. 21817-1 Pa. $4.00

DRAWINGS OF WILLIAM BLAKE, William Blake. 92 plates from Book of Job, Divine Comedy, Paradise Lost, visionary heads, mythological figures, Laocoön, etc. Selection, introduction, commentary by Sir Geoffrey Keynes. 178pp. 8½ x 11.
                                                                                        22303-5 Pa. $4.00

LONDON: A PILGRIMAGE, Gustave Doré, Blanchard Jerrold. Squalor, riches, misery, beauty of mid-Victorian metropolis; 55 wonderful plates, 125 other illustrations, full social, cultural text by Jerrold. 191pp. of text. 8⅛ x 11.
                                                                                        22306-X Pa. $6.00

THE COMPLETE WOODCUTS OF ALBRECHT DÜRER, edited by Dr. W. Kurth. 346 in all: Old Testament, St. Jerome, Passion, Life of Virgin, Apocalypse, many others. Introduction by Campbell Dodgson. 285pp. 8½ x 12¼.   21097-9 Pa. $6.00

THE DISASTERS OF WAR, Francisco Goya. 83 etchings record horrors of Napoleonic wars in Spain and war in general. Reprint of 1st edition, plus 3 additional plates. Introduction by Philip Hofer. 97pp. 9⅜ x 8¼.   21872-4 Pa. $3.50

ENGRAVINGS OF HOGARTH, William Hogarth. 101 of Hogarth's greatest works: Rake's Progress, Harlot's Progress, Illustrations for Hudibras, Midnight Modern Conversation, Before and After, Beer Street and Gin Lane, many more. Full commentary. 256pp. 11 x 14.   22479-1 Pa. $7.95,

PRIMITIVE ART, Franz Boas. Great anthropologist on ceramics, textiles, wood, stone, metal, etc.; patterns, technology, symbols, styles. All areas, but fullest on Northwest Coast Indians. 350 illustrations. 378pp.   20025-6 Pa. $3.75

MOTHER GOOSE'S MELODIES. Facsimile of fabulously rare Munroe and Francis "copyright 1833" Boston edition. Familiar and unusual rhymes, wonderful old woodcut illustrations. Edited by E.F. Bleiler. 128pp. 4½ x 6⅜. 22577-1 Pa. $1.50

MOTHER GOOSE IN HIEROGLYPHICS. Favorite nursery rhymes presented in rebus form for children. Fascinating 1849 edition reproduced in toto, with key. Introduction by E.F. Bleiler. About 400 woodcuts. 64pp. 6⅞ x 5¼. 20745-5 Pa. $1.50

PETER PIPER'S PRACTICAL PRINCIPLES OF PLAIN & PERFECT PRONUNCIATION. Alliterative jingles and tongue-twisters. Reproduction in full of 1830 first American edition. 25 spirited woodcuts. 32pp. 4½ x 6⅜. 22560-7 Pa. $1.25

THE NIGHT BEFORE CHRISTMAS, Clement Moore. Full text, and woodcuts from original 1848 book. Also critical, historical material. 19 illustrations. 40pp. 4⅝ x 6. 22797-9 Pa. $1.35

THE KING OF THE GOLDEN RIVER, John Ruskin. Victorian children's classic of three brothers, their attempts to reach the Golden River, what becomes of them. Facsimile of original 1889 edition. 22 illustrations. 56pp. 4⅝ x 6⅜. 20066-3 Pa. $1.50

DREAMS OF THE RAREBIT FIEND, Winsor McCay. Pioneer cartoon strip, unexcelled for beauty, imagination, in 60 full sequences. Incredible technical virtuosity, wonderful visual wit. Historical introduction. 62pp. 8⅜ x 11¼. 21347-1 Pa. $2.50

THE KATZENJAMMER KIDS, Rudolf Dirks. In full color, 14 strips from 1906-7; full of imagination, characteristic humor. Classic of great historical importance. Introduction by August Derleth. 32pp. 9¼ x 12¼. 23005-8 Pa. $2.00

LITTLE ORPHAN ANNIE AND LITTLE ORPHAN ANNIE IN COSMIC CITY, Harold Gray. Two great sequences from the early strips: our curly-haired heroine defends the Warbucks' financial empire and, then, takes on meanie Phineas P. Pinchpenny. Leapin' lizards! 178pp. 6⅛ x 8⅜. 23107-0 Pa. $2.00

WHEN A FELLER NEEDS A FRIEND, Clare Briggs. 122 cartoons by one of the greatest newspaper cartoonists of the early 20th century — about growing up, making a living, family life, daily frustrations and occasional triumphs. 121pp. 8½ x 9½. 23148-8 Pa. $2.50

ABSOLUTELY MAD INVENTIONS, A.E. Brown, H.A. Jeffcott. Hilarious, useless, or merely absurd inventions all granted patents by the U.S. Patent Office. Edible tie pin, mechanical hat tipper, etc. 57 illustrations. 125pp. 22596-8 Pa. $1.50

THE DEVIL'S DICTIONARY, Ambrose Bierce. Barbed, bitter, brilliant witticisms in the form of a dictionary. Best, most ferocious satire America has produced. 145pp. 20487-1 Pa. $1.75

THE BEST DR. THORNDYKE DETECTIVE STORIES, R. Austin Freeman. The Case of Oscar Brodski, The Moabite Cipher, and 5 other favorites featuring the great scientific detective, plus his long-believed-lost first adventure — 31 New Inn — reprinted here for the first time. Edited by E.F. Bleiler. USO 20388-3 Pa. $3.00

BEST "THINKING MACHINE" DETECTIVE STORIES, Jacques Futrelle. The Problem of Cell 13 and 11 other stories about Prof. Augustus S.F.X. Van Dusen, including two "lost" stories. First reprinting of several. Edited by E.F. Bleiler. 241pp.
20537-1 Pa. $3.00

UNCLE SILAS, J. Sheridan LeFanu. Victorian Gothic mystery novel, considered by many best of period, even better than Collins or Dickens. Wonderful psychological terror. Introduction by Frederick Shroyer. 436pp. 21715-9 Pa. $4.00

BEST DR. POGGIOLI DETECTIVE STORIES, T.S. Stribling. 15 best stories from EQMM and The Saint offer new adventures in Mexico, Florida, Tennessee hills as Poggioli unravels mysteries and combats Count Jalacki. 217pp. 23227-1 Pa. $3.00

EIGHT DIME NOVELS, selected with an introduction by E.F. Bleiler. Adventures of Old King Brady, Frank James, Nick Carter, Deadwood Dick, Buffalo Bill, The Steam Man, Frank Merriwell, and Horatio Alger — 1877 to 1905. Important, entertaining popular literature in facsimile reprint, with original covers. 190pp. 9 x 12. 22975-0 Pa. $3.50

ALICE'S ADVENTURES UNDER GROUND, Lewis Carroll. Facsimile of ms. Carroll gave Alice Liddell in 1864. Different in many ways from final Alice. Handlettered, illustrated by Carroll. Introduction by Martin Gardner. 128pp. 21482-6 Pa. $2.00

ALICE IN WONDERLAND COLORING BOOK, Lewis Carroll. Pictures by John Tenniel. Large-size versions of the famous illustrations of Alice, Cheshire Cat, Mad Hatter and all the others, waiting for your crayons. Abridged text. 36 illustrations. 64pp. 8¼ x 11. 22853-3 Pa. $1.50

AVENTURES D'ALICE AU PAYS DES MERVEILLES, Lewis Carroll. Bué's translation of "Alice" into French, supervised by Carroll himself. Novel way to learn language. (No English text.) 42 Tenniel illustrations. 196pp. 22836-3 Pa. $3.00

MYTHS AND FOLK TALES OF IRELAND, Jeremiah Curtin. 11 stories that are Irish versions of European fairy tales and 9 stories from the Fenian cycle — 20 tales of legend and magic that comprise an essential work in the history of folklore. 256pp. 22430-9 Pa. $3.00

EAST O' THE SUN AND WEST O' THE MOON, George W. Dasent. Only full edition of favorite, wonderful Norwegian fairytales — Why the Sea is Salt, Boots and the Troll, etc. — with 77 illustrations by Kittelsen & Werenskiöld. 418pp.
22521-6 Pa. $4.50

PERRAULT'S FAIRY TALES, Charles Perrault and Gustave Doré. Original versions of Cinderella, Sleeping Beauty, Little Red Riding Hood, etc. in best translation, with 34 wonderful illustrations by Gustave Doré. 117pp. 8⅛ x 11. 22311-6 Pa. $2.50

EARLY NEW ENGLAND GRAVESTONE RUBBINGS, Edmund V. Gillon, Jr. 43 photographs, 226 rubbings show heavily symbolic, macabre, sometimes humorous primitive American art. Up to early 19th century. 207pp. 8⅜ x 11¼.
21380-3 Pa. $4.00

L.J.M. DAGUERRE: THE HISTORY OF THE DIORAMA AND THE DAGUERREOTYPE, Helmut and Alison Gernsheim. Definitive account. Early history, life and work of Daguerre; discovery of daguerreotype process; diffusion abroad; other early photography. 124 illustrations. 226pp. 6⅙ x 9¼.
22290-X Pa. $4.00

PHOTOGRAPHY AND THE AMERICAN SCENE, Robert Taft. The basic book on American photography as art, recording form, 1839-1889. Development, influence on society, great photographers, types (portraits, war, frontier, etc.), whatever else needed. Inexhaustible. Illustrated with 322 early photos, daguerreotypes, tintypes, stereo slides, etc. 546pp. 6⅛ x 9¼.
21201-7 Pa. $5.95

PHOTOGRAPHIC SKETCHBOOK OF THE CIVIL WAR, Alexander Gardner. Reproduction of 1866 volume with 100 on-the-field photographs: Manassas, Lincoln on battlefield, slave pens, etc. Introduction by E.F. Bleiler. 224pp. 10¾ x 9.
22731-6 Pa. $6.00

THE MOVIES: A PICTURE QUIZ BOOK, Stanley Appelbaum & Hayward Cirker. Match stars with their movies, name actors and actresses, test your movie skill with 241 stills from 236 great movies, 1902-1959. Indexes of performers and films. 128pp. 8⅜ x 9¼.
20222-4 Pa. $2.50

THE TALKIES, Richard Griffith. Anthology of features, articles from Photoplay, 1928-1940, reproduced complete. Stars, famous movies, technical features, fabulous ads, etc.; Garbo, Chaplin, King Kong, Lubitsch, etc. 4 color plates, scores of illustrations. 327pp. 8⅜ x 11¼.
22762-6 Pa. $6.95

THE MOVIE MUSICAL FROM VITAPHONE TO "42ND STREET," edited by Miles Kreuger. Relive the rise of the movie musical as reported in the pages of Photoplay magazine (1926-1933): every movie review, cast list, ad, and record review; every significant feature article, production still, biography, forecast, and gossip story. Profusely illustrated. 367pp. 8⅜ x 11¼.
23154-2 Pa. $7.95

JOHANN SEBASTIAN BACH, Philipp Spitta. Great classic of biography, musical commentary, with hundreds of pieces analyzed. Also good for Bach's contemporaries. 450 musical examples. Total of 1799pp.
EUK 22278-0, 22279-9 Clothbd., Two vol. set $25.00

BEETHOVEN AND HIS NINE SYMPHONIES, Sir George Grove. Thorough history, analysis, commentary on symphonies and some related pieces. For either beginner or advanced student. 436 musical passages. 407pp.
20334-4 Pa. $4.00

MOZART AND HIS PIANO CONCERTOS, Cuthbert Girdlestone. The only full-length study. Detailed analyses of all 21 concertos, sources; 417 musical examples. 509pp.
21271-8 Pa. $6.00

THE FITZWILLIAM VIRGINAL BOOK, edited by J. Fuller Maitland, W.B. Squire. Famous early 17th century collection of keyboard music, 300 works by Morley, Byrd, Bull, Gibbons, etc. Modern notation. Total of 938pp. 8⅜ x 11.

ECE 21068-5, 21069-3 Pa., Two vol. set $15.00

COMPLETE STRING QUARTETS, Wolfgang A. Mozart. Breitkopf and Härtel edition. All 23 string quartets plus alternate slow movement to K156. Study score. 277pp. 9⅜ x 12¼.

22372-8 Pa. $6.00

COMPLETE SONG CYCLES, Franz Schubert. Complete piano, vocal music of Die Schöne Müllerin, Die Winterreise, Schwanengesang. Also Drinker English singing translations. Breitkopf and Härtel edition. 217pp. 9⅜ x 12¼.

22649-2 Pa. $5.00

THE COMPLETE PRELUDES AND ETUDES FOR PIANOFORTE SOLO, Alexander Scriabin. All the preludes and etudes including many perfectly spun miniatures. Edited by K.N. Igumnov and Y.I. Mil'shteyn. 250pp. 9 x 12.

22919-X Pa. $6.00

TRISTAN UND ISOLDE, Richard Wagner. Full orchestral score with complete instrumentation. Do not confuse with piano reduction. Commentary by Felix Mottl, great Wagnerian conductor and scholar. Study score. 655pp. 8⅛ x 11.

22915-7 Pa. $11.95

FAVORITE SONGS OF THE NINETIES, ed. Robert Fremont. Full reproduction, including covers, of 88 favorites: Ta-Ra-Ra-Boom-De-Aye, The Band Played On, Bird in a Gilded Cage, Under the Bamboo Tree, After the Ball, etc. 401pp. 9 x 12.

EBE 21536-9 Pa. $6.95

SOUSA'S GREAT MARCHES IN PIANO TRANSCRIPTION: ORIGINAL SHEET MUSIC OF 23 WORKS, John Philip Sousa. Selected by Lester S. Levy. Playing edition includes: The Stars and Stripes Forever, The Thunderer, The Gladiator, King Cotton, Washington Post, much more. 24 illustrations. 111pp. 9 x 12.

USO 23132-1 Pa. $3.50

CLASSIC PIANO RAGS, selected with an introduction by Rudi Blesh. Best ragtime music (1897-1922) by Scott Joplin, James Scott, Joseph F. Lamb, Tom Turpin, 9 others. Printed from best original sheet music, plus covers. 364pp. 9 x 12.

EBE 20469-3 Pa. $7.50

ANALYSIS OF CHINESE CHARACTERS, C.D. Wilder, J.H. Ingram. 1000 most important characters analyzed according to primitives, phonetics, historical development. Traditional method offers mnemonic aid to beginner, intermediate student of Chinese, Japanese. 365pp.

23045-7 Pa. $4.00

MODERN CHINESE: A BASIC COURSE, Faculty of Peking University. Self study, classroom course in modern Mandarin. Records contain phonetics, vocabulary, sentences, lessons. 249 page book contains all recorded text, translations, grammar, vocabulary, exercises. Best course on market. 3 12" 33⅓ monaural records, book, album.

98832-5 Set $12.50

MANUAL OF THE TREES OF NORTH AMERICA, Charles S. Sargent. The basic survey of every native tree and tree-like shrub, 717 species in all. Extremely full descriptions, information on habitat, growth, locales, economics, etc. Necessary to every serious tree lover. Over 100 finding keys. 783 illustrations. Total of 986pp.
20277-1, 20278-X Pa., Two vol. set $9.00

BIRDS OF THE NEW YORK AREA, John Bull. Indispensable guide to more than 400 species within a hundred-mile radius of Manhattan. Information on range, status, breeding, migration, distribution trends, etc. Foreword by Roger Tory Peterson. 17 drawings; maps. 540pp.
23222-0 Pa. $6.00

THE SEA-BEACH AT EBB-TIDE, Augusta Foote Arnold. Identify hundreds of marine plants and animals: algae, seaweeds, squids, crabs, corals, etc. Descriptions cover food, life cycle, size, shape, habitat. Over 600 drawings. 490pp.
21949-6 Pa. $5.00

THE MOTH BOOK, William J. Holland. Identify more than 2,000 moths of North America. General information, precise species descriptions. 623 illustrations plus 48 color plates show almost all species, full size. 1968 edition. Still the basic book. Total of 551pp. 6½ x 9¼.
21948-8 Pa. $6.00

HOW INDIANS USE WILD PLANTS FOR FOOD, MEDICINE & CRAFTS, Frances Densmore. Smithsonian, Bureau of American Ethnology report presents wealth of material on nearly 200 plants used by Chippewas of Minnesota and Wisconsin. 33 plates plus 122pp. of text. 6⅛ x 9¼.
23019-8 Pa. $2.50

OLD NEW YORK IN EARLY PHOTOGRAPHS, edited by Mary Black. Your only chance to see New York City as it was 1853-1906, through 196 wonderful photographs from N.Y. Historical Society. Great Blizzard, Lincoln's funeral procession, great buildings. 228pp. 9 x 12.
22907-6 Pa. $6.95

THE AMERICAN REVOLUTION, A PICTURE SOURCEBOOK, John Grafton. Wonderful Bicentennial picture source, with 411 illustrations (contemporary and 19th century) showing battles, personalities, maps, events, flags, posters, soldier's life, ships, etc. all captioned and explained. A wonderful browsing book, supplement to other historical reading. 160pp. 9 x 12.
23226-3 Pa. $4.00

PERSONAL NARRATIVE OF A PILGRIMAGE TO AL-MADINAH AND MECCAH, Richard Burton. Great travel classic by remarkably colorful personality. Burton, disguised as a Moroccan, visited sacred shrines of Islam, narrowly escaping death. Wonderful observations of Islamic life, customs, personalities. 47 illustrations. Total of 959pp.
21217-3, 21218-1 Pa., Two vol. set $10.00

INCIDENTS OF TRAVEL IN CENTRAL AMERICA, CHIAPAS, AND YUCATAN, John L. Stephens. Almost single-handed discovery of Maya culture; exploration of ruined cities, monuments, temples; customs of Indians. 115 drawings. 892pp.
22404-X, 22405-8 Pa., Two vol. set $9.00

CONSTRUCTION OF AMERICAN FURNITURE TREASURES, Lester Margon. 344 detail drawings, complete text on constructing exact reproductions of 38 early American masterpieces: Hepplewhite sideboard, Duncan Phyfe drop-leaf table, mantel clock, gate-leg dining table, Pa. German cupboard, more. 38 plates. 54 photographs. 168pp. 8⅜ x 11¼.
23056-2 Pa. $4.00

JEWELRY MAKING AND DESIGN, Augustus F. Rose, Antonio Cirino. Professional secrets revealed in thorough, practical guide: tools, materials, processes; rings, brooches, chains, cast pieces, enamelling, setting stones, etc. Do not confuse with skimpy introductions: beginner can use, professional can learn from it. Over 200 illustrations. 306pp.
21750-7 Pa. $3.00

METALWORK AND ENAMELLING, Herbert Maryon. Generally conceded best all-around book. Countless trade secrets: materials, tools, soldering, filigree, setting, inlay, niello, repoussé, casting, polishing, etc. For beginner or expert. Author was foremost British expert. 330 illustrations. 335pp.
22702-2 Pa. $4.00

WEAVING WITH FOOT-POWER LOOMS, Edward F. Worst. Setting up a loom, beginning to weave, constructing equipment, using dyes, more, plus over 285 drafts of traditional patterns including Colonial and Swedish weaves. More than 200 other figures. For beginning and advanced. 275pp. 8¾ x 6⅜.
23064-3 Pa. $4.50

WEAVING A NAVAJO BLANKET, Gladys A. Reichard. Foremost anthropologist studied under Navajo women, reveals every step in process from wool, dyeing, spinning, setting up loom, designing, weaving. Much history, symbolism. With this book you could make one yourself. 97 illustrations. 222pp. 22992-0 Pa. $3.00

NATURAL DYES AND HOME DYEING, Rita J. Adrosko. Use natural ingredients: bark, flowers, leaves, lichens, insects etc. Over 135 specific recipes from historical sources for cotton, wool, other fabrics. Genuine premodern handicrafts. 12 illustrations. 160pp.
22688-3 Pa. $2.00

DRIED FLOWERS, Sarah Whitlock and Martha Rankin. Concise, clear, practical guide to dehydration, glycerinizing, pressing plant material, and more. Covers use of silica gel. 12 drawings. Originally titled "New Techniques with Dried Flowers." 32pp.
21802-3 Pa. $1.00

THOMAS NAST: CARTOONS AND ILLUSTRATIONS, with text by Thomas Nast St. Hill. Father of American political cartooning. Cartoons that destroyed Tweed Ring; inflation, free love, church and state; original Republican elephant and Democratic donkey; Santa Claus; more. 117 illustrations. 146pp. 9 x 12.
22983-1 Pa. $4.00
23067-8 Clothbd. $8.50

FREDERIC REMINGTON: 173 DRAWINGS AND ILLUSTRATIONS. Most famous of the Western artists, most responsible for our myths about the American West in its untamed days. Complete reprinting of Drawings of Frederic Remington (1897), plus other selections. 4 additional drawings in color on covers. 140pp. 9 x 12.
20714-5 Pa. $5.00

How to Solve Chess Problems, Kenneth S. Howard. Practical suggestions on problem solving for very beginners. 58 two-move problems, 46 3-movers, 8 4-movers for practice, plus hints. 171pp. 20748-X Pa. $3.00

A Guide to Fairy Chess, Anthony Dickins. 3-D chess, 4-D chess, chess on a cylindrical board, reflecting pieces that bounce off edges, cooperative chess, retrograde chess, maximummers, much more. Most based on work of great Dawson. Full handbook, 100 problems. 66pp. 7⅞ x 10¾. 22687-5 Pa. $2.00

Win at Backgammon, Millard Hopper. Best opening moves, running game, blocking game, back game, tables of odds, etc. Hopper makes the game clear enough for anyone to play, and win. 43 diagrams. 111pp. 22894-0 Pa. $1.50

Bidding a Bridge Hand, Terence Reese. Master player "thinks out loud" the binding of 75 hands that defy point count systems. Organized by bidding problem—no-fit situations, overbidding, underbidding, cueing your defense, etc. 254pp. EBE 22830-4 Pa. $3.00

The Precision Bidding System in Bridge, C.C. Wei, edited by Alan Truscott. Inventor of precision bidding presents average hands and hands from actual play, including games from 1969 Bermuda Bowl where system emerged. 114 exercises. 116pp. 21171-1 Pa. $1.75

Learn Magic, Henry Hay. 20 simple, easy-to-follow lessons on magic for the new magician: illusions, card tricks, silks, sleights of hand, coin manipulations, escapes, and more —all with a minimum amount of equipment. Final chapter explains the great stage illusions. 92 illustrations. 285pp. 21238-6 Pa. $2.95

The New Magician's Manual, Walter B. Gibson. Step-by-step instructions and clear illustrations guide the novice in mastering 36 tricks; much equipment supplied on 16 pages of cut-out materials. 36 additional tricks. 64 illustrations. 159pp. 6⅝ x 10. 23113-5 Pa. $3.00

Professional Magic for Amateurs, Walter B. Gibson. 50 easy, effective tricks used by professionals —cards, string, tumblers, handkerchiefs, mental magic, etc. 63 illustrations. 223pp. 23012-0 Pa. $2.50

Card Manipulations, Jean Hugard. Very rich collection of manipulations; has taught thousands of fine magicians tricks that are really workable, eye-catching. Easily followed, serious work. Over 200 illustrations. 163pp. 20539-8 Pa. $2.00

Abbott's Encyclopedia of Rope Tricks for Magicians, Stewart James. Complete reference book for amateur and professional magicians containing more than 150 tricks involving knots, penetrations, cut and restored rope, etc. 510 illustrations. Reprint of 3rd edition. 400pp. 23206-9 Pa. $3.50

The Secrets of Houdini, J.C. Cannell. Classic study of Houdini's incredible magic, exposing closely-kept professional secrets and revealing, in general terms, the whole art of stage magic. 67 illustrations. 279pp. 22913-0 Pa. $3.00

THE MAGIC MOVING PICTURE BOOK, Bliss, Sands & Co. The pictures in this book move! Volcanoes erupt, a house burns, a serpentine dancer wiggles her way through a number. By using a specially ruled acetate screen provided, you can obtain these and 15 other startling effects. Originally "The Motograph Moving Picture Book." 32pp. 8¼ x 11.   23224-7 Pa. $1.75

STRING FIGURES AND HOW TO MAKE THEM, Caroline F. Jayne. Fullest, clearest instructions on string figures from around world: Eskimo, Navajo, Lapp, Europe, more. Cats cradle, moving spear, lightning, stars. Introduction by A.C. Haddon. 950 illustrations. 407pp.   20152-X Pa. $3.50

PAPER FOLDING FOR BEGINNERS, William D. Murray and Francis J. Rigney. Clearest book on market for making origami sail boats, roosters, frogs that move legs, cups, bonbon boxes. 40 projects. More than 275 illustrations. Photographs. 94pp.   20713-7 Pa. $1.25

INDIAN SIGN LANGUAGE, William Tomkins. Over 525 signs developed by Sioux, Blackfoot, Cheyenne, Arapahoe and other tribes. Written instructions and diagrams: how to make words, construct sentences. Also 290 pictographs of Sioux and Ojibway tribes. 111pp. 6⅛ x 9¼.   22029-X Pa. $1.75

BOOMERANGS: HOW TO MAKE AND THROW THEM, Bernard S. Mason. Easy to make and throw, dozens of designs: cross-stick, pinwheel, boomabird, tumblestick, Australian curved stick boomerang. Complete throwing instructions. All safe. 99pp.   23028-7 Pa. $1.75

25 KITES THAT FLY, Leslie Hunt. Full, easy to follow instructions for kites made from inexpensive materials. Many novelties. Reeling, raising, designing your own. 70 illustrations. 110pp.   22550-X Pa. $1.50

TRICKS AND GAMES ON THE POOL TABLE, Fred Herrmann. 79 tricks and games, some solitaires, some for 2 or more players, some competitive; mystifying shots and throws, unusual carom, tricks involving cork, coins, a hat, more. 77 figures. 95pp.   21814-7 Pa. $1.50

WOODCRAFT AND CAMPING, Bernard S. Mason. How to make a quick emergency shelter, select woods that will burn immediately, make do with limited supplies, etc. Also making many things out of wood, rawhide, bark, at camp. Formerly titled Woodcraft. 295 illustrations. 580pp.   21951-8 Pa. $4.00

AN INTRODUCTION TO CHESS MOVES AND TACTICS SIMPLY EXPLAINED, Leonard Barden. Informal intermediate introduction: reasons for moves, tactics, openings, traps, positional play, endgame. Isolates patterns. 102pp. USO 21210-6 Pa. $1.35

LASKER'S MANUAL OF CHESS, Dr. Emanuel Lasker. Great world champion offers very thorough coverage of all aspects of chess. Combinations, position play, openings, endgame, aesthetics of chess, philosophy of struggle, much more. Filled with analyzed games. 390pp.   20640-8 Pa. $4.00

SLEEPING BEAUTY, illustrated by Arthur Rackham. Perhaps the fullest, most delightful version ever, told by C.S. Evans. Rackham's best work. 49 illustrations. 110pp. 7⅞ x 10¾.   22756-1 Pa. $2.00

THE WONDERFUL WIZARD OF OZ, L. Frank Baum. Facsimile in full color of America's finest children's classic. Introduction by Martin Gardner. 143 illustrations by W.W. Denslow. 267pp.   20691-2 Pa. $3.00

GOOPS AND HOW TO BE THEM, Gelett Burgess. Classic tongue-in-cheek masquerading as etiquette book. 87 verses, 170 cartoons as Goops demonstrate virtues of table manners, neatness, courtesy, more. 88pp. 6½ x 9¼.
                                                        22233-0 Pa. $2.00

THE BROWNIES, THEIR BOOK, Palmer Cox. Small as mice, cunning as foxes, exuberant, mischievous, Brownies go to zoo, toy shop, seashore, circus, more. 24 verse adventures. 266 illustrations. 144pp. 6⅝ x 9¼.   21265-3 Pa. $2.50

BILLY WHISKERS: THE AUTOBIOGRAPHY OF A GOAT, Frances Trego Montgomery. Escapades of that rambunctious goat. Favorite from turn of the century America. 24 illustrations. 259pp.   22345-0 Pa. $2.75

THE ROCKET BOOK, Peter Newell. Fritz, janitor's kid, sets off rocket in basement of apartment house; an ingenious hole punched through every page traces course of rocket. 22 duotone drawings, verses. 48pp. 6⅞ x 8⅜.   22044-3 Pa. $1.50

CUT AND COLOR PAPER MASKS, Michael Grater. Clowns, animals, funny faces . . . simply color them in, cut them out, and put them together, and you have 9 paper masks to play with and enjoy. Complete instructions. Assembled masks shown in full color on the covers. 32pp. 8¼ x 11.   23171-2 Pa. $1.50

THE TALE OF PETER RABBIT, Beatrix Potter. The inimitable Peter's terrifying adventure in Mr. McGregor's garden, with all 27 wonderful, full-color Potter illustrations. 55pp. 4¼ x 5½.   USO 22827-4 Pa. $1.00

THE TALE OF MRS. TIGGY-WINKLE, Beatrix Potter. Your child will love this story about a very special hedgehog and all 27 wonderful, full-color Potter illustrations. 57pp. 4¼ x 5½.   USO 20546-0 Pa. $1.00

THE TALE OF BENJAMIN BUNNY, Beatrix Potter. Peter Rabbit's cousin coaxes him back into Mr. McGregor's garden for a whole new set of adventures. A favorite with children. All 27 full-color illustrations. 59pp. 4¼ x 5½.
                                                    USO 21102-9 Pa. $1.00

THE MERRY ADVENTURES OF ROBIN HOOD, Howard Pyle. Facsimile of original (1883) edition, finest modern version of English outlaw's adventures. 23 illustrations by Pyle. 296pp. 6½ x 9¼.   22043-5 Pa. $4.00

TWO LITTLE SAVAGES, Ernest Thompson Seton. Adventures of two boys who lived as Indians; explaining Indian ways, woodlore, pioneer methods. 293 illustrations. 286pp.   20985-7 Pa. $3.00

HOUDINI ON MAGIC, Harold Houdini. Edited by Walter Gibson, Morris N. Young. How he escaped; exposés of fake spiritualists; instructions for eye-catching tricks; other fascinating material by and about greatest magician. 155 illustrations. 280pp. 20384-0 Pa. $2.75

HANDBOOK OF THE NUTRITIONAL CONTENTS OF FOOD, U.S. Dept. of Agriculture. Largest, most detailed source of food nutrition information ever prepared. Two mammoth tables: one measuring nutrients in 100 grams of edible portion; the other, in edible portion of 1 pound as purchased. Originally titled Composition of Foods. 190pp. 9 x 12. 21342-0 Pa. $4.00

COMPLETE GUIDE TO HOME CANNING, PRESERVING AND FREEZING, U.S. Dept. of Agriculture. Seven basic manuals with full instructions for jams and jellies; pickles and relishes; canning fruits, vegetables, meat; freezing anything. Really good recipes, exact instructions for optimal results. Save a fortune in food. 156 illustrations. 214pp. 6⅛ x 9¼. 22911-4 Pa. $2.50

THE BREAD TRAY, Louis P. De Gouy. Nearly every bread the cook could buy or make: bread sticks of Italy, fruit breads of Greece, glazed rolls of Vienna, everything from corn pone to croissants. Over 500 recipes altogether. including buns, rolls, muffins, scones, and more. 463pp. 23000-7 Pa. $4.00

CREATIVE HAMBURGER COOKERY, Louis P. De Gouy. 182 unusual recipes for casseroles, meat loaves and hamburgers that turn inexpensive ground meat into memorable main dishes: Arizona chili burgers, burger tamale pie, burger stew, burger corn loaf, burger wine loaf, and more. 120pp. 23001-5 Pa. $1.75

LONG ISLAND SEAFOOD COOKBOOK, J. George Frederick and Jean Joyce. Probably the best American seafood cookbook. Hundreds of recipes. 40 gourmet sauces, 123 recipes using oysters alone! All varieties of fish and seafood amply represented. 324pp. 22677-8 Pa. $3.50

THE EPICUREAN: A COMPLETE TREATISE OF ANALYTICAL AND PRACTICAL STUDIES IN THE CULINARY ART, Charles Ranhofer. Great modern classic. 3,500 recipes from master chef of Delmonico's, turn-of-the-century America's best restaurant. Also explained, many techniques known only to professional chefs. 775 illustrations. 1183pp. 6⅝ x 10. 22680-8 Clothbd. $22.50

THE AMERICAN WINE COOK BOOK, Ted Hatch. Over 700 recipes: old favorites livened up with wine plus many more: Czech fish soup, quince soup, sauce Perigueux, shrimp shortcake, filets Stroganoff, cordon bleu goulash, jambonneau, wine fruit cake, more. 314pp. 22796-0 Pa. $2.50

DELICIOUS VEGETARIAN COOKING, Ivan Baker. Close to 500 delicious and varied recipes: soups, main course dishes (pea, bean, lentil, cheese, vegetable, pasta, and egg dishes), savories, stews, whole-wheat breads and cakes, more. 168pp. USO 22834-7 Pa. $2.00

COOKIES FROM MANY LANDS, Josephine Perry. Crullers, oatmeal cookies, chaux au chocolate, English tea cakes, mandel kuchen, Sacher torte, Danish puff pastry, Swedish cookies — a mouth-watering collection of 223 recipes. 157pp.

22832-0 Pa. $2.25

ROSE RECIPES, Eleanour S. Rohde. How to make sauces, jellies, tarts, salads, pot-pourris, sweet bags, pomanders, perfumes from garden roses; all exact recipes. Century old favorites. 95pp.

22957-2 Pa. $1.75

"OSCAR" OF THE WALDORF'S COOKBOOK, Oscar Tschirky. Famous American chef reveals 3455 recipes that made Waldorf great; cream of French, German, American cooking, in all categories. Full instructions, easy home use. 1896 edition. 907pp. 6⅝ x 9⅜.

20790-0 Clothbd. $15.00

JAMS AND JELLIES, May Byron. Over 500 old-time recipes for delicious jams, jellies, marmalades, preserves, and many other items. Probably the largest jam and jelly book in print. Originally titled May Byron's Jam Book. 276pp.

USO 23130-5 Pa. $3.50

MUSHROOM RECIPES, André L. Simon. 110 recipes for everyday and special cooking. Champignons à la grecque, sole bonne femme, chicken liver croustades, more; 9 basic sauces, 13 ways of cooking mushrooms. 54pp.

USO 20913-X Pa. $1.25

THE BUCKEYE COOKBOOK, Buckeye Publishing Company. Over 1,000 easy-to-follow, traditional recipes from the American Midwest: bread (100 recipes alone), meat, game, jam, candy, cake, ice cream, and many other categories of cooking. 64 illustrations. From 1883 enlarged edition. 416pp.

23218-2 Pa. $4.00

TWENTY-TWO AUTHENTIC BANQUETS FROM INDIA, Robert H. Christie. Complete, easy-to-do recipes for almost 200 authentic Indian dishes assembled in 22 banquets. Arranged by region. Selected from Banquets of the Nations. 192pp.

23200-X Pa. $2.50

Prices subject to change without notice.
Available at your book dealer or write for free catalogue to Dept. GI, Dover Publications, Inc., 180 Varick St., N.Y., N.Y. 10014. Dover publishes more than 150 books each year on science, elementary and advanced mathematics, biology, music, art, literary history, social sciences and other areas.